POLITICAL COMMUNICATION AND COVID-19

This edited collection compares and analyses the most prominent political communicative responses to the outbreak and global spread of the COVID-19 strain of coronavirus within 27 nations across five continents and two supranational organisations: the European Union (EU) and the World Health Organisation (WHO). The book encompasses the various governments' communication of the crisis, the role played by opposition and the vibrancy of the information environment within each nation.

The chapters analyse the communication drawing on theoretical perspectives drawn from the fields of crisis communication, political communication and political psychology. In doing so the book develops a framework to assess the extent to which state communication followed the key indicators of effective communication encapsulated in the principles of: being first; being right; being credible; expressing empathy; promoting action and showing respect. The book also examines how communication circulated within the mass and social media environments and what impact differences in spokespersons, messages and the broader context have on the success of implementing measures likely to reduce the spread of the virus. Cumulatively, the authors develop a global analysis of the responses and how these are shaped by their specific contexts and by the flow of information, while offering lessons for future political crisis communication.

This book will be of great interest to students and researchers of politics, communication and public relations, specifically on courses and modules relating to current affairs, crisis communication and strategic communication, as well as practitioners working in the field of health crisis communication.

Darren Lilleker is a Professor of Political Communication in the Faculty of Media and Communication at Bournemouth University, UK. He is Convenor of the Centre for Comparative Politics and Media Research and teaches across the politics programmes. He has led a range of research projects using qualitative and quantitative methods; and delivered lectures and workshops to students across the world.

Ioana A. Coman is an Assistant Professor at Texas Tech University, USA. She teaches courses focused on public relations, journalism and entrepreneurship. Her research focuses on how different actors engage and interact in risk and crisis communication situations via different platforms, within different contexts and at different levels. Her research has received national and international awards and grants including the Page/Johnson Legacy Scholar (2019 and 2020).

Miloš Gregor is an Assistant Professor at Masaryk University, the Czech Republic. He teaches courses on political communication and marketing, propaganda, disinformation and fake news. Together with Petra Mlejnková, he is a mentor of projects Choose Your Info (Zvol si info) and Fakescape, both dedicated to media literacy awareness. Both projects received awards in the international Peer to Peer: Global Digital Challenge competition.

Edoardo Novelli is an Associate Professor at the University of Roma Tre, Italy. He teaches Political Communication and Media Sociology. His research interests focus on political communication, history of propaganda, electoral campaigns, and on the relationship between politics, media and images. He has been Principal Investigator of international research projects, including the European Election Monitoring Centre, and he is Head of the digital archive of Italian political commercials.

Politics, Media and Political Communication

Titles in this series include:

Communication in Global Jihad

Jonathan Matusitz

Democracy and Fake News

Information Manipulation and Post-Truth Politics

Edited by Serena Giusti and Elisa Piras

Political Communication and COVID-19

Governance and Rhetoric in Times of Crisis

Edited by Darren Lilleker, Ioana A. Coman, Miloš Gregor and Edoardo Novelli

For more information about this series, please visit: https://www.routledge.com
/Politics-Media-and-Political-Communication/book-series/POLMED

POLITICAL COMMUNICATION AND COVID-19

Governance and Rhetoric in Times of Crisis

Edited by Darren Lilleker, Ioana A. Coman,
Miloš Gregor and Edoardo Novelli

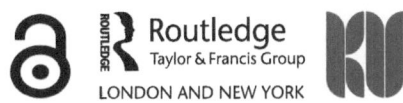

Routledge
Taylor & Francis Group

LONDON AND NEW YORK

An electronic version of this book is freely available, thanks to the
support of libraries working with Knowledge Unlatched (KU). KU is
a collaborative initiative designed to make high quality books Open
Access for the public good. The Open Access ISBN for this book is
9781003120254. More information about the initiative and links to the
Open Access version can be found at www.knowledgeunlatched.org.

First published 2021
by Routledge
2 Park Square, Milton Park, Abingdon, Oxon OX14 4RN

and by Routledge
52 Vanderbilt Avenue, New York, NY 10017

Routledge is an imprint of the Taylor & Francis Group, an informa business

British Library Cataloguing-in-Publication Data
A catalogue record for this book is available from the British Library

Library of Congress Cataloging-in-Publication Data
A catalog record has been requested for this book

ISBN: 978-0-367-63683-8 (hbk)
ISBN: 978-0-367-63679-1 (pbk)
ISBN: 978-1-003-12025-4 (ebk)

DOI: 10.4324/9781003120254

Typeset in Bembo
by Deanta Global Publishing Services, Chennai, India

CONTENTS

Tables   x

Contributors   xi

Foreword   xviii

    Introduction: Political communication, governance and
    rhetoric in times of crisis   1
    Ioana A. Coman, Dalia Elsheikh, Miloš Gregor,
    Darren Lilleker and Edoardo Novelli

CASE STUDIES   **17**

  1 World Health Organisation: The challenges of providing
     global leadership   19
     Darren Lilleker and Miloš Gregor

  2 China: Diversion, ingratiation and victimisation 34
     Menglin Liu and Shan Xu

  3 Japan: New directions for digital Japan   44
     Leslie Tkach-Kawasaki

  4 South Korea: No shutdown, no lockdown   55
     Jangyul Robert Kim and Sera Choi

  5 The United States: Politics versus science?   67
     John M. Callahan

6 The EU: The story of a tragic hero and the 27 dwarfs 79
Dennis Lichtenstein

7 France: An unpopular government facing an unprecedented crisis 88
Pierre-Emmanuel Guigo

8 Australia: A triumph of sorts 99
Fiona Wade

9 Germany: Between a patchwork and best-practice 111
Isabelle Borucki and Ulrike Klinger

10 India: A spectacle of mismanagement 123
Chindu Sreedharan

11 Italy: The frontrunner of the Western countries in an unexpected crisis 132
Edoardo Novelli

12 Spain: Managing the uncertain while facing economic collapse 145
Sergio Pérez Castaños and Alberto Mora Rodríguez

13 Sweden: Lone hero or stubborn outlier? 155
Bengt Johansson and Orla Vigsø

14 The UK: From consensus to confusion 165
Ruth Garland and Darren Lilleker

15 Egypt: Emotive speech masks a complicated reality 177
Dalia Elsheikh

16 Russia: A glass wall 188
Svetlana S. Bodrunova

17 Austria: A ski resort as the virus slingshot of Europe 201
Katie Bates and Lore Hayek

18 Iran: Disciplinary strategies and governmental campaigning 211
Azra Ghandeharion and Josef Kraus

19 Brazil: More than just a little flu   220
    Ícaro Joathan, Andrea Medrado and Thainã Medeiros

20 Norway: From strict measures to pragmatic flexibility   231
    Bente Kalsnes and Eli Skogerbø

21 Iceland: No lockdown and experts at the forefront   239
    Jón Gunnar Ólafsson

22 Ireland: Solid swansong from caretaker government   248
    Dawn Wheatley

23 The Czech Republic: Self-proclaimed role models   259
    Otto Eibl and Miloš Gregor

24 Hungary: Illiberal crisis management   269
    Norbert Merkovity, Márton Bene and Xénia Farkas

25 Poland: Protecting the nation while struggling to maintain
    power   280
    Michał Jacuński

26 Ghana: Political expediency or competent leadership?   292
    Sally Osei-Appiah

27 South Africa: A united front? A divided government   303
    Robert Mattes and Ian Glenn

28 Kosovo: Political crisis, one more challenge alongside
    COVID-19   312
    Dren Gërguri

29 Turkey: Declaring war on an epidemic   323
    Elif Kahraman

30 Political communication and COVID-19: Governance and
    rhetoric in global comparative perspective   333
    Darren Lilleker, Ioana Coman, Miloš Gregor and Edoardo Novelli

TABLES

1.1	WHO chronology	21
2.1	China chronology	37
3.1	Japan chronology	45
4.1	South Korea chronology	57
5.1	US chronology	69
7.1	France chronology	89
8.1	Australia chronology	101
9.1	Germany chronology	112
11.1	Italy chronology	134
12.1	Spain chronology	148
13.1	Sweden chronology	157
14.1	UK chronology	167
15.1	Egypt chronology	178
16.1	Russia chronology	190
17.1	Austria chronology	204
19.1	Brazil chronology	222
22.1	Ireland chronology	250
23.1	Czech Republic chronology	260
24.1	Hungary chronology	271
25.1	Poland chronology	282
26.1	Ghana chronology	295
28.1	Kosovo chronology	314
29.1	Turkey chronology	325
30.1	Comparative data on cases and lockdowns across our sample nations	335

CONTRIBUTORS

Katie Bates is a Postdoctoral Researcher at the Medical University Innsbruck, Austria, and an Honorary Research Fellow in Health Systems at the London School of Hygiene and Tropical Medicine, UK. She has worked across multiple quantitative and qualitative research projects both within academia and as a consultant, including performing monitoring and evaluation for BBC Media Action whose programmes focus on the use of media and communication to improve health, governance and community resilience.

Márton Bene is a Research Fellow at the Centre for Social Sciences – Hungarian Academy of Sciences Centre of Excellence and a Lecturer at Eötvös Lorand University, Hungary. His research focuses on political communication, social media, and politics and political behaviour.

Svetlana S. Bodrunova is a Professor at the School of Journalism and Mass Communications at St Petersburg State University, Russia. She leads the Centre for International Media Research and hosts CMSTW, an annual conference on comparative media studies. She has led six research projects and published two books and over 100 research papers, in Russian and English, on Russian and European journalism, media and politics, social media and ethnicity in communication.

Isabelle Borucki is the Head of the research group on digital party research (DIPART) at the University of Duisburg-Essen, Germany. Her main research areas are digital party politics, governments, political sociology and social network analysis.

John M. Callahan is the Dean of the School of Graduate and Professional Studies at New England College, USA. He is a co-convenor of the German Political Studies Group of the Political Science Association and teaches across the international relations and homeland security programmes, which he also directs. He has participated in a variety of research projects, primarily qualitative in nature, focusing on communication and national security issues and has delivered lectures and workshops to students around the world.

Sera Choi is a PhD Student at Colorado State University, USA. Her research interest falls in crisis, risk and health communication. She is particularly interested in how crisis severity in times of crisis affects post-crisis organisational reputation depending on crisis response strategies.

Ioana A. Coman is an Assistant Professor at Texas Tech University, USA. She teaches courses focused on public relations, journalism and entrepreneurship. Her research focuses on how different actors engage and interact in risk and crisis communication situations via different platforms, within different contexts and at different levels. Her research has received national and international awards and grants including the Page/Johnson Legacy Scholar (2019 and 2020).

Otto Eibl is an Assistant Professor in the Department of Political Science at Masaryk University, the Czech Republic. He teaches courses about political communication and marketing. He also researches the placement of political issues in political space and the communication and marketing strategies of political parties both in and beyond the lead-up to an election. He is a team member of the international research project MAD: Migrants. Analysis of media discourse on migrants in Poland, Great Britain, Ukraine, Albania and the Czech Republic.

Dalia Elsheikh is a Researcher at the Centre for Politics and Media Research at Bournemouth University, UK, and a Fellow of the Higher Education Academy, UK. Before joining academia, she worked as a journalist for more than 16 years including for *Al-Masry Al-Youm*, the first independent newspaper in Egypt, and the BBC in London, UK.

Xénia Farkas is a Junior Research Fellow at the Centre for Social Sciences – Hungarian Academy of Sciences Centre of Excellence and a PhD Student at Corvinus University of Budapest, Hungary. Her main research interest is visual elements of political communication on social media.

Ruth Garland spent 28 years in frontline and leadership roles in public sector strategic communications. She is a Lecturer in Media Cultures at the University of Hertfordshire, UK. Her research focus is on public communication and the relationship between media and politics.

Dren Gërguri is a PhD Candidate and Lecturer in the Department of Journalism in the Faculty of Philology at the University of Prishtina 'Hasan Prishtina,' Kosovo. He has worked as a journalist from 2009. His research interests focus on media-politics relations, political communication, journalism, disinformation/misinformation and media ethics.

Azra Ghandeharion is a Faculty Member at Ferdowsi University of Mashhad, Iran. She is the youngest Associate Professor of English Literature and Cultural Studies in Iran. Her interest in research includes contemporary Middle Eastern art and culture. Her emphasis is on 'Otherness' issues, media studies, body politics and literature of diaspora. She has presented numerous articles in international congresses involving social sciences, humanities and art.

Ian Glenn is a Research Fellow in Communications Science at the University of the Free State, South Africa, and Emeritus Professor of Media Studies at the University of Cape Town, South Africa. He has published widely on literary, cultural and environmental issues and is working on liberal Afropessimism, 1994–2019.

Miloš Gregor is an Assistant Professor at Masaryk University, the Czech Republic. He teaches courses on political communication and marketing, propaganda, disinformation and fake news. Together with Petra Mlejnková, he is a mentor of projects Choose Your Info (Zvol si info) and Fakescape, both dedicated to media literacy awareness. Both projects received awards in the international Peer to Peer: Global Digital Challenge competition.

Pierre-Emmanuel Guigo is an Associate Professor in the History Department at Sciences Po, France. His research has mainly focused on French political communication in a historical perspective. More recently, he also studies satirical TV programmes in a European comparative perspective.

Lore Hayek is an Assistant Professor of Austrian Politics and Civic Education in the Department of Political Science at the University of Innsbruck, Austria. In her research, she focuses on communication strategies of political actors and on the relationship between politics and the media. She has published on personalisation and negativity.

Michał Jacuński is an Associate Professor of Political Science at the University of Wrocław, Poland. His research interest focuses on contemporary political communication and the use of digital media. He has conducted research projects on structural and functional aspects of political parties and on politicians' owned media, on web campaigning and on social media influence.

Ícaro Joathan is a PhD Candidate in Communication at the Fluminense Federal University, Brazil. He is also a journalist at the Federal Institute of Education, Science and Technology of Ceará, Brazil. His interests focus on online election campaigns, negative campaigns, permanent campaigns, political participation on the Internet and public communication.

Bengt Johansson is a Professor in Journalism and Mass Communication in the Department of Journalism, Media and Communication at the University of Gothenburg, Sweden. His research interest is mainly focused on different aspects of risk and crisis communication, political communication and journalism. He is project leader of a project on crisis communication funded by the Swedish civil contingencies agency (MSB) – Crisis Communication and Societal Trust in the Multi-Public Society.

Elif Kahraman is a Lecturer in the Corporate Communications Department at Istanbul University, Turkey. Her areas of interest are public diplomacy, nation branding, political communication and media analysis.

Bente Kalsnes is an Associate Professor in the Department of Communication at Kristiania University College, Norway. Her research interests include political communication, social media, fake news and disinformation. She is part of the research project Source Criticism in an Age of Mediated Disinformation (SCAM) financed by the Norwegian Research Council.

Jangyul Robert Kim is an Associate Professor in the Department of Journalism and Media Communication at Colorado State University, USA. His research interests include issues and crisis communications, public diplomacy, corporate social responsibility, international public relations, health communications and strategic and marketing communications.

Ulrike Klinger is an Assistant Professor of Digital Communication at Freie Universität Berlin, Germany, and Head of the research group on News, Campaigns and the Rationality of Public Discourse at the Weizenbaum Institute for the Networked Society, Germany. Her research focuses on digital public spheres, political communication and digital technologies.

Josef Kraus is an Assistant Professor in the Department of Political Science at Masaryk University, the Czech Republic. He mainly focuses on the region of the Near and Middle East, especially Iran. His emphasis is on Islamic political thought, the role of Iran in the Middle East, religious extremism, and security in the Persian Gulf and Levant. He holds the position of Visiting Professor at Ferdowsi University of Mashhad, Iran, the Al-Hikmah Institute of Qom, Iran and Saints Joseph University of Beirut, Lebanon.

Dennis Lichtenstein is a Postdoctoral Researcher at the Institute for Comparative Media and Communication Studies (CMC) at the Austrian Academy of Sciences in Vienna and the Alpen-Adria-University Klagenfurt, Austria. His habilitation thesis deals with strategic and media communication during international crisis events.

Darren Lilleker is a Professor of Political Communication in the Faculty of Media and Communication at Bournemouth University, UK. He is Convenor of the Centre for Comparative Politics and Media Research and teaches across the politics programmes. He has led a range of research projects using qualitative and quantitative methods and delivered lectures and workshops to students across the world.

Menglin Liu is a PhD Student in the Department of Political Science at the University of California, Davis, USA. She is in the field of American politics and political methodology. Her research interests include state and local governments, voter initiatives, state policy diffusion, interest groups and lobbyists at the local level.

Robert Mattes is a Professor of Government and Public Policy at the University of Strathclyde, UK, and Honorary Professor at the Institute for Democracy, Citizenship and Public Policy in Africa at the University of Cape Town, South Africa. He is co-founder of, and Senior Adviser to, Afrobarometer, a groundbreaking regular survey of public opinion in 35 African countries. His research focuses on the development of democratic attitudes and practices in South Africa and across the continent.

Thainã Medeiros lives in Complexo do Alemão, a group of favelas in Brazil, where he works for Coletivo Papo Reto, a mediactivism collective that uses technologies to provide narratives from a favela perspective and to fight for human rights. He works as a community journalist. Together with other civil society organisations in Complexo do Alemão, he helped set up a Crisis Committee in the favela, mobilising tools that can aid the community in times of hardship.

Andrea Medrado is a Lecturer in Media and Communication at the University of Westminster, UK. She has worked as the Co-Investigator of the eVoices Network and the Co-Chair of the Community Communication Section of the International Association for Media and Communication Research (IAMCR). She was recently elected Vice President of IAMCR. Her research interests include media activism, citizen and community media and the use of technologies by marginalised communities in Global South countries.

Norbert Merkovity is an Assistant Professor in the Department of Political Science at the University of Szeged, Hungary, and part-time Assistant Professor at the National University of Public Service, Hungary. His research interests include political communication and new political communication, attention-based politics and the role of technologies in various political circumstances. He is Chair of the Central and Eastern European Network of the European Communication Research and Education Association (ECREA).

Alberto Mora Rodríguez is a Professor of Political Science at the University of Murcia, Spain. He is a Specialist in Social Research and Quantitative Data Analysis at the Centre for Sociological Research. He is Coordinator of the Masters in Applied Political Analysis, and General Secretary of the Latin American Association of Researchers in Electoral Campaigns. He specialises in political communication and public opinion.

Edoardo Novelli is an Associate Professor at the University of Roma Tre, Italy. He teaches Political Communication and Media Sociology. His research interests focus on political communication, history of propaganda, electoral campaigns, and on the relationship between politics, media and images. He has been Principal Investigator of international research projects, including the European Election Monitoring Centre, and he is Head of the digital archive of Italian political commercials.

Jón Gunnar Ólafsson is a Postdoctoral Researcher in the Faculty of Political Science at the University of Iceland. His recent research focuses on disinformation and social media and he is conducting research on Iceland for the Media for Democracy Monitor (MDM) and the Worlds of Journalism Study (WJS).

Sally Osei-Appiah is a Research Affiliate at the School of Media and Communication at the University of Leeds, UK. Her research interests lie in the areas of gender and political communication, with special focus on mediatisation of politics, African media and journalism, digital campaigning, political news production and visual communication. She is Reviews Editor for the journal *Information, Communication & Society*.

Sergio Pérez Castaños is an Associate Professor in Political Science in the Faculty of Law at Burgos University, Spain, and is Studies Coordinator for the Political Science Degree. He takes part in different research projects both at national and international levels, focusing on political congruence, populist discourse and political communication. He has led the Spanish national section of the European Election Monitoring Centre and is a member of the Spanish Political Science Association Board.

Eli Skogerbø is a Professor in the Department of Media and Communication at the University of Oslo, Norway, and Co-Director of POLKOM – Centre for the Study of Political Communication. She has published widely on media, politics and political communication in the Nordic countries. She is a participant in the project Pandemic Rhetoric: Risk Communication Strategies in a Changed Media Landscape (PAR).

Chindu Sreedharan is a Principal Academic in Journalism at Bournemouth University, UK. He has a particular interest in journalistic storytelling as a means to improve human rights situations and empower marginalised groups. His research focuses on 'abnormal journalisms,' reportage that extends the boundaries of conventional news work. He has led crisis journalism projects in India and Nepal and is Co-Principal Investigator for the Media Action Against Rape.

Leslie Tkach-Kawasaki is an Associate Professor at the University of Tsukuba, Japan. Her research interests include website and social media analysis of Japanese political actors, spanning politicians and political parties to political institutions such as election management boards and local government. In recent years, she has expanded her research interests to incorporate social network and comparative discourse analysis, focusing on renewable energy-related discourse in Japan and Germany in diverse media channels.

Orla Vigsø is a Professor of Media and Communication Studies at the University of Gothenburg, Sweden. His research mainly focuses on visual political communication and crisis communication, but he is also currently working on a study of Swedish political cartoons. He is co-editor of the *Journal of Visual Political Communication*.

Fiona Wade has been a media and communications specialist for over two decades and an adviser to both Liberal and Labor backbenchers in Australia's federal parliament. She has spoken at international and national conferences, is a Visiting Fellow at the University of New South Wales and is Acting Director of Public Affairs and Communications at the Law Council of Australia.

Dawn Wheatley is an Assistant Professor at the School of Communications at Dublin City University, Ireland. She teaches both practical and theoretical subjects to journalism students. Her research interests focus on journalism studies, political communication and social media.

Shan Xu is an Assistant Professor at the College of Media and Communication at Texas Tech University, USA. She is interested in media technologies and especially their effects on well-being and health communication. One of her research interests is the use of real time and longitudinal data (e.g. longitudinal life experience sampling, psychophysiological measures) in conjunction with formal dynamic models to study how media choices are made and the impact of media choices.

FOREWORD

Darren Lilleker, Ioana A. Coman,
Miloš Gregor and Edoardo Novelli

The world is facing an unprecedented test. And this is the moment of truth. Hundreds of thousands of people are falling seriously ill from COVID-19, and the disease is spreading exponentially in many places. Societies are in turmoil and economies are in a nose-dive... We must respond decisively, innovatively and together to suppress the spread of the virus and address the socio-economic devastation that COVID-19 is causing in all regions. The magnitude of the response must match the scale of the crisis – large-scale, coordinated and comprehensive... The message of the report we are issuing today is clear: shared responsibility and global solidarity in response to the impacts of COVID-19. It is a call to action. We must see countries not only united to beat the virus but also to tackle its profound consequences.

(António Guterres, Secretary-General of the
United Nations, 2020)[1]

Guterres' statement to the United Nations on March 17, 2020 was a sound prediction of the impact COVID-19 has had on the world. On December 31, 2019, while many across the world enjoyed fireworks displays to welcome in the new year, news was emerging of a novel coronavirus having been detected in Wuhan province in China. The impact of that virus was at that time unimaginable. Also unimagined was that anyone standing within those crowds might be someone who had visited Wuhan and was now unbeknownst to anyone starting to spread the virus. This stark realisation can only be made with the benefit of hindsight, but by March, COVID-19 was impacting over half the countries across the globe, had become a global health emergency and designated a global pandemic.

Kahn (2020: ix) defines a pandemic as a 'medical and political crisis that requires an understanding of the complex scientific, public health, and public communication capabilities needed for a successful response' and argues that no epidemic has had the impact on health care and economic life that COVID-19 has already had. The COVID-19 pandemic is a very unique crisis for multiple reasons, in particular the speed and scale of the spread. Compared to previous similar outbreaks or pandemics, it demands new, more complex, coordinated efforts, and it seems more than ever, global disaster management (Brandt & Wörlein, 2020). While past similar flu outbreaks (chiefly those in 1889–90, the 1918–20 Spanish flu or the 1957–58 Asian flu) affected countries globally and resulted in high numbers of fatalities, they did not result in global efforts but more localised or national level disaster management and the 2002–4 SARS and 2009 H1N1 epidemics remained limited in scope and measures (Brandt & Wörlein, 2020).

Complicating things further is the fact that the COVID-19 pandemic is accompanied by a veritable *infodemic*. The term was coined by Tedros Adhanom Ghebreyesus, Director-General of the World Health Organisation, in one of his early speeches addressing the COVID-19 crisis, when he said, 'We're not just fighting an epidemic; we're fighting an infodemic' (WHO, 2020). From fake preventive measures and cures, to conspiracy theories; as the world was fighting the COVID-19 global pandemic, a global epidemic of misinformation and disinformation also needed to be tackled as claims spread rapidly through social and mainstream media platforms. It was argued that the infodemic constituted a further serious problem for public health (Zarocostas, 2020).

Finally, in some countries the management of this crisis has been further complicated by its politisation and the fact that contradictory information, or even worse misinformation, came from official sources. What was required for tackling COVID-19 was a united, global approach with consistent messaging across countries with no gaps in communication that could be filled by dubious sources but this was only partially the case.

This book focuses not on the vital work of health professionals in combatting COVID-19 or finding ways of curing victims and vaccinating populations; those works are necessary and will come later. Our work focuses on the also vital area of communication. In order to ensure that citizens (the potential victims of the virus) understand the measures governments are taking, that they as ordinary people need to take, and to trust in the information they receive, there must be effective, coherent and consistent communication. Crisis communications require the clear performance of leadership. The global and national responses need to be coherent and consistent with one another. Information needs to be clearly communicated. Political representatives need to stand together. Measures taken must be seen to be appropriate and timely. Understanding and empathy needs to be shown. Citizens, from monarch, president and parliamentarian to the waiters, bartenders and cleaners, need to be working as one, seen to be facing the same difficulties and having an understanding of one another. Our question is whether the political communication strategies and the way these were implemented laid the groundwork for efforts to be successful.

The work began with a call on Facebook to academics to become involved. The call was a reaction to observing the different approaches taken and the opportunity to explore the divergent national approaches within countries as they faced increases in cases of infections, deaths from COVID-19 and the need to implement quick and decisive measures. Some leaders appeared to be acting too quickly, others were vacillating. Some leaders used a rhetoric of war, others offered empathetic messages of unity. Yet others dismissed the threat, suggesting some form of national exceptionalism.

The call elicited responses from a range of scholars across the field of political communication. It is always difficult to gain a perfect sample of countries and we do not claim this to be the case for this book. What we have are 29 interesting cases. Twenty-seven very different nations, albeit a preponderance of those are European, and the World Health Organisation and European Union. The contributors play to their own strengths and expertise when approaching the topic while adhering to a consistent framework. The case study chapters firstly offer an overview of the political context, this helps us to understand the extent to which the political system was stable and the nature of the polity facing the challenges posed by COVID-19. Secondly, each chapter provides a chronology of the diffusion of COVID-19 within their country, the measures taken and the noteworthy communicational events of the crisis. Thirdly, the chapter provides an analysis of the most important issues which contributed to the successes and failures experienced. The main themes of these are collected within our conclusion where we reflect on the lessons learned for political communication in times of crisis as well as what the crisis teaches us about political communication more broadly.

Unfortunately, this analysis focuses on the first wave of infections alone. The COVID-19 pandemic has proved a moving target. Some countries which faced a first wave of infections early are already experiencing a second wave, and this is reflected within the chronology and analysis of those case studies. Others are not yet out of the first wave, some due to systemic failures in implementing preventative measures, others because the virus arrived there later. Despite these necessary disparities, each narrative offers powerful insights into a range of very different systems and their responses. While the story remains unfinished, it indicates how in each country the scene was set for the management of the pandemic. The first phase of infections represents a time when perceptions of leaders and their performance and perceptions of the threat posed by the virus are defined. There will be further lessons to be learned, but our analysis focuses on a crucial phase: a phase which defined national responses and one which is able to give insights into the ways political leaders deal with crises, how the study of political communication helps explain their successes and failures and to get some, albeit tentative, indications of the correspondence between the strategies implemented and the outcomes.

Note

1 UN Secretary-General virtual press statement on COVID-19 Crisis. Retrieved from: www.un.org/en/un-coronavirus-communications-team/launch-report-socio-economic-impacts-covid-19

References

Brandt, P., & Wörlein, J. (2020). Government crisis communication during the coronavirus crisis: comparing France, Germany, and the United Kingdom. *SciencesPo.fr*. Retrieved from: https://www.sciencespo.fr/cso/fr/content/government-crisis-communication-during-coronavirus-crisis-comparing-france-germany-and-unite.html

Kahn, L. H. (2020). *Who's in charge? Leadership during epidemics, bioterror attacks, and other public health crises.* Second edition. Santa Barbara, CA: Praeger Security International.

WHO. (2020). Director-General's remarks at the media briefing on 2019 novel coronavirus on 8 February 2020. Retrieved from: https://www.who.int/dg/speeches/detail/director-general-s-remarks-at-the-media-briefing-on-2019-novel-coronavirus---8-february-2020

Zarocostas, J. (2020). How to fight an infodemic. *The Lancet*, *395*(10225), 676. https://doi.org/10.1016/S0140-6736(20)30461-X

INTRODUCTION

Political communication, governance and rhetoric in times of crisis

Ioana A. Coman, Dalia Elsheikh, Miloš Gregor, Darren Lilleker and Edoardo Novelli

COVID-19 instigated a global crisis. The fast spread of the virus, the way it overwhelmed health systems in many advanced industrial nations and the immediate demonstration it represented a significant danger to life, forced global and national leaders to consider how to balance the risks to health and society against those of the economy. The measures introduced, which restricted the freedoms of citizens and in most cases involved a complete lockdown of society and the economy, needed carefully considering and communicating. Crisis communication literature provides a framework for how leaders should develop their strategy and perform their role in guiding society. Political communication literature aids an understanding of the wider environment, incorporating analyses of who controls the narrative, how the narrative develops and is shaped by differing actors, and the role played by interactions within the information environment. Political psychology aids an understanding of how citizens receive political communication, how they process messages and what emotions are stimulated by political messages within differing political contexts. In introducing our volume, we draw on these fields of literature. The following sections will firstly cover the core concepts of crisis communication. Secondly, we draw on key concepts from political communication to develop a framework for analysing the communication strategies and practices during the pandemic. Thirdly, we draw on political psychology to develop benchmarks for good practice in ensuring solidarity in fighting COVID-19 prior to providing an overview of how strategy should evolve over the phases of a pandemic, thus providing a framework for analysis to be applied to the data from the case study chapters.

DOI: 10.4324/9781003120254-1

Crisis communication

The crisis and crisis communication literature abound in definitions of crisis, and models of crisis communication and crisis management. Many approach the topic of crisis from an organisational perspective, as opposed to a political perspective, although there are clearly transferable concepts between the corporate and political sphere. This body of literature would largely agree that a crisis represents a 'major occurrence with a potentially negative outcome [etc.]' (Fearn-Banks, 2011: 2, see also Coombs, 2015). Crises can be external events, industrial or consumer actions (strikes or boycott), acts of terrorism or the result of internal failures such as product failure. Whatever the form the crisis takes, they are 'specific, unexpected, and nonroutine events that create high levels of uncertainty and simultaneously present an organization with both opportunities for and threats to its high-priority goals' (Seeger et al., 1998: 239). Crises such as a pandemic are outside of the control of any organisation or nation, but they require 'an immediate response, and may cause harm to the organization's reputation, image, or viability' (CERC, 2014[1]).

A pandemic is perhaps one of the most serious forms of crisis. It is beyond the control of any actor and is inherently complex due to the range and depth of the effects and the need to understand the capabilities required to mitigate the impact (Kahn, 2020: ix). Of central importance, given that both threats and preventative measures need to be communicated to those most vulnerable, is the need 'to inform and alert the public' (CERC, 2014). The Cambridge Environmental Research Consultants (CERC) framework was conceptualised to guide responses to emergency situations and has been employed by the US Center for Disease Control (CDC). It focuses on the simple concept that 'the right message at the right time from the right person can save lives' (Reynolds & Quinn, 2008). Based on lessons learned from previous public health emergencies as well as research insights from different fields (public health, psychology, risk communication etc.), it is meant to help health communicators, emergency responders and organisational leaders to communicate effectively in crisis situations. The key point is that an immediate response is needed because of the unexpected and threatening nature of the health emergency and that communication elements (content, form, timing etc.) could aid resolve the crisis efficiently or prolong and worsen its impact (CERC, 2014).

Eliding with core concepts at the heart of political communication and political psychology, two categories of crisis communication have been identified (Coombs, 2015: 7). Managing information involves the collection, analysis and dissemination of information. Managing meaning, however, involves shaping how people perceive the crisis. The latter process is the most complex. Crisis management spokespersons can unidirectionally disseminate information through traditional (e.g. televised press conferences) and new media (i.e. websites). However, social media allows a plethora of actors to actively engage in crisis communication as consumers, creators and disseminators of information and meaning (Palen, 2008; Perng et al., 2013). A pandemic emerges accompanied by an initial lack of information and high levels of uncertainty, and when the pandemic involves a novel type of virus, it is also accompanied by scientific uncertainty in terms of susceptibility and severity, prevention, treatment etc. (Kahn, 2020). It is thus easy for disagreements over strategy and confusion to emerge between the range of stakeholders engaged in informing stakeholders.

Pandemics also require risk communication, involving communicating information about the potential impact and magnitude to manage expectations and behaviour (CERC, 2014: 7). While in a crisis the effects can be obvious to a community (i.e. in the aftermath of a natural disaster or terrorist attack), risk communication highlights the potential, unseen negative consequences. These may be based on estimates or best guesses, and for areas yet unaffected it can prove difficult to convince the public to comply with restrictive and preventative measures. Risk communication thus adds an additional layer of managing meaning, attempting to govern public perceptions of the level of risk and how to minimise their own risk and that of the wider community.

Political crisis communication

Political communication research suggests the importance of clear leadership during crises, in particular the performance of leadership, media management and control of the narrative within the information environment; these three concepts shape our discussion of how crisis communication can be placed into a political context suitable for understanding the dynamics of communication during the COVID-19 pandemic.

Personalisation

As Kahn (2020: 9) argues, 'Who is in charge during a crisis can have an enormous impact on how many lives are saved or lost. Leaders must make decisions and communicate them effectively to many different groups.' Two models of leadership during crises have been identified (Kahn, 2020): *The Politician Prominence* Model (the politician accepts advice from experts, but keeps the primary decision-making and public communication role) and *The Expert Appointee Prominence* Model (the politician delegates primary decision-making and public communication responsibilities to experts, while providing political support for decisions). The former can lead to personalisation of leadership, involving assuming personal control but also asking the public to place full trust in a leader adopting a presidential or even monarchical character independent of the political system (Webb & Poguntke, 2013). Trust can be a factor of the performance of a particular leader as well as public perceptions of their character (Van Zoonen & Holtz-Bacha, 2000). Hence, during a crisis, the extent to which a leader is able to unite the nation depends on their immediate performance but also on the level of support they command and the longstanding perceptions the public holds of them in terms of their integrity and competence (Renshon, 2000).

The Expert Appointee Prominence Model involves a broader range of spokespersons selected due to their specific roles, expertise and competences. Even when the politician is prominent, experts can be utilised to increase the credibility of government responses, measures implemented and requirements of the public. Within a pandemic, one would expect within this model for virologists to take centre stage, but certain measures would require the presence of other government agencies and groups including, but not limited to, local, federal or national public health agencies, security agencies, emergency service agencies and possibly security services, businesses, healthcare organisations, nongovernmental or supranational agencies or religious organisations.

Mediatisation and media management

Media management is essential for both crisis and risk communication as 'information production and dissemination are critical for crisis preparedness, crisis response, and crisis recovery' (Austin & Jin, 2018: 1). Traditionally, mass media have operated as a bridge between governmental actors communicating about the crisis and their publics, seeking information and interpreting it for their specific audiences (Seeger et al., 1998: 138). Media are argued to fulfil a range of functions during a crisis (Mogensen et al., 2002): providing information; promoting government narratives; emphasising the human interest over political or economic factors; being a source of guidance and consolation; framing coverage based on moral and religious tenets; promoting national values and bringing the nation together to tackle the crisis. The focus of coverage is expected to shift across different stages of the crisis as the official narrative and restrictions on public behaviour changes.

The above suggests political logic dominates and media become subservient to government in the name of the national interest. However, media logic can also assert itself as editors pursue what they believe to be the interests of their own audiences (Stromback, 2008). Media can adopt supportive or oppositional stances to a government in the pursuit of a national or political agenda (Schudson, 2011). When media play a supportive role, the impact is positive for the outcome of the crisis. Research shows mass media help positively change individual behaviours, especially during public health education campaigns (Collinson et al., 2015). However, if the media adopt an oppositional role and competing perspectives enter public discourse, then it can lead to confusion and non-compliance as the public are unsure which position to believe (Lilleker, 2018). Therefore, the role media traditionally plays within a society and its political stance can impact on the ability of a government to shape the narrative.

Media management involves developing a uniformly shared narrative to aid understanding the nature of a crisis. Within political communication literature, this is referred to as framing and if done effectively, can shape both media and public discourse. According to Entman (1993: 52) 'to frame is to select some aspects of a perceived reality and make them more salient in a communicating text, in such a way as to promote a particular problem definition, causal interpretation, moral evaluation, and/or treatment recommendation.' Frames have at least four functions: to define problems, diagnose causes, make moral judgements and suggest remedies (Entman, 1993). As crises make 'people seek causes and make attributions' (Coombs & Holladay, 2004: 97), all actors involved must offer consistent frames which guide understanding. Public opinion, perceptions and impressions about the crisis and the organisation are influenced by media frames; thus how media frame a crisis event, its cause and who is responsible need to be taken into account (Coombs, 2006). During crises, there is a constant negotiation of frames and meanings from actors involved in crisis management (e.g. government/public health officials, etc.), media organisations, oppositional actors, and publics, who are left to make sense out of the differing frames and interpret and reinterpret the crisis and the proposed solutions. The public health model of reporting suggests the frame should focus on the causes of a disease, the risk factors and prevention strategies (Coleman et al., 2011). It also shifts the debate from causes to mitigation and treatment (Coleman et al., 2011). However, when risks are framed as minimal, this can impact policy and public vigilance. Pieri (2019) argues that framing can legitimise ineffective policy interventions: the lack of UK border screening against Ebola was due to it firstly being framed by British media as 'a localised African crisis,' then 'a regional crisis' until finally, it was framed as 'a global security threat.' Furthermore, mass media can sometimes use framing to mediate fear. Theories of fear appeals suggest people will abide by suggested behaviours and preventable measures when afraid. In one study (Zhang et al., 2015: 77) media coverage of H1N1 was found to provoke fear and increase 'levels of perceived knowledge' among the public which lead to 'engagement in the preventive measures.' However, the ability of both governments and mass media to control the narrative has been weakened with the widespread adoption of social media which allows an explosion of pluralism.

A hybrid media information environment

Social media has proven to be problematic as a source of information. Stecula et al. (2020) found during the 2019 US measles outbreak that social media users were more likely to be misinformed about vaccines than those reliant on the mass media. Furthermore, within crisis situations, if official sources do not fill information gaps, high levels of public uncertainty allow the emotional tone to be set on social media (Cmeciu & Coman, 2018). In other words, the narrative becomes controlled by non-official sources. As Utz et al. (2013: 40) argue, 'Social media play in today's societies a fundamental role for the negotiation and dynamics of crises.' Social media platforms offer a direct channel to the public for a range of actors; they can prove to be important sources of information and journalists use them as a means for breaking news due to their immediacy;

have become a space for information seeking and sharing behaviours, as well as healing spaces and are a tool for public responders for organising. On the other hand, social media are also spaces where misinformation and disinformation can spread. During the COVID-19 pandemic, this prompted the WHO to urge governments and media to fight against the 'infodemic.' Therefore, social media provides opportunities for official and alternative narratives to go viral and studies show differing platforms during differing health crises hosting varying levels and density of misinformation (Guidry et al., 2020a, 2020b).

Misleading health information is not a new issue, the term *infodemiology* was coined almost two decades prior to COVID-19 (Eysenbach, 2002). However, it gained increased prominence during this pandemic. During a public health crisis, it is crucial the information environment be science-led, be grounded in policy and health care practice and disseminated to the public through traditional news and social media. However, in an era when trust in expertise has diminished and personal beliefs are employed to filter reality (van Zoonen, 2012) science communication competes for credibility with material prominent purely due to its ability to go viral. The less information and answers science can offer, the greater the space that can be filled with misinformation circulating across social networks. Particularly problematic is the finding that misinformation is shared more often by social media users than verified information (Vosoughi et al., 2018).

Eysenbach (2020) formulates four pillars to fight the infodemic in the context of health care. Firstly, information should transfer from expert (e.g. scholars or doctors) to the public directly so misinterpretation cannot occur, and facts are not influenced by politics, commercial interests, selective reporting, or misunderstanding. Secondly, information must be clearly substantiated with empirical data. Thirdly, information needs to be presented clearly and made accessible to ensure public health literacy (Norman & Skinner, 2006). Fourth and finally, it is important to monitor the information environment and debunk misinformation and rumours.

Thus, political communication research offers clear lessons for crisis communication. Spokespersons must be credible and must develop messages that offer a positive framing of the outcomes of behaviour needed to alleviate the negative effects of the crisis grounded in accessible science while debunking misinformation. Media, in turn, has a crucial role in providing information and judging how to act best in the interests of the whole nation as well as its specific audience without undermining official information and spreading misinformation. Understanding the psychology of populations facing a pandemic helps to explain why these factors are crucial.

Political psychology during pandemics

Initial reports of a new virus emerging in China were 'not a practical warning, but a science fiction movie that had nothing to do with us' (Jetten et al., 2020:

17). The threat posed became apparent later. As the seriousness of the threat pressed governments to implement measures that restrict public freedoms, it was crucial to create a national shared identity which makes compliance a collective endeavour. Jetten et al. (2020) thus argues any behavioural communication needs at its heart a 'we' concept with the public 'shepherded by a paternalistic government' (Jetten et al., 2020: 6). The 'we' concept is a notion of unity created within a culture of we-ness, a culture that 'engenders a sense of common fate and encourages people to join in cooperative efforts' (Greenaway et al., 2020: 54). We-ness provides psychological support through instilling a group-oriented attitude and building emotional intimacy within the community (Yang, 2019). Building a culture of we-ness requires a central unifying figure who can embody 'representing us,' 'doing it for us' and crafting and embedding a sense of us in all communication (Jetten et al., 2020: 25–30). Representing 'us' in particular requires abandoning partisan or ideological positions and all exclusionary notions of society. Doing it for us means leaders cannot be exceptional, practically as well as rhetorically it must be demonstrated that all members of society are 'in it together.' Messages crafted with we-ness embedded emphasise one nation, all in it together, independent of immigration status, race, nationality, religion, creed, gender, sexuality or social status. The unifying leader must represent every single person within the nation's borders. It is argued that this strategy is more likely to ensure we-ness is internalised. This allows social norms (Azjen, 1998) to be established which in turn ensures compliance with preventative measures.

Clearly some leaders, due to their past history, ideological stance or political position can instil unity better than others. Hence some leaders are more trusted by a broader spectrum of a nation's community than others. However, communication can overcome factors that have previously polarised public opinion. Trust can be built through providing clear messages, eradicating errors, confusion or contradiction while also demonstrating empathy, honesty, timeliness, clarity and pathos through communication (Carter et al., 2020: 90–92). Failure to achieve this leads to negative availability bias (Dube-Rioux & Russo, 1988) among those who do not support that leader or their political party which leads to non-compliance. Compliance can be enforced, but voluntary compliance is better. Hence where leaders do not have the full support of a nation, they need to employ nudges while also framing behaviour. Mols (2020: 39) argues that those who are compliant must be framed as heroes and strong, not weak or sheep-like. Positive we-ness creates the conditions where mutual concern and support lead to community resilience. In contrast, exclusivity leads to selfishness and focus on defending smaller societal units – the household rather than the wider community. Selfishness leads to panic buying and hoarding, fearing contact with neighbours and hostility to those in need rather than supporting the isolated and vulnerable (Neville & Reichter, 2020: 74). Framing the struggle against COVID-19 as a national struggle is helped by the fact the virus is an external enemy, although framing it as Chinese has the negative outcome of associating it with anyone who appears South-East Asian (Greenaway et al., 2020: 52).

The adoption of an oppositional stance by members of a community results from failures to institute we-ness and develop a narrative of national unity. Framing COVID-19 as an external threat reinforces national identity and defines we-ness as nationalist. But the values of a nation and understandings of who 'belong' within a nation matter under these conditions (Greenaway et al., 51). Societal divisions and political polarisation lead to partisan-framed behaviours. Perceptions that society is polarised leads to selfishness and a focus on protecting in-groups or smaller societal units rather than we-ness. The more divided societies are, the less likely they will unite in a common cause. Hence, how identity is emphasised, exclusive or inclusive, shapes behavioural responses (Ntontis & Rocha, 2020).

Aside from communicational failures, poverty has been identified as the greatest underlying factor driving non-compliance (Jetten et al., 2020: 7–8), hence measures need to enable compliance. Empathy, as well as indications that measures are effective, reduce stress. Stress can lead to non-compliance among the most economically or virologically vulnerable (Muldoon, 2020). Similarly, the fairness of the rules, their enforcement and all being seen to comply, from leader downwards, prevents disorder. Perceptions of a fairness disparity lead those who feel excluded, less privileged or discriminated against to rebel against their perceived worse deal (Stott & Radbrun, 2020). Discrimination can cut along any societal fissures: haves and have nots, by social class, race or people versus elite, and ultimately lead to disunity. Importantly, feelings of discrimination and exclusion lead people to seek alternative explanations. The COVID-19 pandemic has created an environment ripe for conspiracy theories to flourish and gain traction. Common themes are that the virus was developed deliberately (leading to low trust and fear of a human or state enemy); that the impact is exaggerated to allow greater social control by governments (leading to resistance) or downplayed to benefit others (leading to low trust in authorities). Conspiracy theories are difficult to disprove and are only prevented from spreading when the national leadership instils trust and we-ness.

Crisis phases and communication strategy

Any crisis evolves in phases and it is essential to recognise these, and how strategy should be adapted to each phase. While there can be variance across countries, we would expect a crisis to pass through four main phases: pre-crisis, preparation, crisis and normalisation; the appropriate communication strategy for each is detailed below.

Pre-crisis, build-up phase

If a health crisis is seen as likely, messaging should emphasise internalising information to precondition the audience to the leadership's position related to the impending situation (Lim et al., 2018). New viruses can have a limited global impact, impacting a single nation or region only, which was historically the case with H1N1, SARS and MERS. However, any outbreak should be considered as having the potential to have a global impact, and such a perspective aids preparedness should this be the case (Butler, 2009). Given the uncertainty of health risks, people need to know what is known and what is unknown, and they need to be constantly guided towards behaviour that helps protect their own and others' health. Hence even at the phase when a crisis might unfold it is important for those taking the lead to be first with their communication. The CERC manual (2018) argues, 'Crises are time-sensitive. Communicating information quickly is crucial. For members of the public, the first source of information often becomes the preferred source.'

Within this early phase it is important to control the narrative, if not the information gap can be filled by alternative sources. Public health experts are usually dissatisfied with the way media report health issues, arguing the media focus on the more dramatic stories which gives their audience a distorted view (Coleman et al., 2011). Coverage can also be problematic if information is framed according to prevailing tropes determined by editorial policy, such as partisan or national interests. Hoffman-Goetz, Shannon and Clarke (2003) also argue that the way media cover health issues does not reflect the threats and is usually limited to focusing on mortality. New viruses are often reported as contained in a single area; the media give their audiences the role of passive observer to events happening in a far-off place (Jones et al., 2013). Hence the threat outside of that nation or region is perceived as minimal, with no preparedness despite the globalised nature of the world and the simplicity by which people, and viruses, spread through international travel.

Preparation phase

As build-up continues and a crisis becomes imminent, message emphasis should shift to instruction to prepare publics to respond with specific actions to the crisis. Again, being first is crucial as this allows the identification of a clear point of reference and the construction of a clear narrative. In order to avoid confusion, which can lead to loss of public trust, increased fear and anxiety and obstruction of response measures, coordinated message development and release of information between federal, state and local health officials is critical (Lim et al., 2018). It is also important to have a media management strategy in place as mass media become the main source for consistent trustworthy health information (Schwitzer et al., 2005) and are more important than interpersonal communication in raising awareness (Coleman et al., 2011). Hence the CERC principles highlight that in preparing for an outbreak, official sources must be quick to share information on how to help stop the spread and impact of a disease.

Given people remember the first information they hear during an emergency, this should come from credible sources who will consistently play a leading role: CERC argue the best spokespersons are health experts who can stay ahead of possible rumours, even when the cause of the outbreak or other specifics are unknown. They are also best placed to provide information about the signs and symptoms of the virus, who is most at risk, the treatment and care options, and when to seek medical care. During this phase experts become innately news-worthy as media depend on scientists and doctors when reporting on health and science as they add credibility to journalists' stories (Ramsey, 1999).

While media play a critical role in providing life-saving information, they can also hold government institutions to account reporting for rather than about those affected. Hence governments need to ensure their message, and measures taken, are clearly explained to journalists to avoid reporting that contrasts the original message. Governments must present a solid case for alerting people to the danger of the crisis, allowing journalists to update audiences on develop-ments and provide real life stories to aid understanding across the phases of a pandemic (Gunawardene & Noronha, 2007) and to shape behaviour. But official sources must provide 'localised specific information,' as without this journalists 'can compromise accuracy, perceptions of trust and relevance' (Hannides, 2015: 56) when drawing on a range of sources. Hence close working relationships between media outlets, governments and their nominated experts are crucial for ensuring public preparedness to take measures to protect themselves when a health crisis is imminent.

Crisis phase

When the health crisis hits, communication should remain focussed on instruct-ing, as people need to engage in specific behaviours to get through the crisis. The way government officials develop a narrative or frame to encapsulate the crisis, the government's response and the role the public can play is of crucial impor-tance. Hence official communication needs to provide guidance to the public on how to protect themselves, loved ones and others and build a wider sense of we-ness. Being right and being credible (CERC, 2018[2]) at this stage is crucial: 'Accuracy establishes credibility. Information can include what is known, what is not known, and what is being done to fill in the gaps.' Information should be correct, succinct and not patronising but also empathetic. Communication should be timely, transparent, accurate and science based to build public trust and confidence. There is hence a need to 'minimize speculation, clearly state the strengths and limitations of current data, and avoid over-reassurance of the pub-lic' (Reynolds & Quinn, 2008). Building from the previous phase it is recognised there is an immediate, intense and sustained public demand for information from different actors (healthcare providers, policy makers, news media). Hence, all these stakeholders must work within an integrated framework. CERC principles highlight public health messages and medical guidance should be complemen-tary and not contradictory. They cite the example: 'public health officials should not widely encourage people to go to the doctors if doctors are turning people away and running out of medicine for critically ill people.' Hence everything should always be fact and sense checked as an incorrect message can lead to harmful consequences, lost credibility and the potential loss of trust in future messages. Clinicians need to be a part of the public dialogue answering questions. Five common, avoidable pitfalls emphasised by CERC (2018: 8) are (1) mixed messages from multiple experts; (2) information released late; (3) paternalistic attitudes; (4) not countering rumours and myths in real-time and (5) public power struggles and confusion. These impact negatively on the credibility of official sources, their messages and guidance and lead to negative perceptions towards the governmental response.

Olson and Gawronski (2010) asked, 'Why is it that some authorities, governments/administrations, and even entire regimes emerge from disasters more popular and politically stronger, while most appear to emerge less popular and politically weaker, sometimes fatally so?' Using a framework of "Maslowian Shocks,' they suggested the public estimate a government's disaster response across six dimensions: capability, competence, compassion, correctness, credibility and anticipation. Capability refers to the resources available and mobilised and the extent these are efficient or deficient. Competence refers to the efficient and appropriate application of available resources. Compassion refers to whether communication demonstrates concern for and understanding of victims and their families. Correctness refers to perceptions of honesty in communication, fairness in allocation of resources and transparency in assistance. Credibility refers to the consistent and reliable provision of information. Finally, anticipation asks whether the crisis was avoidable, could better procedures have been in place to aid mitigation and preparedness, what is commonly referred to as disaster risk reduction (Olson & Gawronski, 2010). We argue that these estimations are based on perceptions and relate to three component parts of the response. Firstly, the official messaging, secondly, first-hand experiences and thirdly, second-hand or mediated experiences. These are all cornerstones of a communication strategy which are argued to unite a nation behind measures (Jetten et al., 2020) and are crucial during the crisis phase. Alongside these is emphasising representing us and doing it for us. 'Being quarantined can be disruptive, frustrating, and feel scary. Especially when the reason for quarantine is exposure to a new disease for which there may be limited information.' Hence 'Giving people meaningful things to do calms anxiety, helps restore order, and promotes some sense of control.'[3] Promoting action therefore involves simple, memorable messages that have a heuristic quality, such as 'cover your cough.' These messages need to be promoted in various ways to reach diverse populations (i.e. people with disabilities, different access to information, limited language proficiency etc.). Finally, following the CERC principles, communication must show respect, actively listening to local communities and local leaders and their issues and solutions, acknowledging different cultural beliefs and practices about diseases and not dismissing fears or concerns, giving everyone a chance to talk and ask questions and working with communities in order to adjust behaviours and promote understanding.

Normalisation phase

As the spread of a virus abates, restrictions should be lifted gradually and appropriately without giving an impression of contradiction and causing confusion. The framing narrative of we-ness needs to remain in place to ensure compliance with the revised restrictions and again governments must emphasise they are representing and doing it for 'us' and in the situation with us. As during the crisis phase, clear communication is necessary following those same rules of capability, competence, compassion, correctness, credibility and anticipation.

Conclusion

The above provides a framework for how political communication should be practised during a pandemic, recognising the potential pitfalls and what discourse and rhetoric should be avoided. Of course, this represents a perfect world scenario, however drawing on research in the fields of crisis communication, political communication and political psychology, it is possible to set up this theoretically based straw man. Our 29 case studies will explore the strategies employed within the WHO, 27 nations and the European Union. In our conclusion, we return to these concepts to draw together an analysis of the extent to which nations adhered to this framework, the extent global or supranational organisations provided leadership to enable national leaders and the extent that there is a correspondence between successes and failures and the outcomes across these nations.

Notes

1 https://emergency.cdc.gov/cerc/resources/pdf/cerc_2014edition.pdf
2 https://emergency.cdc.gov/cerc/manual/index.asp
3 www.cdc.gov/media/releases/2020/t0214-covid-19-update.html.html

References

Ajzen, I. (1998). Models of human social behavior and their application to health psychology. *Psychology and Health*, *13*(4), 735–739.
Austin, L., & Jin, Y. (2018). *Social media and crisis communication*. New York: Routledge.
Butler, D. (2009). Swine flu goes global: New influenza virus tests pandemic emergency preparedness. *Nature*, *458*(7242), 1082–1084.
Carter, H., Weston, D., & Amlot, R. (2020). Managing crowds in crises. In J. Jetten, S. D. Reicher, S. A. Haslam, & Cruwys, T. (Eds.), *Together apart: The psychology of COVID-19* (pp. 88–92). London: SAGE.
CERC (2014). https://emergency.cdc.gov/cerc/resources/pdf/cerc_2014edition.pdf
CERC (2018). https://emergency.cdc.gov/cerc/manual/index.asp
Cmeciu, C., & Coman, I. (2018). Twitter as a means of emotional coping and collective (Re) framing of crises. case study: The 'Colectiv' crisis in Romania. *Social Communication*, *4*(2), 6–15.

Coleman, R., Thorson, E., & Wilkins, L. (2011). Testing the effect of framing and sourcing in health news stories. *Journal of Health Communication, 16*(9), 941–954.

Collinson, S., Khan, K., & Heffernan, J. M. (2015). The effects of media reports on disease spread and important public health measurements. *PloS One, 10*(11), e0141423.

Coombs, W. (2006). Crisis management: A communicative approach. In C. H. Botan & V. Hazleton (Eds.), *Public relations theory* (pp. 171–197). Mahwah, NJ: Lawrence Erlbaum Associates.

Coombs, W. (2015). *Ongoing crisis communication. Planning, managing, and responding* (4th ed.). New York: SAGE.

Coombs, W. T., & Holladay, S. J. (2004). Reasoned action in crisis communication: An attribution theory-based approach to crisis management. In D. P. Millar & R. L. Heath (Eds.), *Responding to crisis communication approach to crisis communication* (pp. 95–115). Hillsdale, NJ: Lawrence Erlbaum Associates.

Dube-Rioux, L., & Russo, J. E. (1988). An availability bias in professional judgment. *Journal of Behavioral Decision Making, 1*(4), 223–237.

Entman, R. (1993). Framing toward classification of a fractured paradigm. *Journal of Communication , 43*(4), 51–58.

Eysenbach, G. (2002). Infodemiology: The epidemiology of (mis)information. *American Journal of Medicine, 113*(9), pp. 763–765.

Eysenbach, G. (2020). How to fight an infodemic: The four pillars of infodemic management. *Journal of Medical Internet Research, 22*(6), 1–6.

Fearn-Banks, K. (2011). *Crisis communications a casebook approach.* New York: Routledge.

Greenaway, K. H. (2020). Group threat. In J. Jetten, S. D. Reicher, S. A. Haslam, & T. Cruwys (Eds.), *Together apart: The psychology of COVID-19* (pp. 49–54). London: SAGE.

Guidry, J. P., Coman, I. A., Vraga, E. K., O'Donnell, N. H., & Sreepada, N. (2020a). (S) pin the flu vaccine: Recipes for concern. *Vaccine*, 38(34), 5498–5506.

Guidry, J. P., Meganck, S. L., Perrin, P. B., Messner, M., Lovari, A., & Carlyle, K. E. (2020b). #Ebola: Tweeting and pinning an epidemic. *Atlantic Journal of Communication*, Online https://doi.org/10.1080/15456870.2019.1707202.

Gunawardene, N., & Noronha, F. (2007). *Communicating disasters: An Asia Pacific resource book.* Geneva: United Nations Development Programme.

Hannides, T. (2015). *Humanitarian broadcasting in emergencies: A synthesis of evaluation findings.* London: BBC Media Action.

Hoffman-Goetz, L., Shannon, C., & Clarke, J. N. (2003). Chronic disease coverage in Canadian aboriginal newspapers. *Journal of Health Communication, 8*(5), 475–488.

Jetten, J., Reicher, S. D., Haslam, S. A., & Cruwys, T. (Eds.). (2020). *Together apart: The psychology of COVID-19.* London: SAGE.

Jones, T. M., Van Aelst, P., & Vliegenthart, R. (2013). Foreign nation visibility in US news coverage: A longitudinal analysis (1950–2006). *Communication Research, 40*(3), 417–436.

Kahn, L. (2020). *Who's in charge? Leadership during epidemics, bioterror attacks, and other public health crises.* Santa Barbara, CA: Praeger Security International.

Lilleker, D. (2018). Politics in a post-truth era. *International Journal of Media & Cultural Politics, 14*(3), 277–282.

Lim, R. S. Q., Tan, E. Y., Lim, E. W., Aziz, N. B., & Pang, A. (2018). When a pandemic strikes. In L. Austin & Y. Jin, (Eds.), *Toward the social media pandemic communication model in social media and crisis communication* (pp. 253–266). New York: Routledge.

Mogensen, K., Lindsay, L., Li, X., Perkins, J., & Beardsley, M.(2002). How TV news covered the crisis: The content of CNN, CBS, ABC, NBC and Fox. In B. S.

Greenberg (Ed.), *Communication and terrorism: Public and media responses to 9/11* (pp. 101–120). New York: Hampton Press.

Mols, F. (2020). Behaviour change. In J. Jetten, S. D. Reicher, S. A. Haslam, & T. Cruwys (Eds.), *Together apart: The psychology of COVID-19* (pp. 36–40). London: SAGE.

Muldoon, O. (2020). Collective Trauma. In J. Jetten, S. D. Reicher, S. A. Haslam, & T. Cruwys (Eds.), *Together apart: The psychology of COVID-19* (pp. 36–40). London: SAGE.

Neville, F., & Reicher, S. (2020). Crowds. In J. Jetten, S. D. Reicher, S. A. Haslam, & T. Cruwys (Eds.), *Together apart: The psychology of COVID-19* (pp. 74–79). London: SAGE.

Norman, C. D., & Skinner, H. A. (2006). eHEALS: The eHealth literacy scale. *Journal of Medicine Internet Research, 8*(4), 1–7.

Ntontis, E., & Rocha, C. (2020). Solidarity. In J. Jetten, S. D. Reicher, S. A. Haslam, & T. Cruwys (Eds.), *Together apart: The psychology of COVID-19* (pp. 84–87). London: SAGE.

Olson, R. S., & Gawronski, V. T. (2010). From disaster event to political crisis: A '5C+ A' framework for analysis. *International Studies Perspectives, 11*(3), 205–221.

Palen, L. (2008). Online social media in crisis events. *Educause Quarterly, 31*(3), 76–78.

Perng, S. Y., Büscher, M., Wood, L., Halvorsrud, R., Stiso, M., Ramirez, L., & Al-Akkad, A. (2013). Peripheral response: Microblogging during the 22/7/2011 Norway attacks. *International Journal of Information Systems for Crisis Response and Management (IJISCRAM), 5*(1), 41–57.

Pieri, E. (2019). Media framing and the threat of global pandemics: The Ebola crisis in UK media and policy response. *Sociological Research Online, 24*(1), 73–92.

Ramsey, S. (1999). A benchmark study of elaboration and sourcing in science stories for eight American newspapers. *Journalism & Mass Communication Quarterly, 76*(1), 87–98.

Renshon, S. A. (2000). Political leadership as social capital: Governing in a divided national culture. *Political Psychology, 21*(1), 199–226.

Reynolds, B., & Quinn, S. C. (2008). Effective communication during an influenza pandemic: The value of using a crisis and emergency risk communication framework. *Health Promotion Practice, 9*(4) Supplement, 13–17.

Schudson, M. (2011). *The sociology of news.* New York: Norton & Co.

Schwitzer, G., Mudur, G., Henry, D., Wilson, A., Goozner, M., Simbra, M., & Baverstock, K. A. (2005). What are the roles and responsibilities of the media in disseminating health information? *PLoS Medicine, 2*(7), e215.

Seeger, M. W., Sellnow, T. L., & Ulmer, R. R. (1998). Communication, organization, and crisis. *Annals of the International Communication Association, 21*(1), 231–276.

Stecula, D. A., Kuru, O., & Jamieson, K. H. (2020). *How trust in experts and media use affect acceptance of common anti-vaccination claims.* https://misinforeview.hks.harvard.edu/article/users-of-social-media-more-likely-to-be-misinformed-about-vaccines/

Stott, C., & Radbrun, M. (2020). Social order and disorder. In J. Jetten, S. D. Reicher, S. A. Haslam, & T. Cruwys (Eds.), *Together apart: The psychology of COVID-19* (pp. 93–97). London: SAGE.

Strömbäck, J. (2008). Four phases of mediatization: An analysis of the mediatization of politics. *The International Journal of Press/Politics, 13*(3), 228–246.

Utz, S., Schultz, F., & Glocka, S. (2013). Crisis communication online: How medium, crisis type and emotions affected public reactions in the Fukushima Daiichi nuclear disaster. *Public Relations Review, 39*(1), 40–46.

Van Zoonen, L. (2012). I-Pistemology: Changing truth claims in popular and political culture. *European Journal of Communication, 27*(1), 56–67.

Van Zoonen, L., & Holtz-Bacha, C. (2000). Personalisation in Dutch and German politics: The case of talk show. *Javnost – the Public, 7*(2), 45–56.

Vosoughi, S., Roy, D., & Aral, S. (2018). The spread of true and false news online. *Science, 359*(6380), 1146–1151.

Webb, P., & Poguntke, T. (2013). The presidentialisation of politics thesis defended. *Parliamentary Affairs, 66*(3), 646–654.

Yang, J. (2019). The influence of Korean collectivism on interpersonal communication behaviors. *Journal of the Korea Contents Association, 19*(5), 1–14.

Zhang, L., Kong, Y., & Chang, H. (2015). Media use and health behavior in H1N1 flu crisis: The mediating role of perceived knowledge and fear. *Atlantic Journal of Communication, 23*(2), 67–80.

Case Studies

1

WORLD HEALTH ORGANISATION

The challenges of providing global leadership

Darren Lilleker and Miloš Gregor

Political context

The World Health Organisation (WHO) is a subsidiary agency of the United Nations, established on April 7, 1948, with a remit to advocate for global universal healthcare and coordinate responses to health emergencies. The WHO's reputation rests on the success of projects on which it has provided leadership. It proudly advertises its leading role in eradicating smallpox and the development of a vaccine to combat the Ebola virus, which as a disease transferred from primates to humans and attacks the respiratory and digestive systems and has similarities to COVID-19.

The WHO's ability to oversee global public health relies on effective co-ordination of the World Health Assembly (WHA), a meeting of representatives of the 194 member states as well as securing funding. The WHO's budget, at around four billion dollars a year ($4.8 billion 2020–21),[1] is made up of assessed contributions from member states, based on national GDP and population size, and voluntary contributions; the latter constitute 80% of its budget. The United States, as the most significant contributor, pays in around one hundred million dollars per year in assessed contributions and between one and four hundred million dollars in voluntary contributions, without which the WHO could see its budget contract to one billion dollars.

The ability of the WHO to provide leadership is constrained by an inability to force honest reporting or political compliance with its guidance. It is also hampered by having to balance competing demands, such as between religious teaching and the promotion of safe sex to combat HIV/AIDS. The WHO is also seen as cumbersome, decentralised and bureaucratic, all of which hinders achievement of specific goals on a global scale. The remit of Current Director-General Tedros Adhanom, former Health and Foreign Minister of Ethiopia, is to

DOI: 10.4324/9781003120254-3

improve the WHO's effectiveness in developing better technical and governance partnerships while retaining political independence. COVID-19 highlighted the challenges the WHO faces in providing early alerts, appropriate guidance as well as developing a communication strategy that could reach all nations, their leaders and citizens.

Chronology

From the first case being reported in Wuhan, China on December 31, 2019, by August 28, 2020 there were 24,257,989 cases across all 251 countries recognised by the UN and 827,246 deaths resulting from COVID-19 (https://covid19.who .int/). See Table 1.1.

Analysis

From January 1 to the end of August 2020, the WHO delivered almost a hundred press conferences and briefings. The first official statement on January 23, called on the global community to demonstrate solidarity and cooperation in identifying and tackling the spread, which was then described as only having the potential to be transmitted from human to human. While the WHO cannot create the environment for global solidarity, it had the position to lead the response to COVID-19. In order to do that it must: (1) provide clear, accurate and up-to-date information on the spread, i.e. information on numbers of active cases, human-to-human transmission and mortality rates; (2) identify effective countermeasures to prevent spread and (3) debunk false and misleading information. Our analysis centres on these three key communication areas.

Informing the world

As the agency focusing on health emergencies, the WHO relies on information provided by national authorities. The first occurrence of any disease, number of active cases, infectivity, mortality or source of infection cannot be obtained without cooperation from countries experiencing an outbreak. A problem arises when that country eschews transparency and attempts to restrict information as this constrains the WHO's understanding and ability to develop effective guidance. Unfortunately, this was the case with China at the turn of 2019 and 2020. Information about the first cases of COVID-19 were leaked to the media by whistleblowers, not official communication channels. Moreover, multiple testimonies show China tried to withhold information about the novel coronavirus (Kuo, 2020). China's approach caused several weeks of delay in understanding the threat of COVID-19.

The novel coronavirus outbreak was identified in Wuhan, China, and reported to the WHO representation in China on December 31, 2019. The WHO published a statement informing about a 'pneumonia of unknown cause' on January

TABLE 1.1 WHO chronology

	Date	Global Diffusion of COVID-19	Key official actions	Key communication events
December	31	First case being reported in Wuhan, China.		
January	1		WHO set up IMST (Incident Management Support Team).	Flags a potential threat posed by this new strain of coronavirus by putting the organisation on an emergency footing for dealing with the outbreak.
	4	3 confirmed cases in China.		WHO posted to social media '#China has reported to WHO a cluster of #pneumonia cases – with no deaths – in Wuhan, Hubei Province, China.
	5		Disease Outbreak News includes a risk assessment and advice for public health.	No specific measures for travellers or travel and trade restrictions on China advised.
	10	45 confirmed cases In China. First death reported.	Guidance released stating testing should only be given to those with symptoms.	Technical guidance issued focusing on detecting, testing for and managing potential cases, drawing on experience with SARS and MERS.
	14	50 confirmed cases.		Press briefing and social media posts state no clear evidence of human-to-human transmission.
	22	470 confirmed cases. 9 deaths reported.	Emergency Committee convened to assess whether the outbreak constituted a public health emergency of international concern, no consensus was reached.	Technical advice is issued calling for preparedness for containment, including active surveillance, early detection, isolation and case management, contact tracing and prevention of onward spread.

(Continued)

TABLE 1.1 (Continued)

Date		Global Diffusion of COVID-19	Key official actions	Key communication events
	30	7,912 confirmed cases. 170 deaths reported.	Emergency Committee re-convened, consensus reached that the outbreak constituted a Public Health Emergency of International Concern.	WHO opposes travel restrictions, even on citizens from Hubei province.
February	3	17,478 confirmed cases. 362 deaths reported.	Strategic Preparedness and Response Plan released to help protect states with weaker health systems.	
	11	43,199 confirmed cases. 1,018 deaths reported; 108 in a single day.	Research and Innovation Forum convened to bring together entrepreneurs and funders to help with mitigating the crisis.	
March	11	124,209 confirmed cases. 4,641 deaths reported.	COVID-19 classified as a global pandemic.	
	13	141,073 confirmed cases. 5,486 deaths reported.	COVID-19 Solidarity Response Fund launched to receive donations from private individuals, corporations and institutions.	
	18	209,075 confirmed cases. 9,270 deaths reported; 1,083 in a single day.	WHO and partners launch the Solidarity Trial, an international clinical trial that aims to generate robust data from around the world to find the most effective treatments for COVID-19.	
	20	262,298 confirmed cases. 12,017 deaths reported.	WHO Health Alert for coronavirus launches on WhatsApp.	Media briefing, Director-General (D-G) suggests social distancing measures.

	23	339,301 confirmed cases. 16,634 deaths reported.	WHO and FIFA team up on campaign to kick out coronavirus.	
	25	427,077 confirmed cases. 21,287 deaths reported.	UN launches COVID-19 Global Humanitarian Response Plan to #InvestInHumanity.	
	26	483,727 confirmed cases. 24,147 deaths reported.	Extraordinary Virtual G20 Leaders' Summit on COVID-19.	
	31	767,696 confirmed cases. 40,661 deaths reported.	Report of falsified medical products, including in vitro diagnostics, that claim to prevent, detect, treat or cure COVID-19.	Chatbot launched with Rakuten Viber to help users be informed, learn how to protect themselves, test their knowledge and bust myths.
April	1	842,704 confirmed cases. 44,846 deaths reported.	WHO in Africa holds first 'hackathon' for COVID-19 bringing together entrepreneurs to pioneer creative local solutions and address critical gaps.	
	2	916,160 confirmed cases. 49,811 deaths reported.	COVID-19 Health System Response Monitor created jointly with the European Commission and the European Observatory on Health Systems and Policies to offer cross-country comparisons and track public health initiatives.	
	6	1,228,566 confirmed cases. 72,084 deaths reported.	#BeActive launched campaign with FIFA.	Advice issued on face masks: 'Masks alone cannot stop the #COVID19 pandemic. Countries must continue to find, test, isolate and treat every case and trace every contact.'

(*Continued*)

TABLE 1.1 (Continued)

Date	Global Diffusion of COVID-19	Key official actions	Key communication events
8	1,373,454 confirmed cases 84,303 deaths reported		D-G responds to criticism from US president Trump calling for solidarity and: 'please quarantine politicising COVID-19.'
13	1,787,323 confirmed cases. 116,865 deaths reported.	Expert group forms to collaborate on vaccine development.	
14	1,857,917 confirmed cases. 112,324 deaths reported.	Major update to COVID-19 dashboard https:// covid19.who.int/	
17	12,453 deaths in a single day, the peak of deaths Jan–Aug.		
20	2,321,417 confirmed cases. 167,348 deaths reported.	Launch of text messaging service to provide alert information to those without Internet access.	
24	2,630,691 confirmed cases. 192,482 deaths reported.	Launch of COVID-19 Tools Accelerator: Global Collaboration to Accelerate the Development, Production and Equitable Access to New COVID-19 diagnostics, therapeutics and vaccines.	
30	3,104,568 confirmed cases. 224,724 deaths reported.	D-G convened the third International Health Regulations (IHR) Emergency Committee on COVID-19.	Statement that COVID-19 still represented a Public Health Emergency of International Concern (PHEIC).

(Continued)

May			
4	3,446,082 confirmed cases. 248,061 deaths reported.	D-G addressed leaders from 40 countries from all over the world at a COVID-19 Global Response International Pledging Event, hosted by the European Commission.	
5	3,528,251 confirmed cases. 250,182 deaths reported.	WHO launches the COVID-19 Supply Portal, a purpose-built tool to facilitate and consolidate submission of supply requests.	
10	3,947,799 confirmed cases. 276,633 deaths reported.	WHO sets out considerations in adjusting public health and social measures for workplaces, schools and mass gatherings.	WHO issues interim guidance on contact tracing protocols.
13	4,188,036 confirmed cases. 288,842 deaths reported.	WHO Academy App launched, designed to inform health care workers to help them care for COVID-19 patients and protect themselves.	
15	4,359,238 confirmed cases. 298,925 deaths reported.	WHO released a Scientific Brief on multisystem inflammatory syndrome in children and adolescents.	
18	4,647,626 confirmed cases. 313,233 deaths reported.	The 73rd World Health Assembly, the first ever to be held virtually, adopted a landmark resolution to bring the world together to fight the COVID-19 pandemic.	D-G 'Let our shared humanity be the antidote to our shared threat.'
21	4,918,089 confirmed cases. 324,496 deaths reported.	WHO signed a new agreement with the UN Refugee Agency to support ongoing efforts to protect 70 million+ forcibly displaced people from COVID-19.	

TABLE 1.1 (Continued)

Date	Global Diffusion of COVID-19	Key official actions	Key communication events
29	5,707,599 confirmed cases. 358,565 deaths reported.	Thirty countries and multiple international partners and institutions launched the COVID-19 Technology Access Pool (C-TAP), an initiative to make vaccines, tests, treatments and other health technologies to fight COVID-19 accessible to all.	
June 5	6,516,317 confirmed cases. 388,297 deaths reported.	WHO published updated guidance recommending the wearing of masks to help control the spread of COVID-19.	
13	7,531,572 confirmed cases. 424,627 deaths reported.		WHO reported that Chinese authorities had provided information on a cluster of COVID-19 cases in Beijing.
16	7,918,966 confirmed cases. 436,125 deaths reported.		WHO welcomed initial clinical trial results from the UK that showed dexamethasone, a corticosteroid, could be lifesaving for patients critically ill with COVID-19.
17	8,038,634 confirmed cases. 441,634 deaths reported.	WHO ended trials of hydroxychloroquine as an effective COVID-19 treatment due to poor results.	WHO reminds public to remain vigilant through Mr Bean's Essential COVID-19 Checklist.
26	9,454,484 confirmed cases. 484,313 deaths reported.	The ACT-Accelerator launched its investment case, calling for $31.3 billion over next 12 months to fund diagnostics, therapeutics, vaccines and the health system connector.	

July			
4	10,925,739 confirmed cases. 523,063 deaths reported.	WHO withdraw support for all hydroxychloroquine and lopinavir/ritonavir trials due to poor results.	
6	11,332,503 confirmed cases. 532,381 deaths reported.		WHO shared survey findings, showing that 73 countries have warned that they are at risk of stock-outs of antiretroviral (ARV) medicines as a result of the COVID-19 pandemic.
9	11,879,532 confirmed cases. 545,526 deaths reported.	D-G launches Independent Panel for Pandemic Preparedness and Response (IPPR) to evaluate the world's response to the COVID-19 pandemic.	
13	12,774,911 confirmed cases. 566,681 deaths reported.	'State of Food Security and Nutrition in the World' is published, which forecasted that the COVID-19 pandemic could tip over 130 million more people into chronic hunger by 2021.	
17	13,622,372 confirmed cases. 585,754 deaths reported.	D-G launches updated Global Humanitarian Response Plan for COVID-19 for $10.3 billion to fight the virus in low-income and fragile countries.	
22	14,772,512 confirmed cases. 612,075 deaths reported.	COVID-19 Law Lab launched to provide vital legal information and support for the global COVID-19 response.	
31	17,114,704 confirmed cases. Peak of 293,128 new cases. 668,943 deaths reported	The fourth meeting of the Emergency Committee is held.	News release highlights need for long-term coordinated response.

5. The statement was the first of regular reports on the number of new cases and later, the numbers cured or of those who succumbed to the disease. For these figures, the WHO had to rely on national reports. The speed and credibility of information was thus negatively affected from the outset. The first cases appeared weeks earlier than officially claimed by China and evidence of human-to-human transmission was concealed. Despite having the expertise and capacity to produce its own analysis and recommendations, the WHO had limited access to data at the beginning of 2020. China's political regime kept control over the information and data provided. The WHO was unable to officially confirm human-to-human transmission until January 22, although some information from Chinese doctors indicated the likelihood during the first days of the outbreak and the WHO admitted it was likely on January 14. But it took the identification of cases in Thailand before a definitive statement was made.

Although this delay was due to receiving limited information from China, the WHO received criticism from other states and the media. It was accused of not having a proactive approach, uncritically adopting Chinese statements and providing information belatedly. Hence, during January and February information from the WHO had serious flaws. WHO advice on testing on January 10 stated only those who presented with symptoms should be tested, suggesting there were no asymptomatic carriers.[2] There was also initial uncertainty about person-to-person transmission and the failure at the first meeting of the Emergency Committee on January 22 to reach a consensus on the severity of the global threat made it appear to vacillate. Statements claiming the virus was similar to SARS and MERS, both of which were contained with minimal global disruption, and continued opposition to travel restrictions offer evidence the WHO facilitated the complacency that led to risks being downplayed by national leaders and their health experts. It was only on March 11 that a global pandemic was declared, and nine days later social distancing measures were recommended. By this point, nations had adopted independent approaches, drawing on their own medical experts, to put in place restrictions on travel and social activities. Responding to criticism, Adhanom stated that a global health emergency had been declared on January 30 and some health experts defended the delay in declaring a pandemic as this represented a change in language rather a change in the potential threat (Spinney, 2020). Declaring a pandemic, Adhanom argued in a statement on March 11, was a response to 'alarming levels of inaction' as it was deemed necessary to compel nations to 'detect, test, treat, isolate, trace, and mobilise their people in the response, those with a handful of cases can prevent those cases becoming clusters, and those clusters becoming community transmission.' Criticism thus became muted, and later, only to come from US President Trump who blamed the WHO on many (often contradictory) fronts, for exaggeration of active cases and fatality rates to the belated alerts and, therefore, its responsibility for the pandemic, specifically the situation in the United States (Stevens & Tan, 2020). In response, Trump announced the freezing of US payments to the WHO (Murray, 2020).

However, by that time, the WHO was not a subject of criticism in most other countries. Greater attention was paid to the organisation during the outbreak phase when countries were seeking clear guidance on preventative measures. After the spread of the virus to all continents, the central role of the WHO was to provide global statistics based on data gathered from national authorities and updates on the effectiveness of measures. Further initiatives were introduced but the WHO's focus shifted to the most vulnerable countries as well as refugees. The WHO also sponsored the development of a range of apps and tools to support health workers and people to identify symptoms. The shift in focus demonstrates the WHO sharing good practice, especially from northern hemisphere countries that experienced early outbreaks, but unable to take full leadership for combatting COVID-19 globally or being the sole arbiter of what constituted credible information.

(In)effective measures

Identifying the most effective measures such as travel restrictions and the wearing of face masks equally became challenging. The first advice the WHO offered on international travel came out on January 10, advising the avoidance of close human contact and promoting frequent hand washing. It explicitly stated no restrictions for international traffic were recommended. Updates on January 24–27, 2020 added recommendations for temperature screenings at airports in countries with and without transmission. Later travel advice, published on February 11, saw the WHO repeat it was not recommending any travel or trade restrictions arguing such measures would be effective in the short term only and just in selected cases and cannot be implemented long term. The measures countries should consider were repatriation and quarantine for their citizens residing in affected areas. The WHO continued to advise against travel restriction even when dozens of airline companies suspended or limited flights to China and several countries imposed travel restrictions which came into force from late January (Sang-Hun, 2020). According to the United Nations World Tourism Organisation (UNWTO), by April 6, 96% of all worldwide destinations had introduced travel restrictions and by April 27, 72% had completely closed their borders (UNWTO, 2020). When a responsible restart of international travel became a reality (40% of all countries had eased the restrictions by mid-July), the WHO published updated travel advice on July 30 keeping most of the previous recommendations and containing no recommendation on travel restrictions as retaining the position travel bans had no justification after a virus has spread worldwide. This countered some expert evidence. Chinazzi et al. (2020) showed the epidemic in mainland China would have been delayed by approximately two weeks in the case of 90% travel reductions. The research argued early international restrictions could have helped flatten the curve, mainly in the first affected countries such as Italy, the Republic of Korea and Iran.

Further confusion accompanied the question of whether the wearing of face masks reduced the risk of contagion. Face masks were recommended by many scientific, national and supranational authorities as a public and personal health control measure against the spread of disease. Yet face mask wearing was not promoted by the WHO recommendations. The original interim guidance on January 29 generated confusion when identifying medical masks as the one important protection to limit the spread of COVID-19 but in the same statement noting that use of masks alone is insufficient. The confusion and chaos in the initial recommendation have been criticised (not only) by scholars (Chan et al., 2020). An updated version, released on March 19 stated there was no evidence of the usefulness of face masks for protection; therefore, it was recommended that masks should only be worn by those with a cough, fever or people who have difficulty breathing. Further advice published on April 6 stated mask wearing by healthy people carries potential critical risks but reduced the potential exposure risk to healthy people from those infected but pre-symptomatic. The conflicting evidence has fuelled protest movements opposing mandatory face mask wearing on the grounds they are useless or even counter-productive although these movements are driven as well by political beliefs (Leung et al., 2020). Debates on face masks have continued unabated. Scientific articles have demonstrated any face masks can reduce exposure to respiratory infections, suggesting homemade masks do not provide the same level of protection as medical ones, but can be effective when worn by the majority of a population to protect them from infection by asymptomatic individuals who emit droplets containing the virus (Ma et al., 2020). The WHO stated it recommends an evidence-based approach; however, when providing the list of risks of mask usage, the evidence supporting claims provided by the WHO seems to be missing. The latest update, from June 7, states masks should be used as part of a comprehensive strategy of measures to suppress disease transmission and save lives. Hence with two key preventative measures, travel restrictions and face mask wearing, the WHO has lacked a definitive and clear position.

Rebutting fake news

At the same rate of spread of COVID-19, misinformation and disinformation has gone viral globally, mirroring the challenges society has in controlling what the WHO described as an infodemic (WHO, 2020). The first misleading information appeared in parallel with the initial outbreak of COVID-19. On January 30, the BBC reported on the growing number of conspiracy theories relating to the origin of the virus and misleading advice regarding prevention and cure (BBC, 2020). A frequently circulating story suggested COVID-19 was part of a Chinese (Gertz, 2020) or US (Kurlantzick, 2020) biological weapons programme. *Global Times*, China's state-affiliated tabloid newspaper, published a story claiming the virus was of US origin (Shumei & Lin, 2020) while Iran's supreme leader Ayatollah Ali Kamenei refused US help to fight coronavirus in

March 2020, citing the conspiracy theory that the virus could be US made (Hafezi, 2020).

In late January 2020, conspiracy theories that 5G caused, or helped spread, COVID-19 were shared in Facebook anti-5G groups (Cellan-Jones, 2020). Regardless of the fact that there is no evidence that 5G weakens immune systems or is harmful to humans (Rahman, 2020), that viruses cannot be transmitted by radio waves and COVID-19 has spread to countries without 5G networks, the story gained some credibility. The theory has been debunked by national health authorities, mobile data providers and health experts (Gallagher, 2020). However, a statement by the WHO was slow in being produced.

Another claim, widely shared, advised people to keep their throat moist, avoid spicy food and take vitamin C in order to prevent contagion (Lytvynenko, 2020). The WHO did provide a statement on February 5 stating no treatments, including certain antibiotics, alcohol or herbs, were known to have any palliative effect. The WHO also ended trials of hydroxychloroquine on June 17 due to poor results; however, this seemed belated as Jair Bolsonaro and Donald Trump, presidents of Brazil and the United States respectively, had both extolled the virtues of the drug in preventing infections. On March 21, Trump declared he had completed a two-week course of Hydroxychloroquine and Azithromycin declaring them in a tweet to be 'the biggest game changers in the history of medicine' (Trump, 2020). The WHO launched a Chatbot to aid myth busting and obtain clear factual information; however, it was unable to emerge as the most credible source of information to many, particularly where facts became politicised and among groups who find conspiracy theories compelling (Van Prooijen & Jostmann, 2013).

Conclusion

The WHO should be able to provide global leadership for health emergencies and pandemics. However, the reliance on member states' openness and transparency hinders their ability to be first and be right when identifying the threat posed by a new virus, an issue which is particularly highlighted in the case of COVID-19. The evidence shared by China led to vacillation on the threat posed and so, nations had to develop their own responses to the spread of the virus within their own territories. The declaration of a global health emergency seemed to have limited effect, with the threat downplayed by accompanying questions regarding person-to-person contagion, a failure of the Emergency Committee to reach a consensus on the threat and a refusal to recommend widescale travel restrictions. The failure to have the right information during the early stages meant the WHO had to catch up with state-level approaches and focus on supporting more vulnerable nations who were witnessing the spread of the virus later. Further conflicting advice on the use of face masks opened spaces for a coalition of libertarians and populists to undermine measures to combat contagion. While it is difficult to criticise the WHO for failing to combat the spread of fake news, the lack of credibility due to early vacillation, conflicting recommendations and lack of clarity meant they were not in a strong position to be the primary definers of scientific evidence. These factors highlight not just the weaknesses at the heart of the WHO but weaknesses in the ability of the world to overcome differences and work together when facing a common threat.

Notes

1 The data is obtained from https://www.kff.org/global-health-policy/fact-sheet/the-u-s-government-and-the-world-health-organization/
2 https://apps.who.int/iris/bitstream/handle/10665/330374/WHO-2019-nCoV-laboratory-2020.1-eng.pdf

References

BBC 2020. China coronavirus: Misinformation spreads online about origin and scale. 30 January (https://www.bbc.com/news/blogs-trending-51271037).

Cellan-Jones, R. 2020. Coronavirus: Fake news is spreading fast. *BBC*, 26 February (https://www.bbc.com/news/technology-51646309).

Chan, A. L., Leung, C. C, Lam, T. H., & Cheng, K. K. 2020. To wear or not to wear: WHO's confusing guidance on masks in the COVID-19 pandemic. *The BMJ Opinion*, 11 March (https://blogs.bmj.com/bmj/2020/03/11/whos-confusing-guidance-masks-covid-19-epidemic/).

Chinazzi, M. et al. 2020. The effect of travel restrictions on the spread of the 2019 novel coronavirus (COVID-19) outbreak. *Science* 368(6489), 395–400. doi:10.1126/science.aba9757

Gallagher, R. 2020. 5G virus conspiracy theory fueled by coordinated effort. *Bloomberg*, 10 April (https://www.bloomberg.com/news/articles/2020-04-09/covid-19-link-to-5g-technology-fueled-by-coordinated-effort).

Gertz, B. 2020. Coronavirus may have originated in lab linked to China's biowarfare program. *The Washington Times*, 26 January (https://www.washingtontimes.com/news/2020/jan/26/coronavirus-link-to-china-biowarfare-program-possi/).

Hafezi, P. 2020. Iran's Khamenei rejects U.S. help offer, vows to defeat coronavirus. *Reuters*, 22 March (https://www.reuters.com/article/us-health-coronavirus-iran/irans-khamenei-rejects-u-s-help-offer-vows-to-defeat-coronavirus-idUSKBN21909Y).

Kuo, L. 2020. China withheld data on coronavirus from WHO, recordings reveal. *The Guardian*, 2 June (https://www.theguardian.com/world/2020/jun/02/china-withheld-data-coronavirus-world-health-organization-recordings-reveal).

Kurlantzick, J. 2020. Dictators are using the coronavirus to strengthen their grip on power. *The Washington Post*, 3 April (https://www.washingtonpost.com/outlook/dictators-are-using-the-coronavirus-to-strengthen-their-grip-on-power/2020/04/02/c36582f8-748c-11ea-87da-77a8136c1a6d_story.html).

Leung, N. H. L., Chu, D. K. W., Shiu, E. Y. C, Chan, K-P., McDevitt, J. J., Hau, B. J. P., Yen, H-L., Li, Y., Ip, D. K. M., Peiris, J. S. M., Seto, W-H., Leung, G. M., Milton, D. K., & Cowling, B. J. 2020. Respiratory virus shedding in exhaled breath and efficacy of face masks. *Nature Medicine* 26, 676–680. https://doi.org/10.1038/s41591-020-0843-2.

Lytvynenko, J. 2020. Here are some of the coronavirus hoaxes that spread in the first few weeks. *BuzzFeedNews*, 2 March (https://www.buzzfeednews.com/article/jan

elytvynenko/coronavirus-disinformation-spread?bftwnews&utm_term=4ldqpgc
#4ldqpgc).

Ma, Q. X., Shan, H., Zhang, H. L., Li, G. M., Yang, R. M., & Chen, J. M. 2020.
Potential utilities of mask-wearing and instant hand hygiene for fighting CARS-
CoV-2. *Journal of Medical Virology* 92, 1567–71. doi:10.1002/jmv.25805.

Murray, W. 2020. Trump blames WHO and freezes funding. *The Guardian*, 15 April
(https://www.theguardian.com/world/2020/apr/15/wednesday-briefing-trump
-blames-who-and-freezes-funding).

Rahman, G. 2020. The Wuhan coronavirus has nothing to do with 5G. *FullFact*, 29
January (https://fullfact.org/online/wuhan-5g-coronavirus/).

Sang-Hun, C. 2020. North Korea bans foreign tourists over coronavirus, tour operator
says. *The New York Times*, 21 January (https://www.nytimes.com/2020/01/21/world
/asia/coronavirus-china-north-korea-tourism-ban.html?auth=login-facebook).

Shumei, L., & Lin, W. 2020. US urged to release health info of military athletes who
came to Wuhan in October 2019. *Global Times*, 25 March (https://www.globaltimes
.cn/content/1183658.shtml).

Spinney, L. 2020. Why did the World Health Organisation wait so long to declare
coronavirus a pandemic? *New Statesman*, 12 March (https://www.newstatesman.com
/science-tech/2020/03/why-did-world-health-organisation-wait-so-long-declare-
coronavirus-pandemic).

Stevens, H., Tan, S. 2020. From 'It's going to disappear' to 'WE WILL WIN THIS
WAR.' *The Washington Post*, 31 March (https://www.washingtonpost.com/graphics/
2020/politics/trump-coronavirus-statements/).

Trump, D. 2020. (https://twitter.com/realDonaldTrump/status/12413672399007785
01).

UNWTO 2020. World tourism remains at a standstill as 100% of countries impose
restrictions on travel. (https://www.unwto.org/news/covid-19-world-tourism-
remains-at-a-standstill-as-100-of-countries-impose-restrictions-on-travel).

Van Prooijen, J. W., & Jostmann, N. B. 2013. Belief in conspiracy theories: The influence
of uncertainty and perceived morality. *European Journal of Social Psychology 43*(1),
109–115.

WHO 2020. Novel Coronavirus (2019-nCoV) situation report 13. 2 February (https://
www.who.int/docs/default-source/coronaviruse/situation-reports/20200202-sitrep
-13-ncov-v3.pdf).

2

CHINA

Diversion, ingratiation and victimisation

Menglin Liu and Shan Xu

Political context

China is a one-party system: the Chinese Communist Party (CCP), headed by Xi Jinping since 2012, has been the only legitimate ruling party since 1949. After assuming office, Xi Jinping started touting his vision and interpretation of the 'China Dream,' which was officially defined as the grand rejuvenation of the Chinese nation (Mingfu, 2009). According to Xi Jinping, this means bringing greater prosperity to the Chinese people while elevating China's role in the international community (Kallio, 2015).

The 'China Dream' is believed to have stimulated a new wave of nationalism throughout China.

In addition, public support for the central government has been steadily increasing in recent years. The China Survey 2008, conducted by Texas A&M University, generated one of the latest datasets regarding Chinese citizens' public support for authority at different levels. The approval ratings for central and provincial leaders were as high as 84.4% and 73%, respectively. Among 3,989 respondents, 63.1% of them trusted the country leaders (Li, 2016). On the other hand, with China's economic and educational development, a large number of individuals, especially in advanced provinces, have become more likely to embrace liberal views regarding political institutions and individual freedoms (Pan & Xu, 2018).

Chronology

Start of the epidemic – Wuhan

The first case of COVID-19 was found in Wuhan, the capital of Hubei Province in China, on December 30, 2019. With a population of over 11 million, Wuhan

DOI: 10.4324/9781003120254-4

serves as the transportation hub of China, lying at the intersection of two busy railroads – one connecting the west to the east, and the other linking the north with the south. This makes Wuhan one of the powerhouses of China's economy. With a GDP of 1.484 trillion RMB, or 210 billion USD, Wuhan is in the top ten Chinese cities. As of March 31, China had 81,554 confirmed cases nationwide, with 3,312 reported deaths and 76,238 reported recoveries (National Health Centre).

Timeline and official responses to COVID-19

On the same day the first Wuhan case was discovered, the Hubei Health Commission issued a notice prohibiting individuals from disclosing information about COVID-19 to the general public. On January 1, 2020, the police department summoned eight health care workers who had previously disseminated information (via personal communication, both online and offline) about a potential infectious virus. They were charged with spreading rumours. The accusation against the eight health care workers was reported by the China Central Television (CCTV), which indicated the central government's support for this accusation.

January 11–17, no newly confirmed cases were reported. During this period, two important government bodies met: the Political Consultative Conference and the Third Session of the Hubei Provincial People's Congress. Simultaneously, the Chinese Centre for Disease Control and Prevention (China CDC) activated a second-level public health emergency, indicating the agency's awareness the virus could potentially transmit from person to person. In a bulletin issued on January 16, the Wuhan Health Commission claimed there was no clear evidence of human-to-human transmission, and the possibility was low.

On January 18, Bai Buting Community, in the city of Wuhan, held its annual mass banquet with more than 40,000 families. On the very same day, the Hubei Provincial Spring Festival Gala was held, a celebration which featured the heads of the Hubei government. Later, both the community dinner and the Gala came to stand as symbols of China's mishandling of the outbreak.

On January 20, renowned pulmonologist Zhong Nanshan, who earned international fame for managing the SARS outbreak in China, stated explicitly for the first time that COVID-19 was contagious from human to human, in a nationally televised interview. His statement was confirmed during a China CDC press conference later that day.

On January 21, a news article in *People's Daily* suggested that only open and transparent communication could reduce panic among the public. Two days later, the Chinese Government announced the shutdown of Wuhan and prohibited citizens from leaving the city. As a result, the city's 11 million residents were effectively under quarantine. It was not until April 8 that the Chinese government lifted the lockdown.

By January 29, all 31 provinces in China had activated a first-level public health emergency. The first-level response is only activated when a highly contagious disease is detected and spreads rapidly. According to the National Health Committee, up until January 31 there were 11,791 confirmed cases and 259 deaths nationwide. Finally, on February 13, the head of the Communist Party in Hubei province and the Wuhan communist chiefs were replaced. Table 2.1 briefly summarises the major events.

Analysis

This section focuses on the communicative and messaging strategies used by the Chinese central government during the pandemic, based on two media outlets – *People's Daily* and *Global Times* – owned and managed by the central government. There are two reasons for focusing on these two news outlets as the government's crisis communication. First of all, these news outlets are regarded both by Chinese readers and foreign observers as authoritative statements of official government policy, and are considered the Chinese government's mouthpiece to the people and the rest of the world (Hassid, 2015).Thus, the central government controlled the process of messaging and communicating via news outlets at the national level. Secondly, national news has far more readers than local news agencies, so they were more salient and influential in delivering COVID-19-related messages nationwide. The following sections evaluate the central government's crisis communication via both these media outlets.

The central government's communication strategy

Based on the front pages and editorials of *People's Daily* and *Global Times*, China's central government used two major communication strategies: bolstering and scapegoating (Coombs, 2007). Three specific tactics were implemented to bolster crisis responses and messages from the central government in official news organisations: (1) *diversion* – divert stakeholders' attention from the current crisis to the government's past good work, (2) *ingratiating* – praising stakeholders for their contributions, and (3) *victimisation*, through which crisis managers reminded stakeholders that the organisation itself is a victim of the crisis (Coombs, 2007).

Diversion was one of the most significant tactics in the bolstering strategy. During the pandemic, reminiscing about past achievements was a recurrent topic on the *People's Daily* front pages. For example, on January 31, *People's Daily* reported Xi Jinping's speech to the army and commented that the army had overcome crises such as flooding, blizzards and typhoons. This piece reminded readers the army successfully protected its people over the past decades (*People's Daily*, January 01, 2020). In the same vein, the newspaper spoke highly of the CCP's leadership in past national crises. On February 3, its front page observed that the Chinese people, under the leadership of the CCP, had overcome many

TABLE 2.1 China chronology

	Date	Diffusion of COVID-19	Key official actions.	Key communication events
December	31	The first case was officially confirmed.		
January	1		Eight health care workers were accused by local police of spreading rumours about a potential infectious virus	
	11	No new cases were reported January 11–17.	Political Consultative Conference and The Third Session of Hubei Provincial People's Congress held; CDC activated second-level public health emergency.	
	16			Wuhan Health Commission claimed that there was no clear evidence of human-to-human transmission.
	18		Hubei Provincial Spring Festival Gala was held.	
	20			CDC press conference confirmed Zhong Nanshan's statement that COVID-19 was contagious from human to human, but Wuhan Health Commission claimed that the threat to public health was low.
	21			China's official news outlet suggested that only open and transparent communication could reduce a public pandemic.
	22		The Chinese government announced the shutdown of Wuhan and prohibited citizens from leaving the city.	
	27			Xianwang Zhou, Mayor of Wuhan, responded to complaints about the slow response and mobilisation towards the spread of the virus by saying that local government could only disclose information on infectious disease after being approved by the central government.

(*Continued*)

TABLE 2.1 (Continued)

Date		Diffusion of COVID-19	Key official actions.	Key communication events
	29		All 31 provinces in China had activated the first-level public health emergency response.	*People's Daily* praised ordinary party members for making big sacrifices during the virus outbreak.
	31	11,791 confirmed cases, 259 deaths nationwide.		Xi Jinping's speech to the army was reported by *People's Daily; People's Daily* published 100 scientific facts about COVID-19.
February	2			*Global Times* suggested that it would be wrong to underestimate the CCP's governing capability in the face of crisis; the television press conference of the city of Tianjin was praised by the public.
	3		The head of the Communist Party in Hubei Province and the Wuhan communist chiefs were replaced.	*People's Daily* reviewed past success in overcoming natural disasters and contagious viruses under the leadership of the CCP.
	13		The head of the Communist Party in Hubei Province and the Wuhan communist chiefs were replaced.	
March	12			Lijian Zhao hinted that it might be the US army who brought the epidemic to Wuhan.
	10	80,754 confirmed cases, 3136 deaths.	Xi Jinping made his first visit to Wuhan, the epicentre of the pandemic, since the breakout of the virus.	
	31	81,554 confirmed cases, 3312 deaths.		

struggles and challenges, such as the severe flooding in 1998, SARS in 2003 and the Sichuan earthquake in 2008.

The *Global Times* echoed the *People's Daily* in its editorials regarding the role of the government in fighting COVID-19. For instance, its February 2 editorial attached great importance to China's achievements in coping with SARS 17 years ago, despite the international community being pessimistic about the CCP's governing capacity at that time. The editorial further suggested it would be wrong and short-sighted to underestimate China's capability to deal with this public health crisis, given that China could impose a series of compulsory public policies to curb the spread of the virus – policies which might be impossible to implement in other countries.

Ingratiation was another common tactic used to distract the public from the government's delayed responses. On the second day of Wuhan's lockdown, *Global Times* published an editorial paying tribute to Wuhan citizens. It commented that Wuhan's lockdown decision was the most selfless action since the epidemic, and that people in China should honour and express gratitude to Wuhan. In addition to praising Wuhan, *People's Daily* suggested people from all walks in Wuhan had contributed to fighting COVID-19. For example, on January 29, a front page article praised party members at a company who voluntarily worked overtime to make more face masks, construction workers who worked overnight to build new hospitals in Wuhan and factory workers who worked day and night to make basic protective equipment.

Lastly, the Chinese government blamed other countries and described China as the victim of the pandemic. One of the most salient and controversial issues during the pandemic arose when Lijian Zhao, Foreign Ministry spokesman, tweeted that 'it might be the U.S. army who brought the epidemic to Wuhan. The U.S. owes us an explanation!'[1] This statement placed responsibility for COVID-19 on the United States and implied that China, both the ordinary people and the government, were the victims of this unprecedented pandemic. In early February, *Global Times* also wrote that the US government went too far by banning travel from China since the World Health Organisation (WHO) did not recommend any trade and travel restrictions. By accusing other countries of bringing the virus to China and treating China unfairly, the pro-government news outlets depicted China as a victim. People became more susceptible to the argument that foreign countries were trying to prevent China from getting stronger, especially since the 'China Dream' was largely embraced by Chinese society.

The second strategy, scapegoating, was used to dodge blame. The local and the central governments blamed each other for the initial insufficient and slow response to the pandemic. During an interview for China Central Television, Wuhan mayor Xianwang Zhou responded to criticism of his government's slow response and mobilisation by saying that local government could only disclose information on the infectious disease after being approved by the central government. However, the central government, taking advantage of its own communication platforms, scapegoated its responsibility to the incompetence of local government officials. During a BBC interview, Andrew Marr, China's ambassador to Britain, responded to a question concerning Wenliang Li, the Chinese whistle-blowing doctor who tried to issue the first warning about the deadly coronavirus outbreak. The ambassador said the local not central government, was responsible. He further explained central authorities had sent a team to Wuhan to investigate the death of Wenliang Li. On February 13, personnel changes in both the Wuhan city government and the provincial Hubei government were made public, signalling that it was the incompetence and inefficiency of local authorities that contributed to the slow and chaotic response in the early stages of the crisis.

Crisis and Emergency Risk Communication (CERC)

According to the CERC model, the government should be the *first* to inform the public on what is known and unknown, and to provide health guidance. In China, both local and central governments failed to inform their citizens about COVID-19. On the contrary, they not only silenced healthcare workers who first reported the outbreak of the virus, but they also publicly admonished these healthcare workers. One prominent example involves Wenliang Li, an ophthalmologist who tried to issue a warning about the highly contagious nature of COVID-19. On December 30, he posted messages on social media to his colleagues. However, he was later brought to the police station by the local police and was told to stop making 'false' comments. Seven other healthcare workers were also publicly admonished and silenced.

The second and third principles of CERC require communicating accurate and credible information to the public. Regarding these aspects, the Chinese government performed better in the later stage of the pandemic than in the early stage. During the early period of the pandemic, the government over-reassured the public with inaccurate information. For instance, as late as January 20 the Wuhan Health Commission continued to claim that although person-to-person transmission was possible, the threat to overall public health was low. Later that same day, a team of experts from the National Health Commission reported the opposite. This contradictory information exposed a lack of coordination between the central and the local governments. Poor coordination is likely to confuse the public, further undermine public trust and raise societal anxiety. A similar confusion arose when multiple scientific research institutes reported that various traditional Chinese medicines could help prevent contracting COVID-19. However, these results were later largely debunked.

In the later stage of the pandemic, the Chinese government communicated more accurate information to the public. For instance, the press conference in the city of Tianjin, broadcast on television on February 2, conveyed credible information to the public regarding the prevention and spread of the virus, which was praised by social media users as meticulously logical.

People's Daily also attached importance to overcoming online rumours. On January 28, it ran an article called 'Do Not Let Rumors Get Ahead of Science' on the front page, sending clear information to the public that some popularly disseminated treatments, such as smoking and taking vitamin C, would not help combat the virus. This article also called for caution and rationality when searching for COVID-19 related information online. This exemplifies how official news outlets provided credible information to the masses during the pandemic.

Among the CERC principles, two of them gauge the emotional dimension of communication. According to the CERC framework, an organisation's communication should express both empathy and respect. According to our analysis, official news outlets did show respect for workers at the front line. They frequently mentioned and showed appreciation to healthcare workers, military personnel and factory workers. However, no evidence was found regarding empathy shown to the COVID-19 patients.

CERC also states that communication should promote action, which could be considered a success in China's case. For instance, as mentioned earlier, *Global Times* devoted an editorial expressing gratitude and appreciation to Wuhan citizens for their courage and determination. *Global Times'* comments helped implement the lockdown order and might have quelled dissatisfaction among Wuhan citizens. On January 31, *People's Daily* presented 100 scientific facts about COVID-19 and how to best prevent the spread of the virus. Above all, *People's Daily* recommended wearing masks and specified the correct way of wearing them.

Public interaction and engagement with government communication

Building on the social-mediated crisis communication model (Austin et al., 2012), this section evaluates how society responded to governmental crisis communication by analysing reports produced by one major, relatively independent news outlet in China: CAIXIN.

CAIXIN, a well-known independent news agency in China, serves as an ideal case to analyse the public's response to and interaction with government communication for three reasons. First, it enjoys significant independence from the central government. Thus, it represents an alternative voice to political authority. During the pandemic, CAIXIN assumed the responsibility of analysing and questioning government messages. Second, it reaches a large audience. According to Global Digital Subscription, a report estimating digital-only subscribers to news and magazine media globally, CAIXIN has 300,000 total subscribers: #15 in the world and the only Chinese media outlet in the top 20. In addition, CAIXIN launched a digital version and started official accounts on Weibo and WeChat, two of the most popular social media sites in China. Thirdly, CAIXIN published articles with a variety of opinions on the same topic, sometimes even contradictory ones. Therefore, voices from different sides were heard and broadcast, making it representative of society's response to the government's crisis messaging. For instance, when the public questioned the legitimacy of the local government in hiding important information from the public, CAIXIN ran a comprehensive article analysing the legal boundaries of local authorities.

Throughout the crisis, the government's credibility and legitimacy was at the highest risk when the news of Dr Li's death rippled across the country. Despite censorship, many Chinese people do hold politically liberal views. The death of Dr Li pulled the trigger: the hashtag #wewantfreedomofspeech was created on Weibo, the Chinese version of Twitter, after Dr Li's death was announced at 2 am on Friday, and it had over two million views and more than 5,500 posts in five hours (Li, 2020). Amid fear and calls for justice, based on a variety of current Chinese laws, CAIXIN ran an article to analyse whether the local police department held any authority to admonish Dr Li. Apart from the conclusion that the Wuhan police department's admonishment was not supported by law, they alleged the local authority abused their power and was potentially guilty of serious professional misconduct.

Another topic that generated a lot of public discussion was whether the local government should or was obliged to disclose information and data regarding the virus. CAIXIN observed that, despite complaints against local authorities' delay in informing the public, in light of the current law, local governments were not allowed to reveal information regarding the epidemic. However, the editorial argued local government did fail to make other useful information available to the public, such as health guidance and emergency orders to prevent the spread of the virus. CAIXIN was also involved in the discussion regarding the function of the Red Cross affiliated with the government. It ran a series of op-eds on the role of civil society in collecting and redistributing medical supplies. They called into question the monopoly of the Red Cross and its low efficiency and nepotism, which severely impeded the operation of frontline hospitals. These examples reveal how independent news engaged in public discussion and information transmission during the crisis. Specifically, CAIXIN put controversial social issues into perspective, analysing and questioning governmental messages and actions.

Conclusion

This chapter explored how the Chinese government responded and communicated with the public when the COVID-19 pandemic hit hard, first in one of its megacities (Wuhan) and later nationwide. By analysing two official news outlets in China, we identify three major communicative strategies – diversion, ingratiating and victimisation – utilised by the Chinese central government. The Chinese government failed to communicate openly with its public, which triggered public panic and delayed the containment of the virus. However, the Chinese government also had some success in crisis communication, such as by conveying accurate information to the public in the later phase of the pandemic. The second part of this chapter analyses an independent news outlet in China and how it represented the public's response and interaction with government communication. In sum, this analysis provides insights into crisis communication in China during the COVID-19 pandemic.

Note

1 https://twitter.com/zlj517/status/1238111898828066823?lang=en

References

Austin, L., Fisher Liu, B. and Jin, Y. 2012. How audiences seek out crisis information: Exploring the social-mediated crisis communication model. *Journal of Applied Communication Research*, 40(2), 188–207.

Coombs, W. T. 2007. Crisis management and communications. *Institute for Public Relations*, 4(5), 1–14.

Hassid, J. 2015. *China's Unruly Journalists: How Committed Professionals Are Changing the People's Republic*. Routledge.

Kallio, J. 2015. Dreaming of the great rejuvenation of the Chinese nation. *Fudan Journal of the Humanities and Social Sciences*, 8(4), 521–532.

Li, L. 2016. Reassessing trust in the central government: Evidence from five national surveys. *China Quarterly*, 225, 100–121.

Mingfu, L. 2009. *The Chinese Dream: The Goals, Road and Self-Confidence of China*. Zhongguo Youyi Chuban Gongsi.

National Health Centre, 2020. *New Information about COVID-19 as of March 31st*. www.nhc.gov.cn/yjb/s7860/202004/28668f987f3a4e58b1a2a75db60d8cf2.shtml

Pan, J., and Xu, Y. 2018. China's ideological spectrum. *The Journal of Politics*, 80(1), 254–273.

Yuan, L. 2020. Widespread Outcry in China over death of Coronavirus Doctor. *The New York Times*, 7 February. www.nytimes.com/2020/02/07/business/china-coronavirus -doctor-death.html

3

JAPAN

New directions for digital Japan

Leslie Tkach-Kawasaki

Political context

Shinzo Abe, Japan's prime minister (PM) during the first six months of the pandemic, had been in office for over eight years and has been the longest serving prime minister in Japan. Abe's Liberal Democratic Party (LDP) is the major political party in a coalition majority in the House of Representatives and House of Councillors in Japan's bicameral national Diet, along with the Komeito (Clean Government Party). The most recent elections were held in October 2017 and July 2019, respectively.

In the past eight years, since the LDP returned to office in December 2012 after a brief 3.5-year hiatus, Abe's majority coalition has witnessed the implementation of 'Abenomics' (a series of economic policies espoused by Abe during the 2012 election campaign period), two consumption tax increases (2014 and 2019), enactment of peace and security legislation (2015), and the 'My Number' national registry system (2015). However, cabinet support has been steadily waning since early February (NHK, 2020). At varying times during the COVID-19 pandemic, official decisions, programmes and initiatives made by the Abe administration, the Cabinet Secretariat, and other key decision-making bodies faced criticism from various directions.

The Japanese government took a dual approach to the pandemic, attempting to balance public health concerns with mitigating economic repercussions to ensure recovery. Pursuing an equilibrium between these two objectives took many different forms throughout the course of the pandemic from January to August 2020.

Chronology

The major COVID-19-related events in Japan are summarised in Table 3.1 and can be divided into three main phases.

DOI: 10.4324/9781003120254-5

TABLE 3.1 Japan chronology

Date		Diffusion of cases	Key official actions	Key communication events
January	28	First confirmed Japanese case.	**Start of First Phase:** Cabinet approves specifying coronavirus as a 'designated infectious disease.'	
	30	11 cases.	Novel Coronavirus Response Headquarters is established in the Cabinet Secretariat, Prime Minister's Office.	
	31		Third meeting of Novel Coronavirus Response Headquarters. Entry restrictions go into effect February 1.	
February	1	15 cases.		*Diamond Princess* (*DP*) quarantined.
	3		The *Diamond Princess* arrives in Yokohama and is quarantined. Japanese officials board ship for testing.	
	13	218 cases on the *DP*. First death reported.	Quarantine Act enforcement order changed to allow expanded quarantine activities.	
	14		Novel Coronavirus Expert Meeting established.	
	19	69 cases (not including *DP*)	*DP* quarantine ends, passengers allowed to disembark. Nine government officials who entered *DP* test positive.	
	23			Health Minister Kato announces some *DP* passengers released without testing.
	25		PM (Prime Minister) Abe announces the 'Basic Policies for Novel Coronavirus Disease Control.'	
	27		PM Abe requests school closures from March 2 to early April.	
	28	200 cases.	Hokkaido prefecture declares state of emergency.	

(*Continued*)

TABLE 3.1 (Continued)

Date		Diffusion of cases	Key official actions	Key communication events
March	2	274 cases. 4 deaths.	School closures begin. Companies request employees to 'telework' or 'remote work' from home.	MHLW announces daily subsidy for employees taking time off for childcare.
	10	581 cases.	PM Abe requests cancellation of large-scale events.	Cabinet announces JPY 1 trillion stimulus package and subsidies for freelance workers.
	13	639 cases. 15 deaths.	Legislation allows Abe to declare national 'state of emergency.'	
	19	961 cases.	Hokkaido lifts state of emergency.	
	24			Official announcement of postponement of 2020 Tokyo Olympics and Paralympics.
	25	1,309 cases. 54 deaths.	Tokyo Governor Koike requests citizens to work from home and self-isolate mainly during evenings and weekends.	
April	1	2,502 cases.	PM Abe announces distribution of two cloth masks to each household ('Abenomasks').	Japanese government announces 2-week quarantine for all entrants from April 3.
	6		Abe announces stimulus package including interest-free loans to businesses and a one-off payout of JPY 300,000 for each household.	
	7	4,478 cases. 93 deaths.	**Start of Second Phase**: PM Abe declares state of emergency in seven prefectures until May 6.	
	12		Hokkaido prefectural government announces start of second state of emergency period.	

	Day	Cases/Deaths	Event	
	16	9,362 cases, 190 deaths.	PM Abe declares **national** state of emergency to May 6.	
	20		PM Abe cabinet announces revised stimulus package including JPY 100,000-yen payout per resident.	
May	4	15,369 cases. 536 deaths.	National state of emergency extended to May 31.	
	14	16,240 cases. 697 deaths.	State of emergency lifted in 39 out of 47 prefectures, but remains in major urban areas, Hokkaido and Hyogo.	
	21		State of emergency lifted for Osaka, Kyoto and Hyogo. **Start of Third Phase:**	
	25	16,540 cases. 830 deaths.	National state of emergency ended.	MHWL announced revised 'Basic Policies for Novel Coronavirus Disease Control' recommending new lifestyle changes.
June	2	16,990 cases.	Tokyo Governor Koike warns of possible resurgence in Tokyo.	
	11			'Simplified' plans announced for Olympics postponed until 2021.
	18	17,754 cases.	Voluntary restrictions for cross-prefectural travel lifted.	
	19		Government releases official COCOA contact-tracing app.	
	25	18,209 cases. 968 deaths.	Economic Revitalisation Minister Nishimura announces reorganised Expert Panel.	
July	5	19,820 cases.	Tokyo Governor Yuriko Koike re-elected by landslide.	
	10		Tourism Minister Akaba launches the 'Go to Travel' programme.	
	16	23,656 cases. 985 deaths.	Tourism Minister Akaba announces exclusion of Tokyo residents and people travelling to Tokyo from the 'Go to Travel' campaign.	

The first confirmed case involving a Japanese national was announced on January 28, marking the first of three phases of the pandemic. In late January, establishing centralised legal structures to handle the crisis from the twin perspectives of the health and economic repercussions took centre stage. Throughout February, the quarantine and testing of the *Diamond Princess* cruise ship passengers dominated mass media, and mid-February, the Novel Coronavirus Expert Meeting was established as an advisory panel of medical experts. School closures and work-from-home practices started at the end of February, while throughout March, legal preparations for calling a state of emergency were made by the Abe administration as infectious cases increased. Official announcements in late March postponing the 2020 Tokyo Olympics and Paralympics further underscored the situation's progressing severity.

The 'isolation' phase started with Abe's decision to declare a state of emergency in seven prefectures mainly in the Kanto region on April 7, followed by the national state of emergency declaration on April 16 which was initially to last until May 6. During this period, individuals were 'requested' to self-isolate and work from home. Warnings, but not official bans, against travel during the 'Golden Week' holiday period (end of April/early May) were issued. The state of emergency was lifted gradually through four stages designated by the MHWL (Ministry of Health, Labour and Welfare).

Revised strategies for embarking on a 'new normal' lifestyle as outlined by the MHWL (2020) mark the third phrase from May 25. Infection figures in many prefectures declined and voluntary restrictions for domestic travel were eased. However, from mid-June onwards, a second and more severe wave hit major urban centres such as Tokyo and Osaka, as well as isolated areas such as northern Kyushu. As of mid-July, both Tokyo and Osaka were posting figures higher than in March prior to the national state of emergency period.

Political communication analysis

Political communications and controversies

Throughout the crisis, political communication was centralised and top down, as the Abe administration strived to maintain a balance between health concerns and the economy. Striking a balance between the two proved to be challenging. First, as a means to legally establish centralised control in the early phase of the pandemic at the national level, Abe's Cabinet Secretariat moved swiftly at the end of January to pass legislation identifying the COVID-19 virus as a 'designated infectious disease' under the *Act on the Prevention of Infectious Diseases and Medical Care for Patients with Infectious Diseases* (Asahi Shimbun, 2020a). This designation, along with changing the Quarantine Act enforcement order in mid-February (Umeda, 2020), were key events not only signalling official recognition of the virus as a health risk, but also giving the central government broad legal powers regarding measures such as isolation, quarantines and hospitalisation.

While those legal powers were mandated at the national level, throughout the pandemic period, there were tensions between national and local government in terms of defining powers and legal capabilities. For example, Hokkaido Governor Naomichi Suzuki declared a state of emergency in Hokkaido twice: the first time at the end of February for three weeks, and then again in mid-April prior to the national state of emergency (Kyodo News, 2020b). However, legal provisions for Abe to declare a 'state of emergency' throughout the country were not put in place until March (Asahi Shimbun, 2020b), leading up to the April 7 limited declaration. Furthermore, instead of 'hard lockdowns,' certain powers were given to prefectural governors to request citizens to stay indoors, as well as cancel events and close schools, through the national 'state of emergency' provisions. Furthermore, at the prefectural and municipal levels, local governments could only make 'requests' for individuals to self-isolate or for businesses to reduce their business hours (Japan Local Government Centre, 2020). As the number of cases in urban areas such as Tokyo and Osaka rose during March and then again from mid-June through July, the issue of not being able to legislate business hours at the local level arose repeatedly.

Second, there was controversy concerning the Novel Coronavirus Expert Meeting, the advisory group set up in mid-February to provide medical advice to the centralised Novel Coronavirus Response Headquarters within the Prime Minister's Office (PMO). The initial formation of the panel included infectious disease specialists, as well as policy and legal experts. The main pillars of their recommendations were minimising the burden on the medical system, identifying cluster and contact tracing (as opposed to polymerase chain reaction (PCR) testing), and promoting behavioural changes (Abe, 2020). The panel's recommendation of the '3 Cs' (asking citizens to avoid closed spaces, crowded places and close-contact settings) became a mantra widely disseminated throughout the country.

However, as the pandemic continued, criticism of the panel arose. In addition to the panel's reporting structure and composition, its stance concerning PCR testing, the economic effects of self-isolation and the best practices for carrying out the 3 Cs also came under fire (Takahashi, 2020). In late June 2020, Economic Revitalization Minister Yasutoshi Nishimura announced the panel's reorganisation to include a broader representation of the general public and society, as well as the promotion of former deputy chair Shigeru Omi, chairman of the Japan Community Health Care Organisation, to panel chair (*Japan Times*, 2020a).

During March, the Abe administration's approach to the pandemic started to draw criticism in the Diet. Politicians in the ruling coalition of the LDP and Komeito parties, as well as opposition parties, started discussing possibilities for stimulus packages for both businesses and individuals. In early April, Abe announced the provision of JPY 300,000 (approximately USD 2,700) to the head of each household experiencing economic difficulties, as well as a relief-oriented package for businesses (Nishimura, K. 2020). However, following political pressure and public backlash concerning eligibility, this was revised to JPY 100,000 (approximately USD 900) for each resident (Asahi Shimbun, 2020c).

In addition to the prime minister, who was in the public eye during the first seven months of the pandemic, certain politicians at the national level also took the lead in disseminating political information concerning the crisis. The website of the Prime Minister's Office (www.kantei.go.jp) was updated almost daily with news concerning government responses to the pandemic, as well as summaries of the frequent meetings held by the Novel Coronavirus Response Headquarters. On August 5, Economic Revitalization Minister Yasutoshi Nishimura, the 'face' of the pandemic in terms of public briefings, marked his 100th continuous daily briefing. In addition to Nishimura's briefings, Chief Cabinet Secretary Yoshihide Suga (who became prime minister in mid-September) held press conferences almost daily. In addition to being covered extensively by traditional television companies and featured on the evening news, summaries and YouTube excerpts were also posted on the Abe cabinet website.

Local-level governors were also in the national spotlight at various times during the pandemic. Among them, the most prominent were Tokyo Governor Yuriko Koike and Osaka Governor Hirofumi Yoshimura. Governor Koike, the head of the most populous metropolitan area in the country, shouldered a triple load of dealing with the pandemic's fluctuating infected-status statistics, negotiating the timeline and postponement of the 2020 Olympic and Paralympic Games and fending off rivals in the run-up to the July 2020 Tokyo Gubernatorial election, which she handily won. Through a combination of almost-daily press conferences, social-media use and public-service advertising, Governor Koike was widely praised for her handling of the pandemic within Tokyo. In contrast, the frequent clashes between Governor Yoshimura and the Abe administration (often with Economic Revitalisation Minister Nishimura) focused on granting more authority at the prefectural level to shut down businesses, particularly entertainment establishments (Johnston, 2020).

The internet's critical role

During the period between January and July 2020, internet use increased substantially. First, national, prefectural and local governments used the internet extensively as a means of providing up-to-date information about the pandemic. Information dissemination by government institutions at the national level through the Internet focused mainly on the PMO website (www.kantei .go.jp), the MHLW website (www.mhlw.go.jp) and an official corona-specific website (corona.go.jp) established by the Cabinet Secretariat. An informal survey of their social media accounts in September 2020 suggests some distinct differences in terms of social media use: the corona-specific website posted links to YouTube and Twitter, whereas the other government bodies utilised Instagram and Facebook as well. In terms of popularity, the PMO's office had over a million subscribers to its YouTube channel, compared to slightly over 44,000 for the MHLW and 746 for the corona-specific channels. However, in terms of Twitter popularity, the PMO and MHLW's numbers of followers at 1.3 million and approximately 800,000, respectively were much higher than the 125,400 figure for the corona-specific Twitter account.

Official government information channels also made extensive use of LINE, a free multiplatform software application originally developed for text messaging, phone calls, exchanging photographs and group chats. This application is particularly popular among Japanese youth, and both the PMO and MHLW bodies made extensive use of its features. As of mid-September, the PMO had close to 4 million LINE 'friends.' Furthermore, starting at the end of March, the MHLW periodically distributed pandemic-related public opinion surveys via its LINE account, with results posted on its website as well as LINE's coronavirus-survey website (LINE, 2020).

During the course of the pandemic, e-government services at the prefectural and municipal levels were also expanded. Prefectural websites regularly posted information concerning severity stages, statistics concerning the number of infected people, and available support programmes. Some prefectures such as Ibaraki posted cluster and contact tracing information. Municipal government websites, which were often relatively static prior to the pandemic, became dynamic information hubs, as applications for individual income relief assistance and small-business stimulus programmes, including the 100,000-yen stipend for each individual announced in April, were initially processed at the local level.

Contact tracing was considered an important means for attempting to suppress the spread of the coronavirus, and various apps were developed in Japan with varying degrees of success. Development of the national-level COCOA (Contact Confirming Application) app suffered numerous setbacks, including delays in selecting development partners and software glitches before it became readily available in mid-July (Ishihara & Nagao, 2020). As of July 20, there were 7.69 million downloads of the app (*Japan Times*, 2020b). Apps developed at the prefectural level were also popular, with some featuring registration via QR-codes, LINE or email. Ibaraki prefecture's application featured Amabie, a traditional Japanese folklore character that gained popularity in March and April as a symbolic character of the pandemic in Japan (The *Mainichi*, 2020a).

Throughout the pandemic, social-media platforms also served as an alternative news channel for social commentary, publicity and criticism. During the two-week quarantine period in February 2020, isolated *Diamond Princess* passengers used social media channels such as Facebook and YouTube to communicate their quarantine experience with the rest of the world. Also related to the cruise ship's quarantine situation in mid-February, Kobe University professor Kentaro Iwata criticised how the quarantine was handled by public health officials via a video posted on YouTube, but the video was removed after a short period of time (Kyodo News, 2020a).

Twitter also emerged as a multi-functional alternative information platform. The prime minister's April announcement of the public distribution of two masks per household was the target of Twitter-based criticism with the hashtag #abenomask (*Japan Times*, 2020c). A video distributed in April on Twitter showing Prime Minister Abe playing the guitar and playing with his dog was aimed at popularising self-isolation and 'staying at home' during the 'state of emergency' period. However, there was mixed reaction through Twitter and other media channels to the prime minister's video (*The Mainichi*, 2020b). Also during the 'state of emergency' period, Twitter was used to disseminate information with popular hashtags such as #*shingata korona* (new corona), #*korona ni makenai* (don't lose to corona), #*sutei homu* (stay home) and #*dankai kaijo* (release in stages). Hashtags criticising self-isolation (#*jishuku hantai*, against self-isolation) and public shaming for flouting 'self-isolation' measures (#*jishuku keisatsu*, self-isolation police) also appeared during April and early May.

Finally, as in other countries, rumours and fake news also circulated through various Japanese media channels, including the internet. At the end of February, a photograph showing empty toilet-paper shelves that was distributed through Twitter sparked nationwide panic-buying to the extent industry associations and the national cabinet made announcements to quell the frenzy (Tsuchiya, 2020). Rumours of preventive solutions and cures were also distributed widely in the spring (Kanematsu, 2020), leading the Japanese Consumer Affairs Agency to issue public warnings in the media and on its website. A survey conducted by the Nippon Research Centre during March revealed high trust in television news, newspapers and internet-based news websites, particularly among people in their 50s and older. Younger people, in their teens and 20s, were more likely to use social network services such as Twitter and Instagram, as well as online bulletin board services (Nihon Risachi Senta, 2020). However, the results of a further survey conducted by the Ministry of Internal Affairs and Communications in May showed distinct trends for young people, particularly those in their teens, to disseminate false information without confirming its veracity (Sōmushō, 2020).

Conclusion

While other countries were facing record-high infection numbers during the summer of 2020, at the time of writing in September 2020, Japan was experiencing the downward phase of a second, less severe wave of the virus that had peaked in early August. What did Japan do right? Throughout the pandemic period, policies aimed at the continuous and cautiously balanced approach of focusing on health care and the economy were well publicised and accepted by the public. Criticisms of Japan's low rate of PCR testing were tempered with pointing out the merits of contact tracing and testing only serious cases with an eye to conserving medical resources. Some analysts have pointed to the country's official medical policy of following the 3 Cs (Nishimura, Y., 2020), while the practices of wearing masks in public and observing self-isolation practices may also have played significant roles in curbing the pandemic within Japan.

During the first six months of the pandemic, institutional roles, functions and the use of the internet and social media for political communications evolved greatly. Government institutions at all levels combined and extended their internet-based tools particularly social media, further propelling internet use in a country already famous for its advances in integrating innovative technologies into daily life. Although Shinzo Abe was forced to resign as prime minister for health reasons at the end of August, his successor, Yoshihide Suga, has vowed to continue the Abe administration's approach to managing the pandemic. Over the long term, the COVID-19 pandemic has opened up new possibilities and pitfalls for using the internet in public-sector information dissemination, political communication and social commentary in Japan.

References

Abe, S. (2020). Basic policies for Novel Coronavirus Disease Control summary, 1 July. http://japan.kantei.go.jp/ongoingtopics/_00013.html

Asahi Shimbun (2020a). 'Japan will label coronavirus as infectious disease to fight spread. *Asahi Shimbun*, 27 January.

Asahi Shimbun (2020b). 'Abe Cabinet approves bill to fight coronavirus outbreak. *Asahi Shimbun*, 20 March. www.asahi.com/ajw/articles/13202444

Asahi Shimbun (2020c). Abe orders budget rewrite to add 100,000-yen handouts to all. *Asahi Shimbun*, 16 April. www.asahi.com/ajw/articles/13302380

Ishihara, J., & Nagao, R. (2020). 'Contact-tracing app set to debut in Japan this week. *Nikkei Asian Review*, 16 June. https://asia.nikkei.com/Spotlight/Coronavirus/Cont act-tracing-app-set-to-debut-in-Japan-this-week

Japan Local Government Center (2020). Japan's response to the Coronavirus pandemic. 28 April. www.jlgc.org/04-28-2020/8414/

Japan Times (2020a). Japan to beef up coronavirus panel with local officials and risk experts. 25 June. www.japantimes.co.jp/news/2020/06/25/national/japan-coronavi rus-panel-local-government-risk-experts/

Japan Times (2020b). Downloads of Japan's COVID-19 app slow despite rising infections. 21 July.

Japan Times (2020c). Japan's 'Abenomask' drive tainted by gripes over mold, stains and bugs. *The Japan Times*, 23 April. www.japantimes.co.jp/news/2020/04/23/national/ abenomask-mold-bugs/

Johnston, E. (2020). 'Osaka governor spearheads national effort to enforce business shutdowns over coronavirus. *The Japan Times*, 25 July.

Kanematsu, Y. (2020). Ads touting quack coronavirus cures rampant in Japan. *Nikkei Asian Review*, 9 June. https://asia.nikkei.com/Spotlight/Coronavirus/Ads-touting -quack-coronavirus-cures-rampant-in-Japan

Kyodo News (2020a). Japan disease expert pulls videos blasting situation on virus-hit ship. *Kyodo News*, 20 February. https://english.kyodonews.net/news/2020/02/4b bd92cd4f91-breaking-news-japan-scholar-removes-videos-blasting-situation-on -virus-hit-ship.html

Kyodo News (2020b). Hokkaido declares emergency state again as virus infections grow. *Kyodo News*, 12 April. https://english.kyodonews.net/news/2020/04/3a9aebe957d2 -tokyo-sees-total-coronavirus-infection-cases-top-2000-up-by-166.html

LINE (2020). *Dai gokai shingata korona daisaku no tame no zenkoku chōsa ni gokyōryoku kudasai.* 17 August. https://guide.line.me/ja/coronavirus-survey.html

MHLW (Ministry of Health, Labour and Welfare) (2020). About Coronavirus Disease 2019 (COVID-19). Government Measures 1. *The Basic Policies,* 25 May. www.mhlw.go.jp/stf/seisakunitsuite/bunya/newpage_00032.html#goverment

NHK (2020). *Naikaku shijiritsu.* 12 August. www.nhk.or.jp/senkyo/shijiritsu/

Nihon Risachi Senta (2020). *'Shingata korona uirusu kansenshō no kōdō jōkyō' to yūkō na medeia ni tsuite no chōsa.* 4 April. www.nrc.co.jp/report/200410.html

Nishimura, K. (2020). 'Households to get 300,000 yen in relief for losses from coronavirus. *Asahi Shimbun,* 3 April. www.asahi.com/ajw/articles/13269206

Nishimura, Y. (2020). How Japan beat coronavirus without lockdowns.' *The Wall Street Journal,* July 7. www.wsj.com/articles/how-japan-beat-coronavirus-without-lockdowns-11594163172

Sōmushō (2020). *Shingata korona uirusu kansenshō ni kansuru jōhō ryūtsū chōsa hōkokusho.* 19 June. www.soumu.go.jp/menu_news/s-news/01kiban18_01000082.html

Takahashi, R. (2020). Debate over Japan's virus testing resurfaces amid nationwide outbreak *The Japan Times,* 21 July. www.japantimes.co.jp/news/2020/07/21/national/social-issues/japan-coronavirus-testing-2/

The Mainichi (2020a). Plague-predicting Japanese folklore creature resurfaces amid coronavirus chaos *The Mainichi,* 25 March.

The Mainichi (2020b). Abe's 'stay home' message has fueled anger. *The Mainichi,* 13 April. https://mainichi.jp/english/articles/20200413/p2g/00m/0na/069000c

Tsuchiya, K. (2020). 'Shingata korona to kankeinai toiretto pepa shinausu no kowasa [Fears of toilet paper shortage unrelated to corona virus]. *The Mainichi,* 6 March.

Umeda, S (2020). 'Japan: Cabinet issues orders relating to Infectious Disease Control Act and Quarantine Act. *Library of Congress Global Legal Monitor,* 11 March.

4

SOUTH KOREA

No shutdown, no lockdown

Jangyul Robert Kim and Sera Choi

Political context

South Korea is currently led by its 19th President, Moon Jae-In since 2017. The Moon Government has so far garnered higher approval ratings than any of his predecessors. This is evident in the Minjoo Party of Korea's recent victory in the most recent Parliamentary elections held on April 15, 2020, winning 60% of the National Assembly (180 of 300 seats) (Kim, K.H., 2020). The popularity of the Moon regime continues to skyrocket amidst South Korea's exemplary response to COVID-19.

The Moon Jae-In Government is making great efforts to restore relations with North Korea and establish good relations with China, in contrast with the previous conservative regime that was hostile to the North and favoured relations with the United States (MOHW, 2020a). Additionally, President Moon brokered the peace talks between President Trump of the United States and Kim Jong-Un of North Korea, declaring the Panmunjeom Declaration for Peace, Prosperity and Unification of the Korean Peninsula alongside Kim on April 27, 2018 (Korea.net, 2018).

The South Korean Government has taken an inclusive approach to China and North Korea, while taking a strong stance on Japan. The Moon Government faced criticism from the opposition party because it did not close borders to China, unlike the United States that initially closed its borders to China following the first COVID-19 outbreak (Kim, K. H., 2020). In contrast, the South Korean and Japanese Governments have not been so open to one another. Following the Japanese Government prohibiting entry from South Korea, the South Korean Government immediately reciprocated (Kim, S. H., 2020).

DOI: 10.4324/9781003120254-6

Even though there were policies that were heavily criticised, there are many who welcome and praise Moon's approaches in such areas as anti-nuclear energy, income-driven growth, minimum wage increase, and a 52-hour workweek (Seong, 2019). The legacy of his policies remains open to future evaluation, however.

Chronology

See Table 4.1.

Political Issues in connection with the COVID-19 Emergency

In light of the National Assembly election on April 15, 2020, the rapid spread of COVID-19 has quickly become an even greater political issue. Following the first confirmed case, the South Korean Government took passive measures of self-reporting to quarantine offices upon entry if symptoms were present and if travelling from the Wuhan, China area. This is in contrast to the aggressive measures taken by China's neighbouring country, Taiwan, which banned entry from China (Chen, 2020). South Korea's approach also contrasts with the United States, which had its first confirmed case the same day as South Korea, of which the latter banned entry from China.

Later, as the number of COVID-19 patients increased in South Korea, many experts and opposition parties criticised the government's loose measures and called for an immediate entry ban from China (Kim, H. H., 2020). However, the South Korean Government stood by its stance that it could control the spread of COVID-19. The South Korean Government ultimately decided not to ban entry from China, not only because Xi Jinping of China was scheduled to visit South Korea in April of 2020, but also not to undermine trade and business activity with China (Larsen, 2020). Consequently, COVID-19 confirmed cases increased in South Korea while decreasing in China, leading to a situation in which China banned entry from South Korea.

In addition, there was a clear partisan divide regarding the COVID-19 emergency cash payment for economic revitalisation. Initially, considering the financial sustainability of the government, the top 30% income bracket were to be excluded from receiving the relief payment and then all qualified citizens received up to 1 million Won (approx. 830 US dollars) (Roh, 2020). The opposition party criticised it as a political act, given the timely announcement one day before the April 15 election, but later changed its position that it was necessary to pay emergency relief to all citizens. Eventually, the government decided to give all citizens a relief payment but an option to receive a 15% tax exemption instead to those who declined to receive the subsidy (Kwak, 2020). This decision yet faced another criticism from the opposition party that the option would be testing the morality of the people.

TABLE 4.1 South Korea chronology

Date		# of Cases	Key official actions	Key communication events
January	20	1	**Start Phase 1**. Infectious disease alert status moved from level 1 (blue) to level 2 (yellow).	The first briefing was held, to continue twice daily, broadcast and streamed live; information shared included confirmed cases, deaths, and technological developments etc.
	23	1	Central Disaster and Safety Countermeasures Headquarters (CDSCHQ) was established.	
	27	4	Infectious disease alert status increased to level 3 (orange).	
	31	7	KCDC and Korean Association for Clinical Trial Quality Management established and verified real-time COVID-19 tests (Real Time RT-PCR) with increase in test speed and efficiency, resulting with confirmatory tests within 6 hours.	
February	1	12	The government required those who entered South Korea or those who overlap with confirmed cases to install the 'COVID-19 Self-Isolator Safety Protection App.' Supplied 720,000 masks for high-risk workplaces.	
	2	15	14-day self-isolation mandated for people who had had contact with patients with positive test results for COVID-19.	
	4	16	COVID-19 contact tracing mobile application was made available on Google store (i.e. Corona Doctor).	
	12	28	A self-diagnosis mobile application became available to the public, allowing users to monitor health conditions and find available information such as finding testing clinics by using the 1399 line.	

(Continued)

TABLE 4.1 (Continued)

Date	# of Cases	Key official actions	Key communication events
23	602	**Phase 2.** Infectious disease alert status moved to level 4 (red).	Prescriptions and consultation meetings were provided virtually by physicians.
26	1,261	The first drive-through testing station was launched by the local government in Goyang City. Buddhist Orders and the Catholic Church stop services, and most Protestant churches switched to online worship.	
March 10	7,513	**Phase 3.** The start of all school levels, from kindergarten to high school, deferred to March 23.	
22	8,897		Launched an 'enhanced social distancing campaign.'
23	8,961		CDSCHQ and KCDC started regular briefings online. Reporters asked questions through 'KakaoTalk,' and the top five most important were answered.
April 20	10,674	CDSCHQ eased social distancing restrictions based on situational occurrences.	
27	10,738	Smart self-isolation management enhancement tools using information and communication technology (ICT) were implemented.	Individuals who violated quarantine guidelines required to wear 'reliable wristbands' to track them during their isolation period.
May 4	10,801		The government hosted the first web seminar on 'K-Protection' with health and medical experts.
5	10,804		200th briefing reached.
June 10	11,902 cases; 276 deaths		Quick Response (QR) registration requirements for entertainment facilities mandated.

As many countries also provided emergency relief funds in response to the COVID-19 pandemic, the South Korean Government's decision cannot simply be seen as a political act of charity. It was also found that those who received the subsidy have somewhat contributed to revitalising the local economy. However, contrary to the government's expectations, an insignificant portion (less than 1%) of the population declined the subsidy and donated to relief efforts (KBS, 2020).

Social issues in connection with the COVID-19 emergency

The political parties also differed in opinions on the cause of COVID-19 in South Korea. While the opposition party claimed that it had been a result of the failure to ban entry from China, the ruling party blamed Sincheonji (a cult church), considered a Christian heresy (Kim, S. B., 2020). Their reason was the confirmation of COVID-19 cases among Shincheonji members originating from Wuhan.

In addition, the South Korean Government urged people to refrain from external activities as COVID-19 spread, instead of forcing people not to gather. Complying with government guidelines, Buddhist Orders and the Catholic Church stopped regular worship and gatherings, and most Protestant churches switched to online worship on February 26 (Steger, 2020). However, some Protestant churches kept in-person worship on Sundays, leading to conflict with the government and local residents (Do, 2020).

Schools and day-care centres have also postponed starting a new academic semester, causing trouble for working parents. Universities have postponed openings as well, later moving to online courses, causing many tuition-refund-requests from dissatisfied students (MOHW, 2020a).

Uses and role of social networks and the web

South Korea is one of the most internet-savvy countries in the world. Notable points in South Korea's response to COVID-19 are the cooperation between the government and the private sector, effective role distribution and mutual complementation (MOHW, 2020b). The South Korean response, from the government to the private sector level, has gained attention from all over the world.

Web-based quarantine management and contact tracing

First, the government required those who entered South Korea or those who overlap with confirmed people to install the 'COVID-19 Self-Isolator Safety Protection App' which was available on February 12 (MOHW, 2020c). This app allows people to self-report their body temperature and health situation twice a day, which a dedicated public official then immediately checks for symptoms and anomalies and takes necessary actions immediately if there are any unusual features (MOHW, 2020c). Moreover, as soon as the quarantined person leaves the quarantine location, an alarm notifies the dedicated public official immediately (Kim, W. J., 2020).

Active use of COVID-19-related apps for the general public

In addition to the government, citizen developers and corporations have also actively assisted by launching COVID-19 related apps to help prevent the spread of the virus (Park, H. I., 2020). Popular portals such as Naver and Kakao created COVID-19 maps providing real-time status updates. Among the mobile apps, on February 4, the app 'Corona Doctor' was launched and even recommended by the Google store. This app shows COVID-19-related information including confirmed case information, contact tracing, testing sites and quarantine hospitals (*Corona Doctor APK*, 2020). The 'Corona 100m' app, developed on February 11, sends a notification when the user is within 100m of a location visited by a confirmed case. When a user types in a location in the 'Coronaita' app, it notifies the user of nearby places frequented by confirmed cases and shows the risk value of the user for the given location (Park, H. I., 2020). Compared to the launch of COVID-19 contact tracing apps by Apple and Google in May 20 (Landi, 2020), these apps have been used in South Korea since mid-February (Kim, K. J., 2020; MOHW, 2020c). Moreover, citizen developers and startups have developed apps that share mask purchase information, such as GoodDoc Mask Scanner, Mask Reminder, Wear Mask and Let's Buy Masks in March (Lee, 2020).

Other key considerations

A hero is born in times of crisis. Once again, South Korean doctors and nurses from other regions freely volunteered to go to Daegu, the epicentre of the pandemic, at the risk of becoming infected themselves (Park, K. B., 2020). This reminds of the many civilian divers who voluntarily went to the sinking area and participated in rescue efforts following the sinking of MV Sewol. As in nations worldwide, the true heroes of this pandemic are the frontline healthcare workers. In addition, many landlords have voluntarily cut or even refused to accept rent from their tenants (Han, 2020).

Analysis

Leadership and a point of reference

South Korea has dealt with multiple outbreaks of pandemics including MERS and SARS. Moreover, it has become increasingly common for the general population to wear facial masks on a regular basis, due to the yellow dust and fine particles (PM10 and PM2.5) coming from China annually. Conversely, through these experiences, it was possible for the South Korean Government to effectively respond to COVID-19.

On January 23, three days after the first COVID-19 case was confirmed, the South Korean government established the Central Disaster and Safety Countermeasures Headquarters (CDSCHQ). CDSCHQ consists of the heads of 17 government departments, including the Ministry of Health and Welfare, the Korean Centres for Disease Control and Prevention (KCDC) and the Ministry of Food and Drug Safety (MFDS) (COVID-19, Republic of Korea, 2020). In the event of a national crisis, the prime minister assumes the leading role.

The South Korean Government enacted its National Crisis Management System immediately after the crisis and raised the alert level from level 1 (blue) to level 2 (yellow) (MOHW, 2020c). The government then required all individuals entering South Korea within 14 days after visiting Wuhan, China, to submit the health questionnaire and report to a quarantine officer if experiencing fever or respiratory symptoms. On January 27, the government raised the alert level from level 2 (yellow) to level 3 (orange) and held meetings with private companies to discuss decisions to produce diagnostic kits (MOHW, 2020b). The government also increased the number of COVID-19 testing sites and encouraged mask production.

In addition, CDSCHQ officially briefed the public about the status of COVID-19 and the government's response and actions twice a day since January 20 – broadcast and streamed live (MOHW, 2020d). They shared not only basic data such as the number of confirmed cases and deaths, but also leveraged advanced technology and apps to keep the public informed and prepared. They further utilised the government's social media channels to actively communicate with the public and encouraged private app developers and startups to create mobile apps through supporting web cloud services.

The South Korean Government's COVID-19-related announcement was thoroughly conducted through CDSCHQ only. The Minister of Health and Welfare (Park Neung-Hoo), Head of the Centres for Disease Control (Jung Eun-Kyung) and the Deputy Minister of Health and Welfare (Kim Kang-Lip) made the announcement. As all three of the experts are doctors related to health and welfare, they had the ability and experience to answer reporters' questions immediately.

In particular, the honest and diligent work demonstrated by Jung Eun-Kyung, head of the KCDC, was highlighted by many global news media. From her saying 'I sleep over an hour' while her hair visibly greyed from not having the time to go to the salon, to a strong message saying, 'Virus can't beat Korea' (Walker, 2020), as these messages were spread through social media, the South Korean Government continued to earn the people's trust. This was supported by a 16%

increase in the government trust among a poll of south Koreans from January to April (Edelman, 2020).

Main actors

The South Korean Government, through CDSCHQ, consistently communicated with the public. The official announcements were delivered in real time to the public, not only through traditional media such as newspapers and broadcasts, but also through government social media. Portal sites (e.g. Naver and Daum) played an equally important role in distributing COVID-19-related data and resources in real time and cooperated as much as possible to help people follow the government's guide.

In addition, scientists and health communications experts echoed the same messages to fortify the government's announcement, adding credibility and trust to the government's messages. The South Korean Government recommended wearing a mask from the beginning.

It cannot be said that the South Korean Government has responded well since the early days of COVID-19. Nevertheless, ultimately, it can be said that South Korea's quarantine policy has been successful, as shown by the low number of confirmed cases and related deaths compared to other countries. Most importantly, the critical main actors were those who believed in the government's messages, and voluntarily practised social distancing and mask-wearing, despite there being no active government coercion such as a nation-wide shutdown. Without the diligent voluntary participation and cooperation from the people, it would have been impossible to prevent the rapid spread of COVID-19 while maintaining daily, normal life.

Was the expert guidance used consistently and clearly?

The most important group of South Korean experts in COVID-19 response consists of government officials, such as Jung Eun-Kyung, head of the KCDC, who has experienced similar crises in the past and gained valuable professional knowledge. Of course, other expert groups such as the Korean Medical Association weighed in as well, but the information provided by the voice of CDSCHQ had the most significant influence on the behaviour of the people.

The South Korean Government deserves praise in its efforts to communicate consistently and transparently throughout its COVID-19 response. Many were optimistic in the early days regarding the detrimental effects of COVID-19, not too dissimilar from the initial reactions of President Trump of the United States and Prime Minister Abe of Japan. However, as the situation became severe, the South Korean Government responded rapidly and was able to curb COVID-19 as a result. In particular, the South Korean Government's real-time notification on the status of confirmed cases and the movement of those people through smartphones played a major role in preventing a more dramatic spread of COVID-19.

Was the action that was required clearly justified and in line with a clear objective?

The message of the government and the people's participation did not always perfectly match. Despite the government's preaching of voluntary segregation and social distancing, the implementation was not always clear and followed. For example, while schools shifted to delays and online classes, private institutions remained open, leading to an ironic situation where students went to the private academies instead of to schools. While public libraries, museums and sports facilities closed, private gyms, restaurants and stores remained open. In addition, clubs, karaoke rooms and pubs all remained open, leading to negative side effects. In particular, young people ignored the government's repeated warnings, and frequented clubs/bars, eventually leading to confirmed cases in a club in Itaewon. As a result, the government has become increasingly strict, and then reiterated social distancing and voluntary quarantining.

In some Western countries such as France, there was criticism that South Korea's response violated privacy rights (Xu & Lee, 2020). However, it should be viewed from the point that while these countries enforced stay-at-home orders and greatly reduced economic activities, South Korea was able to maintain daily and economic activities throughout the pandemic.

The misinformation environment

Not all information provided by the government had been consistent. The government had always recommended wearing masks, but not as strong as it does today. As COVID-19 confirmed cases increased, the government strongly recommended wearing a mask.

The government (MFDS)'s announcement of what mask to wear was inconsistent however. Lee Eui-Kyung, the Minister of the MFDS, first announced in a press release, 'it is desirable to wear a 'KF94' or 'KF99' grade masks to prevent new COVID-19 infection' (Kim, D. C., 2020), but later added 'KF80,' dental masks and droplet masks to the list as the weather warmed.

Conclusion

It can be said that the efforts of the South Korean Government experiencing the first-ever COVID-19 pandemic are still overall successful. In particular, its 'no shutdown, no lockdown' stance to ensure the least disruption to the lives of the people has been commended as an exemplary prevention and response model that has since been introduced in other countries. The success of the South Korean response model are due to the following: (1) increasing the production of diagnostic kits as soon as COVID-19 occurred, (2) instituting creative testing methods such as drive-through and walk-through to test a large number of people efficiently and rapidly, (3) taking on the costs of testing and treatments so that everyone can receive proper care, (4) all of the public voluntarily wearing masks to suppress the transmission of COVID-19 as much as possible, (5) the ability of the South Korean Government to secure a consistent mask production capability through past experiences with fine dust/particles from China, SARS and MERS, (6) the dedication of the frontline workers, public officials and volunteers and lastly, (7) despite privacy concerns, effectively managing confirmed cases through smartphone apps in real time.

From a communications perspective, it should be highly evaluated that the South Korean Government immediately responded to COVID-19 by (1) quickly forming CDSCHQ, and carrying out consistent and transparent communications, (2) earning the people's trust through consistent communications from experts such as the head of the KCDC, Jung Eun-Kyung, (3) utilising both traditional and social media effectively to communicate with the public and (4) supporting private experts and startups to develop relevant apps and using such apps. At the same time, it remains regretful that the Moon Jae-In Government (1) sent confusing messages regarding mask-wearing guidance, (2) lacked consistency in social distancing implementation and (3) announced the relief funds the day before the National Assembly elections.

References

Chen, C. (2020). Taiwan bans entry of all Chinese nationals as Wuhan virus surges. *Focus Taiwan* https://focustaiwan.tw/society/202002050025, https://focustaiwan.tw/society/202002050025

Corona Doctor APK (2020). *APK.tools.* https://apk.tools/

COVID-19, Republic of Korea (2020). *COVID-19 Response.* http://ncov.mohw.go.kr/en/baroView.do?brdId=11&brdGubun=111

Do, J. G. (2020). Despite COVID-19, some churches keep worship on Sunday. *Khan.* http://news.khan.co.kr/kh_news/khan_art_view.html?artid=202002281702001&code=960100

Edelman (2020). *Edelman Reliability Index Survey.* https://www.edelman.kr/newsroom/2020-trust-barometer-spring-update-press-release

Han, J. H. (2020). Daegu citizens help and protect each other 'Reduction of rent.' *Ohmynews.* www.ohmynews.com/NWS_Web/View/at_pg.aspx?CNTN_CD=A0002615161&CMPT_CD=P0010&utm_source=naver&utm_medium=newsearch&utm_campaign=naver_news

KBS (2020). *Emergency Relief Fund Donation Reaches 28.2 Billion Won for a Month.* http://world.kbs.co.kr/service/news_view:sp.htm?lang=k&Seq_Code=357339&board_code=91&page=1

Kim, D. C. (2020). COVID-19 and the responses of government, media and the citizens. *Daily Pharm.* http://m.dailypharm.com/News/263283

Kim, H. H. (2020). Contradictory in response to China. *Hankyung.* www.hankyung.com/politics/article/202003062270i

Kim, K. H. (2020). In the 21st general election, the birth of 'Super Yeo-dang' (total). *Yonhap News.* www.yna.co.kr/view/AKR20200416031200001?input=1195m

Kim, K. J. (2020). Rising apps as COVID-19 expands. *MK*. www.mk.co.kr/news/bu siness/view/2020/03/245260/

Kim, S. B. (2020). Democratic party blames Shincheonji, Republican party blames China. *Khan*. http://news.khan.co.kr/kh_news/khan_art_view.html?artid=2020 02252243005&code=910402

Kim, S. H. (2020). `Eye for eyes` the immigration restrictions. *MK*. www.mk.co.kr/ne ws/politics/view/2020/03/239675/

Kim, W. J. (2020). 'Self-isolator App'… 'an alarm when one leaves the quarantine location.' *YTN*. www.ytn.co.kr/_ln/0103_202003071800539230

Korea.net (2018). *Panmunjom Declaration on Peace, Prosperity and Reunification of the Korean Peninsula* [Press Release]. www.korea.net/Government/Current-Affairs/National-Affairs/view?subId=641&affairId=656&pageIndex=1&articleId=3412

Kwak, H. J. (2020). If you donate emergency relief payment…15% tax exemption instead. *Seoul Shinmun*. www.seoul.co.kr/news/newsView.php?id=20200429500077 &wlog_tag3=naver

Landi, H. (2020). Apple and Google launch contact tracing API for COVID-19 exposure. *Fierce Healthcare*. www.fiercehealthcare.com/tech/apple-and-google-launch-covid-19-exposure-notification-api

Larsen, M. S. (2020). South Korea's President tried to help China contain the Coronavirus. *Foreign Policy*. https://foreignpolicy.com/2020/03/09/moon-jae-in-china-coron avirus-impeachment-south-korea-president/

Lee, J. E. (2020). Launched app service to notify the sale of masks. *Newsis*. https://newsis. com/view/?id=NISX20200311_0000951057&cID=13001&pID=13000

Ministry of Health and Welfare (MOHW) (2020a). *COVID-19 Response Meeting Presided* [Press release]. www.mohw.go.kr/eng/nw/nw0101vw.jsp?PAR_MENU_ID=1007 &MENU_ID=100701&page=1&CONT_SEQ=352978

Ministry of Health and Welfare (MOHW) (2020b). *Diagnosis of COVID-19 Accelerated through Public-Private Cooperation* [Press release]. www.mohw.go.kr/react/al/sal030 1vw.jsp?PAR_MENU_ID=04&MENU_ID=0403&page=1&CONT_SEQ =352571&SEARCHKEY=CONTENT&SEARCHVALUE=%EC%A7%84%EB% 8B%A8%ED%82%A4%ED%8A%B8

Ministry of Health and Welfare (MOHW) (2020c). *IMS Meeting for Novel Coronavirus* [Press release]. www.mohw.go.kr/eng/nw/nw0101vw.jsp?PAR_MENU_ID=1007 &MENU_ID=100701&page=1&CONT_SEQ=352865

Ministry of Health and Welfare (MOHW) (2020d). *Regular Briefing on COVID-19* [Press release]. www.mohw.go.kr/react/al/sal0301vw.jsp?PAR_MENU_ID=04&MENU _ID=0403&page=8&CONT_SEQ=354363

Park, H. I. (2020). COVID-19 popular app. *Chosun Ilbo*. https://biz.chosun.com/site/da ta/html_dir/2020/02/28/2020022803239.html?utm_source=naver&utm_medium =original&utm_campaign=biz

Park, K. B. (2020). I'm going to Daegu to stop COVID-19. *Kookje Shinmun*. www.k ookje.co.kr/news2011/asp/newsbody.asp?code=0300&key=20200227.99099010504

Roh, J. M. (2020). Se-Kyun Jung 'The importance of COVID-19 Emergency Disaster Support.' *Media Today*. www.mediatoday.co.kr/news/articleView.html?idxno=2 06655

Seong, H. Y. (2019). Three tasks to be solved by President moon. *Hankyoreh*. www.hani .co.kr/arti/politics/polibar/916433.html, www.hani.co.kr/arti/politics/polibar/916 433.html

Steger, I. (2020). How religion is playing a role in the spread of coronavirus in Korea. *Quartz*. https://qz.com/1808390/religion-is-at-the-heart-of-koreas-coronav

irus-outbreak/, https://qz.com/1808390/religion-is-at-the-heart-of-koreas-coronav
irus-outbreak/

Walker, S. (2020). Thank God for calm, competent deputies. *The Wall Street Journal.*
www.wsj.com/articles/in-the-coronavirus-crisis-deputies-are-the-leaders-we-turn-
to-11585972802

Xu, A., & Lee, J. (2020). Gov't rebuts French lawyer critical of Korea's COVID-19
response. *Korea.net.* www.korea.net/NewsFocus/Society/view?articleId=184727

5

THE UNITED STATES

Politics versus science?

John M. Callahan

Political context

The US government first became aware of the novel coronavirus outbreak as a potential pandemic and national security issue on or around January 1, 2020. At that time, impeachment proceedings were under way in the US Congress, and steps were being taken to end a trade war that had been underway between the United States and China. In early January, the United States came very near to a war with Iran, a situation in which the strategic restraint of the administration was under significant attack by the media and the Democrat-controlled House of Representatives.

By the end of February and early March, when cases of the virus were publicly announced in the United States, the impeachment crisis was over, and that, combined with the end of the trade war and the avoidance of a new Middle East conflict put the Trump administration in a relatively good position, in fact, with higher polling numbers than at any previous time.

Indeed, political eyes were focused on the Democratic Party, which was in the throes of attempting to find a candidate to challenge Trump for the presidency in 2020, and seeing the mainstream party select former Vice President Joseph Biden as their candidate, in spite of mediocre debate performance and a primary race that was still in contention.

In short, the administration and the American people were focused on the upcoming election and an economy that continued to drive forward for the third straight year of Trump's Presidency. The media reported events in Wuhan, but coronavirus was not a recurring news item until mid- to late-February, understandably when Americans overseas and on cruise ships began to be infected, and focus increased when the virus seriously affected Italy. This chapter examines the period of January 1 to May 31. By the end of May, protests and unrest

DOI: 10.4324/9781003120254-7

surrounding the death of George Floyd at the hand of a Minnesota Police officer eclipsed COVID-19 as the main news story in the United States.

Chronology

See Table 5.1.

Analysis

It is perhaps unsurprising that the initial responses to the COVID-19 outbreak originated from the Centers for Disease Control and Prevention (CDC), as it was, at that point, a foreign crisis. Furthermore, the Trump administration had a series of significant issues to deal with in January and February, ranging from impeachment hearings to brinkmanship with Iran. Nevertheless, the President was quick to comment on the crisis and attempted to build confidence by painting the impact of the virus and the US response in a positive light.

That effort began in January, with Trump's (2020a) speech in Davos, and his prediction that should the virus spread to the US, it would be handled 'Very Well'. Later in the month, in Michigan, he touted international cooperation, saying, 'Now we're working very strongly with China on the coronavirus, that's a new thing that a lot of people are talking about. Hopefully, it won't be as bad as some people think it could be' (Trump, 2020b). On February 25, in a speech in India, Trump continued to take an optimistic tone, saying the coronavirus was 'well under control' and that there were 'very few people with it' (Lemire, 2020). Larry Kudlow, White House economic adviser, said in an interview with CNBC that the virus was contained in the United States, and the economic impact would be minimal.

However, on that day, the CDC announced that it expected community spread of the virus. 'It's not so much a question of if this will happen anymore but rather more a question of exactly when this will happen and how many people in this country will have severe illness,' said Dr Nancy Messonnier, director of the CDC's National Center for Immunization and Respiratory Diseases (Boboltz, 2020). This would not be the last time that messages from leaders and scientists were in conflict. Nevertheless, the White House ended February in an upbeat mood, with Trump (2020c) stating,

> We've taken the most aggressive actions to confront the coronavirus. They are the most aggressive taken by any country. And we're the No. 1 travel destination anywhere in the world, yet we have far fewer cases of the disease than even countries with much less travel or a much smaller population.

February would prove to be the calm before the storm for coronavirus.

TABLE 5.1 US chronology

Month	Date	Diffusion of COVID-19	Key Official Actions	Key Communication Events
January	5		CDC issues warning to travellers to Wuhan.	
	6		CDC activates Incident Management System (IMS).	
	17			CDC COVID-19 IMS holds its first press conference.
	21	First case confirmed in Seattle, Washington.		
	22			President Trump speaks to the media at the World Economic Forum in Davos.
	29		A White House-level task force is set up, directed by Health and Human Services Secretary Alex Azar.	
	30			Trump commented further on the virus at a political rally in Warren, Michigan.
	31	Total for January – one known case, no deaths.	The United States suspends entry to foreign nationals from mainland China, US public health emergency declared, backdated to Jan 27.	
February	2			President Trump justifies decision to exclude travel from China on Fox News (Hannity, 2020).

(Continued)

TABLE 5.1 (Continued)

Month	Date	Diffusion of COVID-19	Key Official Actions	Key Communication Events
	4		The Department of Homeland Security announced all flights into the United States containing travellers originating in China must route through selected airports with enhanced screening procedures.	
	6	First American dies in Wuhan.		
	7		The United States pledged 100 million dollars in aid to China to fight the virus.	
	24		The White House requested 1.25 billion dollars of additional funds to combat COVID-19.	
	25	First US military member infected in South Korea.		Trump speaks to the media while in India. The CDC predicts community spread likely.
	26		Whistleblower reveals personnel treating Americans evacuated from Wuhan lacked personal protective equipment (PPE) or proper training.	President Trump announced Vice President Mike Pence would lead the US response, defends decision to close the border.
	29	The victim in Seattle became the first American to die. February totals: 1 dead, 68 known infections.	Travel restrictions expanded to include Italy and South Korea. The Food and Drug Administration took steps to expand testing availability.	The White House makes a Press Statement expressing confidence in the response.

March		
2	Federal Reserve announces emergency rate cut.	In a daily press briefing, President Trump has first significant divergence with Dr. Fauci.
4	The Securities and Exchange Commission (SEC, 2020) announces a regulatory relief package for companies impacted by the virus.	
6		President Trump visited CDC headquarters in Atlanta, announced he did not plan to cancel travel and social gatherings in America (Baker, 2020).
10		President Trump speaks about testing.
11	The White House announced travel bans on 26 European countries for 30 days. Low interest loans to impacted small businesses and mitigation strategies for states designated hotspots of infection announced.	The World Health Organisation declares that COVID-19 is a global pandemic.
12		Trump announces crisis response measures.
13	The COVID-19 virus is declared a US national emergency. Restrictions increased on Americans returning from abroad. House of Representatives reach agreement with White House on *Families First Coronavirus Response Act* (FFCRA) relief bill. The Dept of Defence announces travel ban for civilian employees.	
15	The CDC recommended gatherings of 50+ people be cancelled for 2 months.	
17	The White House recommends 15 days of social distancing across the United States.	

(*Continued*)

TABLE 5.1 (Continued)

Month	Date	Diffusion of COVID-19	Key Official Actions	Key Communication Events
	18		President Trump signed an executive order to activate the *Defense Production Act* to force production of necessary items. However, he did not implement the act at that time (Dzhanova, 2020).	
	20			In the White House Daily briefing, President Trump sparred with Dr Anthony Fauci over the potential efficacy of malaria drugs against COVID-19. Trump said he was going with 'gut feelings' on the issue (Alonso-Zaldivar, 2020).
	24			Trump discusses reopening the United States on Fox News.
	29		Trump signed the FFCRA, injecting two trillion dollars into the economy.	
	31	**116,415 cases, 3,806 dead.**	14% of employed population filed for unemployment, worst rate since the Great Depression.	
April	3		The CDC issues new guidance on face masks.	
	11	The United States has highest number of COVID-19 deaths, deaths reported in all 50 states.		
	15		Protests erupt in four states against stay-at-home orders.	

16	The White House urges states to plan for reopening.
20	Georgia, South Carolina and Tennessee announce reopening plans. By end of May, all 50 states have announced such plans.
23	Additional relief funding announced for hospitals hit hard by the virus.
27	Warnings of food shortages and supply chain breakdowns follow news the virus had spread to several meat processing facilities.
	US economy shrank by 4.8% in first quarter of 2020, worst since the 2008 great recession.
	President Trump attends his last daily media appearance of this period.
30	Federal distancing restrictions expired.
	1,061,028 cases, 57,137 dead.
May	
11	The Food and Drug Administration approve Remdesivir to treat hospitalised patients.
15	15 states announce reopening plans, following international norms.
	Trump: major speech about the search for a vaccine.
25	George Floyd died in police custody in Minneapolis, Minnesota.
29	**1,774,034 cases, 97,959 dead.**
	White House announces the United States would withdraw from the WHO, claiming the organisation was dominated by China and not working in the interests of all members.

Crisis response and federalism

Initially, the CDC and White House were clearly in the driving seat of the US response to the crisis. However, as the crisis grew, the perception of leadership became more bifurcated as the crisis became politicised. The nature of US disaster response mechanisms also worked against a perception of centralised response. The Department of Homeland Security's National Response Framework mandates that the leading role in crisis management be at the lowest level possible. So, as COVID-19 spread, and the number of infections and hotspots grew, the state governors became more central to the crisis response. This caused significant friction and politicised every act. Any shortage of supplies, however temporary, was blamed on the Federal Government, even in cases in which state resources were not fully utilised. The most public example of this was the open feud between President Trump and New York Governor Andrew Cuomo. Each held daily press conferences, and a key feature of those press conferences was them bashing each other. Of note is that the two, actually close, associates from Mr. Trump's career in New York, were in nearly constant communication and often warned each other before each daily bashing. Internal dissension also came to exemplify the response, particularly between the political White House team and the scientists, most notably Dr Anthony Fauci, discussed in more detail below.

Trump's efforts to communicate federal economic responses were decisive and positive throughout the crisis. Beginning with the travel bans, by March this included financial stimulus. On March 12, in an oval office speech which justified the bans, President Trump said,

> Using emergency authority, I will be instructing the Treasury Department to defer tax payments, without interest or penalties, for certain individuals and businesses negatively impacted. This action will provide more than $200 billion of additional liquidity to the economy. Finally, I am calling on Congress to provide Americans with immediate payroll tax relief. Hopefully, they will consider this very strongly. We are at a critical time in the fight against the virus. We made a lifesaving move with early action on China.
>
> *(Trump, 2020d)*

The issue of reopening, which Trump began discussing as early as late March, put him once again in conflict with the state governors over who actually had the right to make such decisions. On March 25, in an interview with Fox News, Trump expressed hope the country would be able to reopen by Easter, April 12, stating, 'You will have packed churches all over our country, I think it would be a beautiful time and it is just about the timeline that I think is right' (Leonardi, 2020). Trump altered his Easter prediction and extended social distancing by a further two weeks, though he predicted by June 1, the country would be 'well on the way to recovery' (Smith, 2020). On May 15, Trump announced 'Operation Warp Speed,' which proposed to provide funding and support such that a vaccine might be developed by the end of 2020 (Duster, 2020). He also encouraged Americans to enjoy the upcoming Memorial Day holidays, as death rates seemed to be slowing around the country.

Media and social media

Any crisis taking place in the Trump administration is guaranteed to include a robust social media component. Consistent with crisis communication practices, key decisions and proclamations were made via social media channels. The President, as was the custom by this point in his Presidency, made significant announcements and statements via Twitter, and he continued his practice of engaging in media sparring contests both in his press availabilities and in his social media communications.

A bigger concern and lesson from the COVID-19 response is the open warfare that continues between the Trump administration and the traditional media. The administration entered office in a state of war with two major print outlets, the *Washington Post* and the *New York Times*, as well as CNN and MSNBC among the television media networks. This has led to a complete polarisation over his actions, and an increasing number of actions taken specifically to speak to the Republican Party base and to take symbolic actions which, even when proven wrong or when undone, still speak to Trump's base.

A key example of this was Trump's personal attendance at the daily White House COVID-19 task force press conferences in April and May. Although Trump had appointed Vice President Pence as Task Force Leader, he insisted on taking the stage along with Pence, Dr Fauci and other experts. The results were mixed. On some days, Trump's optimism and bravado carried the day. On others, the briefings and subsequent Twitter storms and post-briefing debates between the participants negated the benefits of the informational briefings.

'Good science' and 'bad science' – politicised science

Americans are well-known science sceptics (Reints, 2020), which is interesting considering that they are also known as tech fetishists believing technology can solve all problems. The greatest scepticism seems to come when technology is said not to work. This happened early in the COVID-19 crisis, when statements from the World Health Organisation (WHO), CDC and even Dr Anthony Fauci, Director of the National Institute of Allergy and Infectious Diseases, suggested face masks were not an effective defence against the spread of COVID-19. Simultaneously, organisations ranging from hospitals to state governments were begging for more masks for first responders and hospital personnel. On April 3, the CDC reversed its guidance, recommending use of face masks, and providing grist for the rising tide of speculation regarding CDC and WHO motives

(Dwyer, 2020). This was a split narrative that collapsed under its own weight. In hindsight, it was obvious that the anti-mask messaging campaign was designed to try to secure masks for the first responders. However, the distrust generated by that campaign continues to the present day.

The struggle between President Trump and the scientific community grew in intensity as the crisis went on. On March 2, Trump suggested a vaccine might be ready for distribution in three to four months, a statement that was clarified by Dr Anthony Fauci, who said that it normally took at least a year for successful vaccine development. This was the first of a series of intense, but relatively genteel disagreements between the two. Fauci ceased to be included in the daily press briefings weeks before Trump himself stopped attending at the end of April.

Neither social media or politics are good vehicles for science. Nearly every statement of any scientific body had its discreditors on one side or another of the political divide. Whether it was a debate over the efficacy of Hydroxychloriquine or Rendesevir against the virus, or masks, or how the virus spreads and what it does to victims of various age groups, every issue was debated bitterly on traditional and social media and in the halls of power in Washington. When President Trump began taking Hydroxychloriquine in May, he argued it was a preventative; health experts stated it only had some benefit to patients who had already suffered from the virus. Beginning on March 10, the issue of testing became another political and scientific hot potato. At the press briefing, Trump (2020e) said, 'when people need a test, they can get a test. When the professionals need a test, when they need tests for people, they can get the test. It's gone really well.'

Finally, the goals of the response effort seemed to change, or morph. In early March, there was unified discussion of the concept of 'flattening the curve'; slowing the spread of the virus to a rate which could be handled by existing medical facilities. By May, talk of flattening the curve faded from discussion. The effort had essentially succeeded, but because the discussion ended, the concept was forgotten.

Conclusion

The COVID-19 crisis highlighted several factors which have become hallmarks of American political communications in recent decades. Disagreement between branches of government, especially when led by different political parties, is nothing new. However, conflicting messaging among the departments of the executive branch, has reached a peak in the Trump administration, with the President and key administration officials frequently publicly disagreeing on key messages. By the same token, a series of structural and personality-driven issues led to a lack of consistency on key messaging points, such as when and how long to social distance, when states could close and reopen, if masks should be worn etc.

Trump's public responses began by downplaying the threat of COVID-19; however, that changed in February when the threat became clear and the virus entered the United States Trump, political and scientific experts and leaders all communicated frequently on the growing crisis but often recommended divergent responses. Hence the COVID-19 crisis, is still ongoing, and, perhaps, worsening. It may not be the greatest public health crisis in US history, but it will certainly be known as the most disruptive at political and economic levels. The lessons it teaches are those which every crisis teaches; that clear, consistent and confident decisions and communications are vital to any crisis response. It was these lessons that were patently not learned when facing the COVID-19 pandemic.

References

Alonso-Zaldivar, R. (2020). 'Trump vs Fauci: President's gut sense collides with science.' *Associated Press*, March 20. https://apnews.com/432a37435f28015e8b45eeff710cd254

Baker, P. (2020). 'Trump says "People Have to Remain Calm" amid Coronavirus outbreak.' *The New York Times*, March 6. www.nytimes.com/2020/03/06/us/polit ics/trump-coronavirus-cdc.html

Boboltz, S. (2020). 'CDC urges Americans to prepare for Coronavirus spread.' *Huffington Post*, February 26. www.huffpost.com/entry/cdc-warns-americans-coronavirus-spread_n_5e556b10c5b63b9c9ce47a7c.

Duster, C. (2020). 'Trump administration's "Operation Warp Speed" identifies 14 vaccines to focus on.' *CNN*, May 4. www.cnn.com/2020/05/04/politics/operation -warp-speed-coronavirus-vaccines/index.html.

Dwyer, C. (2020). 'CDC now recommends Americans consider wearing cloth face coverings in public.' *National Public Radio*, April 3. www.npr.org/sections/coro navirus-live-updates/2020/04/03/826219824/president-trump-says-cdc-now-reco mmends-americans-wear-cloth-masks-in-public.

Dzhanova, Y. (2020). 'Trump invoked the defense production act. Here's how he can use its powers.' *CNBC*, March 20. www.cnbc.com/2020/03/20/trump-invoked-the-def ense-production-act-heres-how-he-can-use-its-powers.html.

Hannity, S. (2020). 'Interview with President Trump.' *Fox News*, February 2.

Lemire, J. (2020). 'Trump says coronavirus "very well under control" in US.' *ABC News*, February 25. https://abcnews.go.com/Business/wireStory/trump-coronavirus-contr ol-us-69201209.

Leonardi (2020). '"Beautiful thing": Trump hopes to see "packed churches" on Easter Sunday.' *The Washington Examiner*, March 24. www.washingtonexaminer.com/news/ beautiful-thing-trump-hopes-to-see-packed-churches-on-easter-sunday.

Reints, R. (2020). 'People are becoming increasingly skeptical of science, report finds.' *Fortune*, March 20. https://fortune.com/2019/03/20/state-of-science-report/

SEC (2020). 'SEC provides conditional regulatory relief and assistance for companies affected by the Coronavirus Disease 2019 (COVID-19).' *U.S. Securities and Exchange Commission*, March 4. www.sec.gov/news/press-release/2020-53.

Smith, A. (2020). 'Trump extends social distancing guidelines to April 30, predicts "great things" by June 1.' *NBC News*, March 29. www.nbcnews.com/politics/donal d-trump/trump-extends-social-distancing-guidelines-april-30-predicts-great-thing s-n1171536.

Trump, D. (2020a). 'Trump speaks in Davos, addresses the world economic forum.' *Fox News*, January 26. www.foxnews.com/politics/trump-speaks-in-davos-addresses-the -world-economic-forum-live-blog.

Trump, D. (2020b). 'Remarks by President Trump at a USMCA celebration with American workers | Warren, MI.' *www.whitehouse.gov*, January 30. www.whitehouse. gov/briefings-statements/remarks-president-trump-usmca-celebration-american -workers-warren-mi/.

Trump, D. (2020c). *Remarks to the Media*. February 29. www.whitehouse.gov/briefings -statements/remarks-president-trump-vice-president-pence-members-coronavirus- task-force-press-conference-2/.

Trump, D. (2020d). *Remarks by President Trump in Address to the Nation*. March 11. www.w hitehouse.gov/briefings-statements/remarks-president-trump-address-nation/.

Trump, D. (2020e). *Remarks by President Trump After Meeting with Republican Senators*. March 10. www.whitehouse.gov/briefings-statements/remarks-president-trump-m eeting-republican-senators-2/.

6

THE EU

The story of a tragic hero and the 27 dwarfs

Dennis Lichtenstein

Political context

Within the institutional framework of the European Union (EU), the European Commission (EC) shares its executive power with the heads of states and governments in the European Council (EUCO). Both institutions have had new leaders since December 2019 – the German conservative Ursula von der Leyen (EC) and the Belgian liberal Charles Michel (EUCO). Since von der Leyen's presidency was the result of technocratic negotiations in the EUCO, her selection was highly contested in the European Parliament (EP), as well as in the media.

For von der Leyen, the COVID-19 crisis was an early and, perhaps, term-defining test. While her attempts to balance emancipation from, and cooperation with, the EUCO have been carefully observed, the EC's role in crisis management is generally challenging. Although the EC has developed crisis management capacity in the last few decades, it operates within 'a system under construction' (Larsson et al., 2009: 6). The EC's role has been described as a mediator or consensus builder that must deal with 'an unclear division of competences between the national and European levels' (Boin et al., 2013: 3). Its main tasks are to enable close cooperation between member states, coordinate their contributions and add value to existing national capacities without taking over and encroaching on national sensibilities.

Strong and successful European crisis management became a pressing task early in 2020 as COVID-19 hit the EU during a general legitimation crisis resulting from internal struggles during the euro and migration crises, Brexit and the emergence of authoritarian tendencies in Hungary and Poland (Dinan et al., 2017). In autumn 2019, no more than 42% of EU citizens had a positive view of the EU, with significant differences between the member states (European Commission, 2019).

DOI: 10.4324/9781003120254-8

Chronology

The first case of COVID-19 in an EU country was announced on January 24, 2020 in France. Since then, the virus has spread rapidly between and within the member states. By early September, more than 2.2 million infections, and more than 181,000 deaths, have been reported in the EU and the United Kingdom (ECDC, 2020). The number of infections varied between the member states, and national governments reacted at different speeds and with varying strategies (see the case study chapters). While EU institutions failed to provide an early and coherent strategy for crisis management, EU countries unilaterally closed their borders within the Schengen area and initially banned exports of protective equipment, refusing to show solidarity with other member states (Paun & Deutsch, 2020).

The EC's crisis management approach was implemented in January and February 2020 with efforts to support the member states, in line with the EC's legal competences and use of established instruments. On January 9, the EC's Directorate-General for Health and Safety activated its Early Warning and Response System to enable the member states to share information on infections and crisis management measures.[1] The EC also used the EU Civil Protection Mechanism to assist member states with the repatriation of their citizens from abroad. Other major initiatives were to combine forces for procuring medical equipment on the global market and rapid support for research on the COVID-19 virus. In line with the EC's competences in foreign policy and emergency services, it offered support for China and announced a 232-million-euro aid package for global preparedness for the virus (European Commission, 2020b).

The EC's activities increased after being provided, on March 6, with a mandate by the EUCO to take further steps to respond to the COVID-19 crisis. Von der Leyen's coronavirus response team consisted of the EU commissioners for the key issues of health, borders, mobility and macroeconomy. Major efforts in the EC's crisis management strategy concerned medical research, support for national health systems, the stabilisation of the European market and national economies, and global cooperation to contain the virus. For financing large parts of their crisis management activities, the EC made 40 billion euros available from the European Investment Bank.

With regard to medical research, the EU invested 80 million euros to support the German vaccine developer CureVac (March 16) and another 48.5 million euros, from the Horizon2020 programme, in research teams (March 31). It also established a platform for scientific exchange and created a strategic RescEU stock for medical equipment (March 19, 457 million euros). While duties on medical devices and protective equipment from third countries were suspended (April 3), the EC enabled the member states to access the European Stability Mechanism (ESM), provided the funds are used for health purposes (April 9). Further investments aimed to support the national health systems, with 2.7 million euros from the EU Emergency Support Instrument (April 14) and 10 million euros for masks for health workers in 17 member states (May 8). Starting on May 4, the EU participated in the international donor marathon, within the so-called Global Response Strategy, by contributing 1.4 billion euros to fund the joint development and global delivery of coronavirus diagnostics, treatments and a vaccine (May 12). Efforts to establish guidelines for mobile data apps to fight the pandemic have, so far, not resulted in the development of a European app or common standards for national apps.

Further major efforts followed the goal to stabilise the member states' economies and develop an economic recovery strategy. Through the suspension of the eurozone's Stability and Growth Pact, EC and EU finance ministers allowed for higher national public deficits, which increased the flexibility of national finance policies (March 23). This was supplemented by the European Central Bank (ECB), which announced a 750-billion-euro bond purchase programme to avoid speculation against highly indebted countries (March 18) and extended the programme with another 600 billion euros on June 4. Moreover, the EC offered a one billion euro guarantee for credits for small and medium-sized companies (April 6) and a banking package to facilitate lending (April 28). The EC also initiated the SURE programme, with a 100-billion-euro loan guarantee to support short-time work in the member states. To promote economic recovery, a German-French initiative proposed a 500 billion euro fund for making non-repayable grants available to EU countries (May 18). To finance the fund, the EU will be allowed to take on debt, which can be seen as a step towards closer economic integration. Von der Leyen extended this plan with an additional 250 billion euros for credit, calling the 750-billion-euro fund Next Generation EU (May 27). After intense negotiations, the Next Generation EU plan gained acceptance in the EUCO even though the amount of grants was cut down to 390 billion euro (Herszenhorn et al., 2020a).

During the response to the crisis, both medical and economic help were strongly related to the EU internal market. On March 16, the EC provided rules for border management to ensure the free movement of goods and critical workers, despite the closure of borders, and to facilitate cross-border treatment of patients and deployment of medical staff. The EU introduced green lanes to ensure the flow of goods (March 23). It provided road maps for a coordinated reopening, including the lifting of travel restrictions, which was practised in June. Crisis management also focused on customer and passenger rights, support for the agri-food sector, and humanitarian aid. At the end of March, the EU announced a 40-billion-euro aid package for Syrian refugees and vulnerable groups in Iraq, Jordan and Lebanon (European Commission, 2020b).

Analysis

Throughout the COVID-19 crisis, the EU has been confronted with high expectations for a strong and solidary approach to EU crisis management (Hüther et al., 2020; Maas & Scholz, 2020). The EC's ability and freedom to act, however, depends on the nation states' engagement, their willingness to cooperate and their ability to find compromises (Hammargård & Olsson, 2019). This forces the EC to balance leadership with negotiations outside the limelight and it must be considered as one reason why, during the initial months of the COVID-19 crisis, the EC failed to provide an early, strong and coherent crisis response. Instead, it gave the impression of being unprepared and underestimating the situation. Relying on experts from the Platform for European Preparedness Against Emerging Epidemics, at the end of January the EU health commissioner, Stella Kyriakides, saw only a moderate threat and gave assurances that the EU would be ready to meet the virus outbreak (Foote, 2020). At the same time, the EC president did not mention the virus in her speech on the EU's role in the world at the World Economic Forum in Davos.

The EC was reserved in public communication, even after the number of infections increased, national governments closed their borders and export bans resulted in confrontations between the member states. In consequence, the EC faced strong criticism, in particular from the EU's most seriously affected countries, such as Italy. In light of the initially uncoordinated and nation-based approach to crisis management, national leaders from France, Spain and Italy – all countries with high numbers of COVID-19 cases, intense economic problems and societal tensions – highlighted the danger of populism and Euroscepticism spreading in their populations. They called the crisis a 'moment of truth' (Macron, 2020), 'the most difficult moment for the EU since its foundation' (Sanchez, 2020), and the possible 'end of Europe' (Conte, 2020). As the magazine *Politico* concluded, the EC's silence reflected the dominance of national competences in health policy and demonstrated the EU had 'relatively limited power during public health emergencies' (Herszenhorn et al., 2020b).

The EC's communication increased and gained coherence after it had received a mandate from the EUCO and established the coronavirus response team in March 2020. Using public statements, such as speeches, op-eds in European newspapers, the EC's website and social media platforms, as the main instruments of communication, the EC deployed two main frames known from political crisis communication literature (e.g., Coombs, 2020; Nord & Olsson, 2013). The EC attempted to encourage solidarity and cooperation between member states and constructed the crisis as a chance for the modernisation of the EU (renewal and hope frame). Providing information on the EU's crisis management actions and its costs, the EC used a managerial frame. This frame emphasised leadership and legitimised the EC's role and policies in crisis management. The EC's crisis communication was supported by the EP and the ECB, whereas different national interests in the EUCO diminished its message consistency.

Following the goal to encourage solidarity and cooperation, von der Leyen openly addressed deficits in the EU's early approach to crisis management and was engaged in restoring its public image. She condemned the unilateral closure of borders and the refusal to show solidarity considering the lack of medical supplies and equipment. As she put it: 'When Europe really needed to be there for each other, too many initially looked out for themselves. When Europe really needed an "all for one" spirit, too many initially gave an "only for me" response' (von der Leyen, 2020b). This criticism of national governments was combined with apologies directed at EU citizens, empathy with their sorrows and worries and a praising of citizens' solidarity. Promising that the EU would bring its citizens through the crisis, von der Leyen encouraged them 'to stand up for Europe' (von der Leyen, 2020d) and called for unity. She also frequently praised cooperation between the member states in public statements and emphasised the need for close cooperation (e.g. European Commission, 2020a). Von der Leyen (2020b) warned national governments not to weaken fundamental rights and democratic values in their management of the crisis but carefully avoided blaming individual governments. Western EU countries' governments, on the other hand, openly criticised emergency legislation in Hungary and Poland and demanded the exclusion of the Hungarian Fidesz party from the European People's Party in the EP.

Motivational appeals for solidarity and unity culminated in the promise of modernisation of the EU. Von der Leyen framed the COVID-19 crisis as a historic moment that requires responsible and courageous behaviour and entails major opportunities for the EU. She created the notion of a strong democratic 'new Europe' in a new world, in which politics and the principles of globalisation will change, and politics and societies will overcome old divisions and disputes (von der Leyen, 2020c). In doing so, she stressed that the COVID-19 crisis offers an opportunity for the development of a more resilient, green and digital Europe. In a speech at the EP, she concluded, 'I know that tomorrow Europe's soul will shine brighter than ever before' (von der Leyen, 2020d). This hope and renewal frame was, however, not grounded by policy plans or a roadmap for its realisation. On social media, the EC and EP contributed to her messages with motivational campaigns that also emphasised solidarity and unity (#StrongerTogether, #UnitedAgainstCoronavirus and #EuropeansAgainstCovid19). Social media campaigns gave voice to citizens and civil society as well as to medical doctors, EU politicians and representatives from companies. In addition to showing empathy and awareness for societal problems, the social media campaigns provided legal information about consumer rights and gave citizens hygiene guidance and lifestyle tips for social distancing. EU politicians acted as role models in practising solidarity and hygienic measures.

The EC's commitment to motivate citizens to support the EU was accompanied by strong attempts to legitimise its role and policy development during crisis management by deploying a managerial frame. While the EC regularly described its role as a consultant or coordinator and its measures as an add-on to national crisis management, in its online communication it provided a constant flow of information about, and words of praise for, EU measures. In addition, the EC used the crisis to promote its main projects, the Green Deal and digitalisation. With its visions for the future of Europe, the EC claimed a leading role in the management of the crisis and contributed to its image as an innovator in the development of the EU. For this purpose, the EC's framing of the COVID-19 crisis stressed problems and solutions that are within the EU's competences.

In the EC's framing, the COVID-19 crisis is a European economic crisis first and a global health crisis second. Framing the crisis as a 'global challenge' resulted in calls for 'massive and coordinated global action' (von der Leyen & Michel, 2020) from the entire international community, in which the EU represents its member states' interests. In addition, framing the crisis as a 'European economic crisis' stressed the EU's main competence in economic policy and its role as a protective power for the common market and its financial stability. On its website and social media, the EC regularly conveyed information about investments aimed at supporting member states' economies. Public statements, for instance from the EC vice-president, Margrethe Vestager (2020), emphasised the value of the internal market as a key instrument in crisis management.

Von der Leyen (2020a), demonstrating leadership, gave the strong promise that there would be no half-measures and 'we are ready to do everything that is required.' Her position was in line with the President of the ECB's bond purchase programme that – inspired by Mario Draghi's famous statement during the euro crisis – was interpreted as Christine Lagarde's 'whatever it takes moment' and welcomed by southern EU countries' leaders (Sciorilli Borrelli, 2020). Strong leadership was also demonstrated by calling EU investment a Marshall Plan for Europe and the EU budget, which was used for investment, the 'mothership of our recovery' (von der Leyen, 2020d). Highlighting its leading role in the management of the economic crisis, the EC also called on the member states to provide a future EU budget that has firepower and can generate the necessary investment (von der Leyen, 2020c). These efforts were complemented on social media with strategies to generate trust in economic and health-related EU measures (#EUTakeTheInitiative and #GlobalResponse) and express demands for a Green Deal, coordinated action and a large EU budget.

The EC's ability to act as an economic crisis manager was limited by national competences in finance policy and budget decisions. In the EUCO, national interests and disagreements concerning the financing of the EU recovery strategy also prevailed (Herszenhorn et al., 2020a). The call by nine southern EU governments for Coronabonds, in a joint letter to the EUCO president, Charles Michel, (Wilmès et al., 2020) was openly rejected by Germany and the so-called frugal four, Austria, Sweden, Denmark and the Netherlands (later joined by Finland), who claimed financial aid from the ESM. The proposed Next Generation EU fund divided member states in the EUCO since the issue has reawakened fundamental conflicts on EU finance policy and the deepening of economic integration. In this struggle, the EC received support from the ECB and members of the EP, who criticised the EC's lack of executive and budgetary power and called for a strengthening of its capacity to act (Panetta, 2020). However, during this time of dispute, the German Federal Constitutional Court judged that, with its bond purchase programme during the euro crisis, the ECB had exceeded its competences. Even though the court declared that the decision 'does not concern any financial assistance measures taken by the EU or the ECB in the context of the current coronavirus crisis' (The Federal Constitutional Court, 2020), it was used as an argument against the EC's economic policy in public debates. In contrast to this, the German president of parliament Wolfgang Schäuble (2020) called for using the crisis to push for EU economic union.

Conclusion

The EU's response to the COVID-19 crisis aimed to motivate citizens and member states for unity and emphasised its efforts for a strong and determined crisis management. While the EU and the EP engaged in extensive online communication, the EU's role in the COVID-19 crisis was discussed critically in the media of the member states. This was not only due to the EC's weak leadership at the beginning of the crisis but also due to media attention directed at national leaders highlighting their disunity. The EU, thus, failed to exploit the pandemic to overcome its legitimation crisis. Any changes during the economic recovery period that follows will depend on unity and cooperation in the EUCO. Polls indicate that most EU citizens (57%) were not satisfied with the solidarity between member states or EU crisis interventions (52%). The majority of EU citizens, however, noticed the EU crisis management (74%) and is supportive of a bigger budget for the EU to overcome the pandemic (56%) and for more competences for the EU to deal with future crises (68%) (European Parliament, 2020). Regarding the EC's crisis management capacities, the COVID-19 crisis and the acceptance of von der Leyen's Next Generation EU recovery plan resulted in an extension of the EC's fiscal competences.

Note

1 All measures in EU crisis management are documented on the EC's websites (European Commission, 2020b).

References

Boin, A., Ekengren, M., & Rhinard, M. (2013). *The European Union as Crisis Manager. Patterns and Prospects.* Cambridge University Press.

Conte (2020). Italy's Conte Warns of EU Collapse Ahead of Crucial Financial Talks. *Politico*, Brussels, 9 April. www.politico.eu/article/italys-conte-warns-of-eu-collapse-ahead-crucial-financial-talks-coronavirus/

Coombs, W. T. (2020). Political Public Relations and Crisis Communication. A Public Relations Perspective. In J. Strömbäck & S. Kiousis (Eds.), *Political Public Relations. Concepts, Principles, and Applications.* Routledge.

Dinan, D., Nugent, N., & Paterson, W. E. (Eds.). (2017). *The European Union in Crisis.* Macmillan Education.

ECDC (2020). COVID-19 Situation Update for the EU/EEA and the UK. www.ecdc.e uropa.eu/en/cases-2019-ncov-eueea

European Commission (2019). Standard Eurobarometer 92 – Autumn 2019. Public Opinion in the European Union, First Results. https://ec.europa.eu/commfrontoffic e/publicopinion/

European Commission (2020a). Coronavirus: Commission Statement on Consulting Member States on the Proposal to Extend State Aid Temporary Framework. Brussels, 27 March. https://ec.europa.eu/commission/presscorner/detail/en/STATEMENT _20_551

European Commission (2020b). Timeline of EU Action. https://ec.europa.eu/info/live -work-travel-eu/health/coronavirus-response/timeline-eu-action_en

European Parliament (2020). Uncertainty, EU, Hope. Public Opinion in Times of COVID-19. Brussels. www.europarl.europa.eu/at-your-service/files/be-heard/e urobarometer/2020/public_opinion_in_the_eu_in_time_of_coronavirus_crisis/re port/en-covid19-survey-report.pdf

Foote, N. (2020). EU 'Well Prepared' to Deal with Coronavirus, Says Health Expert. *EURACTIV.com*, Brussels, 24 January. www.euractiv.com/section/health-consumer s/news/eu-well-prepared-to-deal-with-coronavirus-says-health-expert/

Hammargård, K., & Olsson, E.-K. (2019). Explaining the European Commission's Strategies in Times of Crisis. *Cambridge Review of International Affairs*, *32*(2), 159–177. https://doi.org/10.1080/09557571.2019.1577800

Herszenhorn, D. M., Bayer, L., & Momtaz, R. (2020a). Takeaways from the EU Budget and Recovery Deal. *Politico*, Brussels, 7 July. www.politico.eu/article/5-takeaways -from-the-eu-budget-mff-and-recovery-deal-coronavirus/

Herszenhorn, D. M., Paun, C., & Deutsch, J. (2020b). Europe Fails to Help Italy in Coronavirus Fight. *Politico*, Brussels, 5 March. www.politico.eu/article/eu-aims-bet ter-control-coronavirus-responses/

Hüther, M., Bofinger, P., Dullien, S., Felbermayr, G., Schularick, M., Südekum, J., & Trebesch, C. (2020). Europe Must Demonstrate Financial Solidarity. Op-ed in Newstatesman and Other. *EUROPA Medica*, 30 March. www.iwkoeln.de/en/press/ gastbeitraege/beitrag/michael-huether-europe-must-demonstrate-financial-solidarit y.html

Larsson, P., Hagström Friesel, E., & Olsson, S. (2009). Understanding the Crisis Management System of the European Union. In S. Olsson (Ed.), *Crisis Management in the European Union. Cooperation in the Face of Emergencies* (pp. 1–16). Springer.

Maas, H., & Scholz, O. (2020). A Response to the Corona Crisis in Europe Based on Solidarity. *Op-ed in Les Echos (France), La Stampa (Italy), El País (Spain), Público (Portugal) and Ta Nea (Greece)*, 4 April. www.auswaertiges-amt.de/en/newsroom/ news/maas-scholz-corona/2330904

Macron, E. (2020). Transcript: 'We Are at a Moment of Truth.' *Financial Times*, London, 17 April. www.ft.com/content/317b4f61-672e-4c4b-b816-71e0ff63cab2

Nord, L. W., & Olsson, E.-K. (2013). Frame, Set, Match! Towards a Model of Successful Crisis Rhetoric. *Public Relations Inquiry*, *2*(1), 79–94. https://doi.org/10.1177 /2046147X12464205

Panetta, F. (2020). Joint Response to Coronavirus Crisis Will Benefit All EU Countries. *Politico*, Brussels, 21 April. www.politico.eu/article/joint-response-coronavirus-crisis -benefit-all-eu-countries/

Paun, C., & Deutsch, J. (2020). Health Ministers Squabble Over Face Masks at Coronavirus Talks. *Politico*, Brussels, 7 March. www.politico.eu/article/health-mini sters-squabble-over-face-masks-at-coronavirus-talks/

Sanchez, P. (2020). Spain Calls for Action from Europe as Daily Death Toll Rises Again. *The Guardian*, London, 26 March. www.theguardian.com/world/2020/mar/29/sp ain-poised-to-tighten-coronavirus-lockdown-after-record-daily-toll

Schäuble, W. (2020). Die Zukunft Europas. Aus Eigener Stärke [The Future of Europa. Through Our Own Strength]. *Frankfurter Allgemeine Zeitung*, Frankfurt a.M., 5 July. www.faz.net/aktuell/politik/inland/gastbeitrag-wolfgang-schaeuble-aus-eigener-st aerke-16846887.html?GEPC=s3&premium=0x7be8371ad4a8e50d67660d00e3e86c 61#void

Sciorilli Borrelli, S. (2020). ECB Rises to Expectations with Massive Bond-Buying Move. *Politico*, Brussels, 19 March. www.politico.eu/article/the-ecb-rises-up-to-e xpectations-launches-massive-bond-buying-program/

The Federal Constitutional Court (2020). ECB Decisions on the Public Sector Purchase Programme Exceed EU Competences. *Press Release 32/2020*, Brussels, 5 May. www.b undesverfassungsgericht.de/SharedDocs/Pressemitteilungen/EN/2020/bvg20-032. html

Vestager, M. (2020). Statement by Executive Vice-President Margrethe Vestager on State Aid Measures to Address the Economic Impact of COVID-19. Brussels, 13 March. https://ec.europa.eu/commission/presscorner/detail/de/STATEMENT_20_467

Von der Leyen, U. (2020a). Statement by President von der Leyen at the Joint Press Conference with President Michel, Following the EU Leaders' Videoconference on COVID-19. Brussels, 17 March. https://ec.europa.eu/commission/presscorner/detail /en/STATEMENT_20_483

Von der Leyen, U. (2020b). Statement by President von der Leyen on Emergency Measures in Member States. Brussels, 31 March. https://ec.europa.eu/commission/ presscorner/detail/en/statement_20_567

Von der Leyen, U. (2020c). Speech by President von der Leyen at the European Parliament Plenary on the European Coordinated Response to the COVID-19 Outbreak. Brussels, 26 March. https://ec.europa.eu/commission/presscorner/detail /en/SPEECH_20_532

Von der Leyen, U. (2020d). Speech by President von der Leyen at the European Parliament Plenary on the EU Coordinated Action to Combat the Coronavirus Pandemic and its Consequences. Brussels, 16 April. https://ec.europa.eu/cyprus/ne ws/20200416_1_en

Von der Leyen, U., & Michel, C. (2020). Joint Statement by President von der Leyen and President Michel Following the G20 Leaders' Videoconference. Brussels, 26 March. https://ec.europa.eu/commission/presscorner/detail/en/STATEMENT_20_537

Wilmès, S., Macron, E., Mitsotakis, K., Varadkar, L., Conte, G., Bettel, X., Costa, A., Janša, J., & Sánchez, P. (2020, 25 March). Joint Letter of 9 European Leaders to Charles Michel. www.governo.it/sites/new.governo.it/files/letter_michel_2020 0325_eng.pdf

7

FRANCE

An unpopular government facing an unprecedented crisis

Pierre-Emmanuel Guigo

Political context

When the pandemic hit France, the country was in the middle of municipal elections planned for March 15 and 22. French president Emmanuel Macron, a centrist, elected in 2017 and his government, led by the centre-right Edouard Philippe, were already weakened by their unpopularity. One year before, the government faced protests from a social movement called the 'yellow vests' for several months. In December and January 2019–2020, the longest strikes in French history challenged retirement reforms initiated by the President. Hence, these municipal elections were a crucial electoral deadline, the first after the 2017 presidential election, and just two years before the next presidential race. That explains why government concerns regarding COVID-19 were raised late. On January 21, Agnès Buzyn, the Health Minister, declared the risks of propagation of the virus in the population 'weak.' On February 16, she resigned just one month before the lockdown, to be replaced as LREM (the President's party) candidate for the Parisian council by the former candidate, Benjamin Griveaux, who had been discredited when intimate videos surfaced online.[1]

Chronology

See Table 7.1.

Analysis

When President Macron announced the closure of all schools and universities on Thursday March 12, the French population was largely flabbergasted. Four days later, the lockdown was enlarged to the whole population. In the midst of

DOI: 10.4324/9781003120254-9

TABLE 7.1 France chronology

Date		Diffusion of the COVID-19	Key official actions	Key communication events
January	21			Health Minister Agnès Buzyn declares that the risk of propagation of the virus is 'weak.'
	24	First cases in France.		
	31		Beginning of the French citizens repatriation.	
February	1		France is the last country of the Schengen space to maintain connections with China.	
	8	Five new cases in High Savoy. The border with Italy remains open.		
	14	Death of the first patient in France.		
	16			The Health Minister Agnès Buzyn resigns to become candidate for mayor of Paris.
	17–21	Large evangelical meeting in Mulhouse, half the participants become infected which rapidly spreads across the territory.		
	23		French government launches epidemic plan.	

(Continued)

TABLE 7.1 (Continued)

Date		Diffusion of the COVID-19	Key official actions	Key communication events
	26	Death of the first French victim.		
	27	New cluster of cases in the Oise department, where repatriated citizens landed earlier.		
	29	More than 100 new cases detected.		
March	4			The government spokesperson declares schools won't be closed, 'we cannot stop life in France.'
	5	3 more deaths.		
	6			The President goes to a theatre representation and declares, 'Life goes on.'
	9		Gatherings of 1,000+ persons are banned.	
	12		All schools and universities to close. Homeworking is promoted and exceptional measures of partial unemployment taken. Maintenance of the municipal elections.	First TV speech of the President since the beginning of the crisis. He declares that coronavirus is 'the most serious health crisis France has experienced in a century.'
	14	4,500 people infected, 91 deaths.	Prime Minister declares that all 'non-essential' public spaces to close at midnight.	

15		First round of municipal elections. 21 million voters go to the polls. But 55% of electors have decided to abstain.	
16	6,000+ cases confirmed and 150 deaths.	All borders close, unnecessary travel banned. Second round of municipal elections postponed. Masks are reserved for health personnel.	At 8 pm, the President makes a new TV address. He repeats 6 times 'we are at war.' The lockdown announced to be from noon the next day.
17		One million people leave the Parisian region. At noon, the lockdown starts.	French population spontaneously starts to applaud every 8 pm for the medical professions.
18	More than 9,000 cases and 200 deaths.		The Minister of Economy declares 'all employees whose businesses are still open must continue to go there.'
19			600 doctors file a complaint against former Health Minister Agnès Buzyn and Prime Minister Edouard Philippe for negligence and state lies.
22	16,000 cases and 674 deaths.	State of emergency becomes law. Government can take all necessary measures without the Parliament authorisation.	

(Continued)

TABLE 7.1 (Continued)

Date		Diffusion of the COVID-19	Key official actions	Key communication events
	24	More than 1,000 deaths.		
	25			The government spokesperson declares masks are not necessary for ordinary citizens.
	27		PM extends lockdown until April 15.	
	30	3,000+ deaths; 20,000+ hospitalised.		
April	6	For the first time, deaths in retirement homes are taken into account adding 2,400 to the total.		
	7	More than 10,000 deaths recorded.		
	13	20,000 deaths in France.	The lockdown is extended until May 11.	New TV address by the President.
	20	More than 23,000 deaths.		
	28		The Prime Minister announces that the end of the lockdown will be adapted to each department. Until the beginning of June, all travel of more than 100 km is forbidden.	

May	5	More than 25,000 deaths.
	11	Lockdown lifting ('deconfinement') starts in France. Green and red zones are set up. In the red zone for Paris, suburbs and the northern part of the country, parks and beaches remain closed. All travel over 100 km remains forbidden until June.
June	2	Shops and restaurants can reopen in the green zone. All travel permitted without restrictions. The second round of municipal elections is organised for the June 28.
	22	Shops, restaurants and bars can reopen in the whole country.
	28	Major defeat for presidential party at the municipal elections. But Prime Minister Edouard Philippe is reelected Mayor of Le Havre. Agnès Buzyn obtains only 13% of the votes in Paris.

municipal elections, with an unpopular government, COVID-19 had been a minimal consideration until Macron's speech.

In this chapter, we will see how the government reacted to the crisis. Then we will focus on the obsessive media coverage and then we will study the 'rally round the flag effect' initiated by the President. This study will analyse the television appearances made by the President, the Prime Minister, the Health Minister, the General Health Director and the government spokesperson. The media coverage of the crisis is analysed using the data base of the National Audiovisual Institute.

An unexpected crisis

When the novel coronavirus was identified in China at the end of December, all French political parties were concentrated on preparation for the municipal elections planned for March 15 and 22. The resignation of Health Minister Agnès Buzyn to become candidate for mayor of Paris shows the low attention paid by political elites to the impending crisis. The new Health Minister, Olivier Véran, made multiple reassuring interventions, explaining several times that the French Health System was ready to deal with the virus and downplaying the danger, considering coronavirus as a 'simple flu,' countering the alarm calls of doctors and specialists. One week before the lockdown, to reassure the population, the President visited a theatre and declared 'life goes on.' When the spread of the virus reached 4,000 after March 9, Macron finally made the declaration on March 12 announcing the closure of all schools and universities, but insisted the first round of the municipal elections would go ahead the next Sunday. Two days later, the Prime Minister (PM) extended the closure to all unnecessary public spaces, but municipal elections were still scheduled. Finally, on March 16, the President explained all unnecessary travels would be forbidden for two weeks from the next morning, without using the word 'confinement' (lockdown). This left the public response open to interpretation.

The government seemed surprised by the crisis. Even the alarm calls from Italian doctors and journalists did not elicit a reaction. Moreover, the restriction measures seemed contradictory, with the government deciding to close public spaces but not cancelling municipal elections, despite requests from the medical profession. Confusion was exacerbated by contradictions between the President's statements and the statements by the government. From March 12, the President's speeches aimed at uniting and reassuring the population, but without explaining any concrete measures. These presidential announcements often had to be completed by the Prime Minister in a subsequent television speech or the Security Minister's declarations giving details of the closures, lockdown and travel restrictions. This distribution of tasks continued in the period of lockdown. On April 13, Emmanuel Macron gave a television address announcing the end of the lockdown on May 11, without explaining how. Two weeks later, the Prime Minister, during a speech at the Assembly, gave the concrete details of the lifting of lockdown ('deconfinement'), how it would differ within each region and which travel restrictions would remain in place. Even inside the government, completely different messages were communicated. While the Prime Minister, the Health Minister and the Security Minister advocated for a strict respect of lockdown, the Minister of Economy and the Minister of Agriculture argued for continued economic activity. The spokesperson, Sibeth N'diaye, who was responsible for explaining and justifying government policy, in fact made several mistakes. She stigmatised professors 'who are not working' despite the pedagogical continuity launched by the Education ministry using digital platforms. And then she explained that masks are not necessary, because French people 'don't know how to use them properly.' At the same time, all medical experts urged the government to order masks, which were in short supply, and the World Health Organisation reminded of the necessity to wear masks to prevent the spread of the virus. The communication by government was also questioned by former Health Minister Agnès Buzyn, who declared on March 17 in the newspaper *Le Monde* that she urged the Prime Minister and President to take necessary measures at the end of January and to cancel municipal elections. Just after these revelations, 600 doctors filed a complaint against the government. The confusion in the government positions and contradictory declarations encouraged a general distrust which was reinforced by media coverage. According to the IFOP barometer for the *Journal du dimanche* (Sunday newspaper) 55% of the population trusted the government to face the crisis on March 20. By April 2, trust had fallen to 47%, and fell again to 38% one week later.

Obsessive media coverage

The crisis generated unprecedented media coverage from the television and press. As with the political reaction, we see the same pattern of delayed focus. French media are largely nation-focused, hence the first peak of coverage happened on January 24 when the first two cases were declared on the French territory.

According to *La revue des médias* (the magazine published by the Audiovisual National Institute), coverage exploded after the death of the first French COVID-19 victim on February 26, coverage that also covered the lockdown measures taken by the Italian government. From that moment, more than 50% of the airtime of news channels was dedicated to the COVID-19 crisis. The 24h television news channels dedicated almost all its programmes to COVID-19: 75% between March 16–22 (Bayet & Hervé, 2020a). The audience of the main television channels, particularly during the 8 pm news, exploded with 15 or 20 million viewers, rather than the 4–5 million in ordinary times. Average time spent in front of the television by the French people increased from 3.29 hours to 4.41 hours per day. The television audience increased particularly among the teenagers and young adults (15–24 years old): +65%.[2]

Press analyses confirms this tendency. The number of mentions exploded at the beginning of March, with unprecedented press coverage according to a Tagaday study. Each day 19,000 articles were dedicated to the coronavirus from

March 17. This is more than three times more than for the preceding national crisis: the yellow vest protests (6,000 mentions). And twice the coverage for the election of Emmanuel Macron in 2017.[3]

The news channels and online media were certainly those focusing the most on the crisis. With this focus on COVID-19, even the first round of the municipal elections went unnoticed. The media coverage can be split into three periods. The first days of the crisis to the beginning of the lockdown saw journalists remaining descriptive about the rise of infections, the number of deaths and the measures taken by the government. Some days after the start of the lockdown (particularly from March 19), criticism of government from the medical profession became increasingly prominent in press and television reports. With the end of the lockdown (May 11), media returned to a descriptive style, explaining and commenting on the technical measures taken by the Prime Minister to reopen shops and public spaces.

Social networks saw significant public solidarity emerging in the face of the virus (retail of masks and visors) and support for the medical profession. After social media users called on others to applaud the medical profession at 8 pm, the meeting became viral each day in the whole country for several weeks.

Traditional channels (TF1, France 2, France 3, M6) adapted some entertainment programmes (television series, films and shows) to the crisis. They also created new televised programmes; for instance, France 2 broadcast classic movies (mainly French comedies of the 1960s and 1970s with Louis de Funès) each afternoon from the first week of lockdown in order to entertain people, with great audience success. But, like news channels, they gave more importance to news and current affairs. The 8 pm television news broadcasts were extended (almost an hour instead of 30 minutes), and the morning programmes were dedicated to debates and interviews regarding COVID-19. These programmes, in particular, mainly focused on polemics by doctors and other medical professionals attacking the government's actions.

The big winners of the focus on COVID-19 were doctors and medical experts, who were interviewed perpetually on television channels. Some of them were employed full time to participate in debates and to answer questions (by Twitter or phone) of citizens on the virus and the situation (Gerald Kierzek on TF1, the main French television channel, Damien Mascret on France 2 and Brigitte Milhau on CNEWS). They were not chosen for their competence in virology (for instance, Damien Mascret is a sexologist), but because they were used to being on television giving medical advice.

An infatuation emerged around the personality of one infections specialist, Professor Raoult and his treatment: hydroxychloroquine. Director of the medical centre of Marseille, he suggested in January the use of this cheap medicine in online videos which gained a huge audience (7 million views). Television journalists remained sceptical and gave minimal coverage to his work; some even presented him as a charlatan. But he rapidly became a very popular figure (600,000 followers on Twitter for an account created on March 25!). According to a poll, 59% of the French people considered his treatment to be effective against the virus.[4] When Emmanuel Macron visited Marseille on April 9, he took time to meet Professor Raoult. The use or not of hydroxychloroquine became a national debate, with significant coverage by the media. The news magazine *Paris Match* dedicated three articles and a cover to Professor Raoult and on the News channel BFM-TV, hydroxychloroquine was cited 35 times per hour by the end of March (Bayet & Hervé, 2020a). Some doctors called for the authorisation of use of hydroxychloroquine, bolstered when Donald Trump revealed on May 19 that he was taking hydroxychloroquine as a preventive treatment.

This prominence of medical experts also meant criticism of the government was given significant airtime and weight. Leaders of doctors' unions were often interviewed on television and criticised the lack of preparedness of the government for the crisis and denounced the absence of protective equipment. Jean-Paul Hamon, President of the Doctors' Federation, appeared on several television channels and stated, 'the government will be held accountable.' Political scientist Guillaume Bigot went so far as to say that the government must answer for crimes against humanity. On social networks these attacks against the government were particularly viral. The anger at the government was reinforced after the government authorised large retail stores to sell masks. After the lack of masks available to medical professionals at the beginning of the crisis, several millions of masks appeared mysteriously in shops.

An upset rally round the flag

In such a crisis, public opinion usually backs the President and government. This 'rally round the flag effect' is well known (Mueller, 1970). In recent French history such a phenomenon was witnessed, benefitting François Hollande around the 2015 terrorist attacks (Guigo, 2019). Despite his unpopularity, Hollande gained 20% popularity in polls just after the attacks. At the beginning of the COVID-19 crisis, we saw the same unity behind the President. Emmanuel Macron gained around 10% in polls (8% for Odoxa, 13% for IFOP[5]).

The French President tried to appear as the State's father using war vocabulary to frame the crisis. In his second television intervention, he repeats 6 times: 'this is war.' He chose to continue visits to hospitals and ordinary citizens facing the virus. But strong criticism from the medical profession against the actions of government caused a decline in the President's popularity in May (a 7-point decrease). Polls also indicate significant distrust of the actions of the government. On the other hand, the Prime Minister benefitted from the crisis (46% approved his politics according to IFOP, May 5). More discreet and rigorous, Edouard Philippe built trust with the citizens. He appeared the only one to take the crisis seriously from the beginning. His sobriety reassured the population. Journalists highlighted more and more the conflict between the Prime Minister and the President and even a rivalry. Two years before the presidential election, Philippe was seen by some as ambitious enough to stand for the presidency himself. This seems confirmed by Philippe's resignation just after the second round of the municipal elections (July 3) and the choice for the new prime minister was a then-unknown personality, former adviser of Nicolas Sarkozy: Jean Castex.

Conclusion

As per a large part of the population, the French government was surprised by the COVID-19 crisis. It needed time to take appropriate measures and develop a clear communication strategy. The French president Emmanuel Macron tried to gather the population around the flag but failed to build trust in his actions. Criticisms by medical professionals of the government approach were widely broadcast by the media, particularly by news channels and the social networks. Only the prime minister, developing a more discrete and precise communication approach when explaining the practical measures taken for implementing and lifting lockdown seemed to nurture public trust. Appearing as a new rival for President Macron, Edouard Phillippe had to resign after the municipal elections. Thus, two years before the presidential election, the COVID-19 crisis contributed to weakening the government and reshuffled the cards for the next elections.

Notes

1 Benjamin Griveaux had to resign as candidate to become Mayor of Paris, after the diffusion on the internet of a sex tape he sent to his mistress.
2 www.mediametrie.fr/fr/le-public-et-les-medias-un-lien-renforce-pendant-le-c onfinement#:~:text=BFM%20TV%2C%20CNews%2C%20LCI%20et,info%20est %20multipli%C3%A9e%20par%20trois.
3 *Le Journal du Dimanche*, March 21, 2020.
4 IFOP for *Le Parisien*, April 5, 2020.
5 *Le Journal du Dimanche*, May 1, 2020.

References

Bayet, A., & Hervé, N. (2020a). Information à la télé et coronavirus : l'INA a mesuré le temps d'antenne historique consacré au COVID-19, *La Revue des médias*. https://la revuedesmedias.ina.fr/etude-coronavirus-covid19-temps-antenne-information

Guigo, P.-E. (2019). La communication médiatique des présidents de la république française en période d'attentats (1985–2016). *Le Temps des médias*, 32, pp. 20–37.

Mueller, J. (1970). 'Presidential popularity from Truman to Johnson. *American Political Science Review*, 64, pp. 18–34.

8

AUSTRALIA

A triumph of sorts

Fiona Wade

Political context

At the 2019 federal election, Australian politics confounded opinion polls and pundits. Victory was handed to a government that trailed in every opinion poll across the country and had lost its majority in the House of Representatives due to defections and by-election losses. The 'miracle' result (Crabb, 2019) returned the Liberal–National coalition government with a slim majority in the House and transformed Prime Minister (PM) Scott Morrison's authority within his party and the country, signalling a rebirth of a sitting prime minister and the salvation of a troubled government.[1]

Fresh from victory, Morrison's government spent the following months frittering away the public's goodwill. They lacked a discernible policy programme, were divided over climate policy and tainted by scandal over its pork-barrelling of community sport funding grants which claimed a ministerial scalp. But it was Morrison's mishandling of the summer bushfires, and his ill-timed family holiday to Hawaii, a trip his office initially denied he had taken, that raised doubts about whether his campaign skills could translate into effective governing.

In January, Newspoll[2] recorded a massive hit to Morrison's personal approval rating, with Morrison being overtaken as preferred leader by the opposition's Anthony Albanese. This trend continued in February.

However, in the new all-encompassing COVID-19 reality, by March, Morrison's approval had regained momentum, only to surge ahead in April, as he presided over a series of momentous health and economic-related responses to the pandemic.

Timing, in short, can be everything in politics.

DOI: 10.4324/9781003120254-10

Chronology

Like a leaky tap, the first COVID-19 infections began to appear, slowly, from the end of January. Over the following two weeks, cases climbed to 15. From mid-April, there was a sustained and relatively low number of new cases reported daily, with an easing of restrictions occurring from May 8. See Table 8.1.

The COVID-19 pandemic remains an evolving situation and the Australian Government's response involves a diverse range of activities and measures undertaken by a variety of Australian Public Service departments and agencies.

The enacting of the *Biosecurity Act* 2015 (Cth)[3] allows federal, state and territory governments to exercise coercive laws that potentially interfere with personal liberties, unheard of in a liberal society. Non-compliance attracts significant penalties, and limited review mechanisms are available. State and territory governments also have their own *Public Health Acts*,[4] with enforcement the responsibility of state and territory police forces. But while leaders have been consistent in calling for strict social distancing rules, commitment to enforce has differed, with ACT police taking an 'inform and educate'[5] approach, while New South Wales (NSW) calls for those contravening restrictions to be reported to Crime Stoppers.[6]

Government monitoring of the movements of an individual is an anathema to Australians and their way of life. Yet, there was tacit acceptance of the government's introduction of the COVIDSafe app. Used for 'contact tracing,' location monitoring and assessing the extent to which social distancing and mobility restrictions are being observed, the somewhat lacklustre public outcry indicated a perception that public health benefits outweighed concerns of personal privacy, security and potential risk of harm.

Early public health messaging was unclear. From traditional news outlets to social media, people were made even more anxious by the mix of confusing and competing information. Fear drove panic buying of household staples; compounded by access to global news reports of events occurring in other countries. A spike in the number of racist attacks was reported across the country, with Chinese restaurants, Chinese tourists and Chinese Australians being targeted both online and in the street.

The establishment of a National Cabinet by the Prime Minister[7] was designed to promote a co-operative federalism, and deliver a consistent national response to COVID-19 with the governments of the country speaking with one voice. But this was never going to be easy, given the differing needs of the state and territories to that of the federal government.

The PM has been consistent in citing the economic implications of COVID-19, and Australians in turn are worried whether a post-pandemic Australian society will be more selfish, in recession and will have an overburdened health system.[8] With the rates of unemployment skyrocketing in April, the highest jobless rate since October 2001,[9] such uncertainty is warranted. Governments have rolled out stimulus packages at a level unheard of since the global financial crisis.

TABLE 8.1 Australia chronology

Date		Diffusion of COVID-19	Key official actions	Key communication events
January	1	Unofficial infection starts.	Chief Medical Officer (CMO) receives notification from WHO regarding pneumonia cases in Wuhan.	
	5		No new cases with virus believed to be transmitted from animals to humans.	
	19			Australian media begins to report on virus.
	20	Human–human transmission confirmed.		
	22		Incident response centre set up.	
	23		Sydney screens arrivals from Wuhan.	First joint PM and CMO press conference.
				By the end of May, the PM will have given over 150 pressers, speeches and interviews on COVID-19.
	25	First case detected.		
	29	7ᵃ cases.	Australians evacuated from Wuhan.	
February	1	12 cases.	Border to China closed.	
	27		PM announces national pandemic.	
	29	24 cases.	Travellers from Iran quarantined.	Daily press conferences begin with PM and CMO in Canberra.

(Continued)

TABLE 8.1 (Continued)

Date		Diffusion of COVID-19	Key official actions	Key communication events
March	1	First COVID-19 death.		
	3	33 cases.		Panic buying begins.
	5	57 cases, 2 deaths.	Travellers from Korea quarantined.	
	7			CMO announces no need for face masks.
	11		$2.4 billion health plan to fight virus.	Actors Tom Hanks and Rita Wilson test positive in Queensland.
	12	122 cases, 3 deaths.	Financial assistance – $17.6 billion.	
	13	140 cases, 3 deaths.	National Cabinet formed.	Minister for Home Affairs, the Hon Peter Dutton MP tests positive.
	14			'Help Stop the Spread and Stay Healthy' national media campaign launched.
	15	298 cases, 5 deaths.	Gatherings >500 banned, cruise ships banned.	
	16		Supermarkets limit staple items.	
	17		All arrivals to self-isolate. Stricter social distancing. Work from home.	
	18		*Biosecurity (Human Biosecurity Emergency) (Human Coronavirus with Pandemic Potential) Declaration 2020* enacted.	PM calls hoarding of supplies 'un-Australian.'
	19	510 cases, 6 deaths.		Ruby Princess docks – 2700 passengers and crew disembark with no quarantine.
	20		2020 Federal Budget deferred. Borders closed to non-citizens. Strict social distancing. Mandatory quarantine for all arrivals.	

Date	Cases/deaths	Measures	Media/Info
21			Crowds defy social distancing on beaches.
22		$66 billion assistance package.	Twitter calls for ABC Health reporter Norman Swan to be CMO.
23	**Peak of new daily cases**	Bars, clubs, cinemas, casinos and gyms closed. Takeaway only.	
24		Courts cease face-to-face hearings.	
25		Travel banned to all countries.	Launch of text campaign.
26		Restaurants, cafes, auctions, open houses closed. Five people allowed at weddings, ten at funerals.	
27		Shops close.	
29		$1.1 billion for mental health, domestic violence.	Official coronavirus info app launched.
30	3966 cases, 16 deaths.	$130 billion JobKeeper. Military deployed to conduct COVID compliance checks. No more than 2 people allowed to gather.	
April 2	4979 cases, 21 deaths.	Childcare becomes free.	
5	5687 cases, 34 deaths.		COVID-19 daily infographic launched by Department of Health.
7			Toilet paper shortage reported in the media.
9		$27 million for indigenous, regional arts.	
13			Newmarch Aged Care Home becomes second-deadliest cluster.
15	6203 cases, 54 deaths.	Special Commission of Inquiry into the Ruby Princess established.	

(Continued)

TABLE 8.1 (Continued)

Date		Diffusion of COVID-19	Key official actions	Key communication events
	23	6645 cases, 71 deaths [20 from the Ruby Princess].		
	24		Testing becomes available for everyone.	
	26			'Stay COVID free, do the three' campaign and COVIDSafe tracing app.
May	1		Roadmap for staged return endorsed by National Cabinet.	
	5		$205 million for aged care.	
	8		Three-step plan to the easing of restrictions.	
	15		$48.1 National Mental Health and Wellbeing.	
	22	7079 cases, 100 deaths.		Launch of mythbusting page.
	29	7139 cases, 103 deaths.	$131.4 for public hospitals	
June	6			Black Lives Matter protests.
	15		Courts begin staggered face-to-face hearings.	
	29	7686 cases, 104 deaths.		Celebrity chef Pete Evans on *60 Minutes* claiming there is no pandemic.

[a] Coronavirus (COVID-19) current situation and case numbers, Department of Health, Commonwealth of Australia, www.health.gov.au/news/health-alerts/novel-coronavirus-2019-ncov-health-alert/coronavirus-covid-19-current-situation-and-case-numbers.

With provisions for the jobless, help for employers to cover part or all of their employees' wages, assistance for small businesses – it doesn't cover the short-term employed, those in the arts, on student visas, non-citizens and thousands of workers paid in cash.

COVID-19 has altered civic and social life, with face-to-face community and social interaction moving online. A myriad of online communities from WhatsApp neighbourhood groups, invitation only Facebook pages, parenting, and sports groups, to gardening and cookery forums emerged. Zoom, Skype and Microsoft teams replaced business meetings, courts instigated electronic methods to file and witness documents, while school and university teaching moved online. In the performing arts, artists adapted existing materials, luring users with digitised archives, virtual tours and streaming performances, and literary festivals have moved online. But lockdown has not promoted a new form of congeniality for everyone, with rates of domestic violence[10] and calls to mental health hotlines increasing.[11]

Analysis

Political science literature suggests that in a crisis a leader must, '"ramp up" their performance…the tasks of leadership requires more than organising an effective response. Leaders must build and support transboundary collaboration and transnational institutions that can effectively deal with the borderless nature of contemporary crisis' (Boin et al., 2016: 1).

Set against this benchmark, Morrison had difficulty gaining traction, given his disastrous leadership during the bushfires and the subsequent lack of public confidence in his authority. He also had to navigate the intricacy of a federated political system, which provides three levels of government that, in principle, work together to deliver the services needed to run the country, but in reality, is fraught with individual agendas and priorities.

Underneath the overarching federal parliament sits six states which, together with two self-governing territories, all have their own constitutions, parliaments, governments and laws. And if that is not enough, there are over 500 councils that sit within the states that oversee local community services. Although there is delineation over who does what, state and territory interests often clash with those at the federal level.

Morrison made it clear to the nation that decisions would be made in accordance with the medical advice.[12] Australia's Chief Medical Officer (CMO), Dr Brendan Murphy, became the PM's unlikely wingman in a series of daily press conferences, providing the PM with the optics required.

Theoretically, there was a clear structure to the dissemination of information. The Australian Health Protection Principal Committee (AHPPC), the key – decision-making body for health emergencies and comprising all state and territory chief health – officers and chaired by the CMO, provide the medical advice. The CMO reports to the PM, who then presides over National Cabinet.

The PM assumed the position of primary government spokesperson, but a range of spokespeople have been made available during the outbreak, including all federal, state and territory Health Ministers and Chief Health Officers, dependent on the stage of the outbreak and the aim of communications. When the focus of the message is related to events and activities in a specific jurisdiction, the spokesperson was determined by that state or territory.

All clear cut in theory, but in practice, not so black and white.

The ongoing challenge faced by the public has been to understand why the public advice seemed to disagree with itself and why federal and state governments were saying different things. The reasons for the differences were simply thanks to the fundamentals of federalism, but the resulting friction did nothing to shore up public confidence in either the PM or the Premiers during the early days of the crisis.

There was confusion and panic in the community about social distancing measures, lockdown and school closures. Words such as hotspot and cluster entered the vernacular. The Premiers broke ranks, making public statements before the National Cabinet met, resulting in many Australians struggling to comprehend the range of announcements.

The conflicting messaging over schools is a prime example, with the CMO and the PM maintaining a position that schools should remain open,[13] in contrast to the Premiers, who announced that schools should close, but could remain open for parents who are essential workers.

The PM advocated for schools to stay open for two reasons. First, because the CMO said there was no compelling medical evidence to close schools and second, because keeping schools open makes it possible for parents to go to work. With the welfare of the economy being a concern of the Commonwealth (in contrast to education which is the concern of the State), the PM's objective was to keep people in work, and therefore less reliant on government benefits.

A wide range of information has been made available since the outbreak of the pandemic. The federal, state and territory governments moved to position themselves as authoritative sources, while enlisting the cooperation of key spokespeople in the non-government sector (e.g. university academics, the Australian Medical Association), important for building confidence in the response strategies. According to recent surveys. Australians concerned about the virus have been consuming more news than ever before (Park et al., 2020), relying on television news as a primary source of information.

The press conference, held in the courtyard of the federal parliament in Canberra, emerged as a central communication tool, providing a platform for the PM to propagate announcements from National Cabinet. The live broadcasts, livestreams and coverage of these press conferences showcased the role of the political journalist in asking questions and seeking clarification. These journalists, members of the Federal Parliamentary Press Gallery, with their access to the government were thus positioned as leaders in the dissemination of the federal government's message, with state political reporters providing the state and territory narrative.

But the PM's early handling of the crisis was messy, not helped by 10 pm media conferences and the release of unpolished and conflicting messaging that did little to calm and reassure the public. It was not long before the information gap was being filled by the ABC's Dr Norman Swan, the national broadcaster's medical and health commentator. Extremely critical of the government's handling of the virus, Swan advocated for more stringent measures. Accolades came from across mainstream and social media channels, with Swan 'perceived as being Australia's medical voice of reason as the COVID-19 pandemic has swept the nation' (Graham, 2020).

Popular former commercial TV and radio host, Dr Karl Kruszelnick, with degrees in medicine and biomedical engineering, and one of Australia's 100 National Living Treasures, also added to the media narrative but without the same impact as Swan. Heard predominantly on commercial radio, Dr Karl (as he is affectionately known) has been critical of the lack of government spending on vaccine development.

Mainstream media outlets have been turning to scientists and health experts to stay up to date with the rapidly changing situation. Head of the Kirby Institute's Biosecurity Programme at the University of New South Wales, Professor Raina MacIntyre, has been a media favourite, used to explain complex virology in everyday language. Often the single female in a sea of grey-suited men, her calm and measured responses have resonated calm and empathy.

Consistent and informative government communication with the public, through the media and other sources, has shaped the way the public has gauged the perception of risk. The dissemination of up-to-date, consistent and accurate information about the status of the disease outbreak overseas and in Australia served to alert people to the risk and help them make more informed decisions about work, travel and other activities.

The public awareness campaign was launched in March. Using television streaming services, social media and news services, the key principles applied included:

- Openness and transparency;
- Accurate risk communication, including where there was uncertainty;
- Consistent, clear messages;
- Regular, timely provision of tailored information;
- Early release of public messages;
- Use of social media where appropriate;
- Flexible selection of methods appropriate to the situation at the time and
- Use of a wide range of communication methods to reach a broad audience.

The opposition and other critics claim that the government was too slow to educate the public on how to prevent the spread of the virus through hygiene and social distancing measures.

When the campaign did launch, the integrated marketing campaign included videos, posters, social media tiles and radio podcasts, with audiences directed to the Department of Health webpage for up-to-date information.

The main messaging called for Australians to:

- Stay 1.5 metres away from others;
- Wash hands regularly for 20 seconds with soap and water;
- Avoid touching your face and
- If sick, stay at home.

Following the release of the COVIDSafe tracing app, the campaign was updated, again pointing to the Department of Health website as the authority and calling Australians to 'Stay COVID Free, Do The 3,' referring to the washing of hands, maintaining physical distancing and uploading the COVIDSafe app.[14]

Using online media as a dissemination tool for information and misinformation illustrates technology, such as the internet, is a 'double-edged sword,' particularly social media, where information and misinformation travel fast. Throughout the pandemic, federal, state and territory governments have battled the dissemination of misleading rumours and conspiracy theories on the origin of the virus, paired with fearmongering, racism and conspiracy theories.

The PM publicly urged Australians to stop believing unverified content circulated on the internet and through text messages, following reports that an online post, claiming to be based on information from an Australian government cabinet briefing, was going viral. Upon investigation, it was found that the post was a direct copy of a Malaysian government announcement, only with Australia inserted into the text.

There was an emergence of fake government departments with online accounts peddling disinformation, for example the 'Department of Diseasology Paramatta,' which necessitated hasty counter action by legitimate government agencies. Misinformation has also been disseminated by public influencers with vast social media followings – such as lifestyle gurus and politicians, causing the CMO to call for non-medical experts to not give medical advice to the public. For instance Alan Jones, one of the most powerful radio broadcasters in the country, insisted most people would get a 'mild illness,'[15] claiming that COVID-19 was the 'health version of global warming'[16] while on Fox Footy, Eddie McGuire suggested the spread of the virus, which is 'just the flu'[17] could be slowed by warmer weather. Meanwhile, former federal politician Bronwyn Bishop claimed on Sky television, that the Chinese government had unleashed the virus to kill off the weak in their community.[18] *60 Minutes* aired a programme featuring celebrity chef and former *MasterChef* judge Pete Evans[19] promoting coronavirus conspiracy theories, leaving some die-hard fans of the chef ecstatic, and others horrified.

The government's clear objective has been to 'flatten the curve' of cases, and to minimise the impact of COVID-19 on the economy. Utilising draconian measures within the *Biosecurity Act* to curb citizen interaction has been the government's trump card. But inconsistency and confusion of early messaging made it difficult for the risk to resonate, especially with younger Australians, who flouted social distancing rules and descended upon the beaches in the balmy autumn weather.

While the future remains uncertain, the change in Morrison's political fortunes continues, as he emerges from the lockdown as a unifying figure almost unrecognisable from the man who lost control of the narrative during the bushfire crisis. Instead he is winning over a public that appears to be warming to his new look collaborative, centrist leadership.

Notes

1 Morrison took over the prime ministership on August 24, 2018, after a party room vote stripped Prime Minister Malcolm Turnbull of the leadership. Turnbull had previously ousted out Tony Abbott as Prime Minister in 2015.
2 Newspoll (2020), *The Australian*.
3 Op.cit.
4 *Public Health Act 2010* (NSW); *Public Health and Wellbeing Act 2008* (Vic); *Public Health Act 2005* (Qld); *Public Health Act 1997* (ACT) *Emergency Management Act 2005* (WA); *Notifiable Diseases Act 1981* (NT); *Public Health Act 2011* (SA); *Biosecurity Act 2019* (TAS).
5 Canberrans urged to continue COVID 19 compliance, May 19, ACT policing.
6 Government of New South Wales.
7 Media Release, March 13, 2020.
8 Saeri, A.; Slattery, P.; Smith, L. (April 8, 2020) More Australians are worried about a recession and an increasingly selfish society than about coronavirus itself, Monash University.
9 Employment and Unemployment, Australian Bureau of Statistics, Commonwealth of Australia.
10 The Courts launch COVID-19 list to deal with urgent parenting, April 26, 2020, Family Court of Australia.
11 Beyond Blue Ltd (2020).
12 Media Release, January 23, 2020, Parliament House Canberra.
13 Press Conference transcript, March 24, 2020, Parliament House Canberra.
14 COVIDSafe app campaign resources (2020), Commonwealth of Australia.
15 Alan Jones addresses coronavirus pandemic (March 17, 2020).
16 Siedel, J. (March 18, 2020) Alan Jones 'dangerous' coronavirus theory, *The Chronicle*.
17 Tyeson, C. (March 20, 2020), Eddie McQuire, Not a Doctor, Rattled off Dangerous Coronavirus Lies on live TV Last Night, *Pedestrian*.
18 Toilet paper panic (March 9, 2020) *Media Watch*, ABC.
19 Bond, N. (June 8, 2020) Pete Evans' boasts he played 60 Minutes Australia like a 'game of chess.'

References

Australian Bureau of Statistics (2020). *Employment and Unemployment, Australia, Canberra.* www.abs.gov.au/employment-and-unemployment
Beyond Blue Ltd (2020). https://coronavirus.beyondblue.org.au/

Boin, A., Hart, P., Stern, E. & Sunderlius, B. (2016). *The Politics of Crisis Management: Public Leadership under Pressure.* Cambridge University Press, UK.

Bond, N. (2020). Pete Evans' Boasts He Played 60 Minutes Australia Like a 'Game of Chess.' *news.com.au*, 8 June, www.news.com.au/entertainment/tv/current-affairs/p ete-evans-sneaky-move-against-60-minutes/news-story/ea5871fdd49dd6093791109 13598a41a

Commonwealth of Australia (2020). *COVIDSafe App Campaign Resources.* www.health .gov.au/resources/collections/covidsafe-app-campaign-resources

Commonwealth of Australia (2020). *Biosecurity (Human Biosecurity Emergency) (Human Coronavirus with Pandemic Potential 2020.* www.legislation.gov.au/Details/F2020L002 66

COVIDSafe App Campaign Resources (2020). *Commonwealth of Australia.* www.health .gov.au/resources/collections/covidsafe-app-campaign-resources

Crabb, A. (2019) With a 'Miracle' Election Result, Scott Morrison Has the Mandate to Do Whatever He Likes – So What Will it Be? *ABC*, 19 May, www.abc.net.au/ news/2019-05-19/annabel-crabb-election-result-2019-scott-morrison-mandate/1 1127994

Department of Health (2020). *Coronavirus (COVID-19) Current Situation and Case Numbers, Australia, Canberra.* www.health.gov.au/news/health-alerts/novel-coronav irus-2019-ncov-health-alert/coronavirus-covid-19-current-situation-and-case -numbers

Family Court of Australia (2020). *The Courts Launch COVID-19 List to Deal with Urgent Parenting.* 26 April, www.familycourt.gov.au/wps/wcm/connect/fcoaweb/about/ne ws/mr260420

Graham, J. (2020). 'ABC medical expert and Coronacast host Dr Norman Swan tested for COVID-19,' The Young Witness www.youngwitness.com.au/story/6703192/dr -norman-swan-tested-for-coronavirus/

Jones, A. (2020). Alan Jones Addresses Coronavirus Pandemic. *2gb*, 17 March, www.2gb .com/alan-jones-addresses-coronavirus-pandemic/

Newspoll (2020). *The Australian.* www.theaustralian.com.au/nation/newspoll

Park, S., Fisher, C., Lee, J. Y. & McGuinness, K. (2020). *COVID-19: Australian News and Misinformation.* www.canberra.edu.au/research/faculty-research-centres/nmrc/p ublications/documents/COVID-19-Australian-news-and-misinformation.pdf

Saeri, A., Slattery, P. & Smith, L (2020). *More Australians Are Worried about a Recession and an Increasingly Selfish Society Than about Coronavirus Itself.* Monash University. 8 April, https://lens.monash.edu/@politics-society/2020/04/08/1380008/more-australian s-are-worried-about-a-recession-and-an-increasingly-selfish-society-than-about-c oronavirus-itself

Siedel, J. (2020). Alan Jones 'Dangerous' Coronavirus Theory. *The Chronicle*, 18 March, www.thechronicle.com.au/news/alan-jones-dangerous-coronavirus-theory/397481 4/

Tyeson, C. (2020). Eddie McQuire, Not a Doctor, Rattled off Dangerous Coronavirus Lies on Live TV Last Night. *Pedestrian*, 20 March, www.pedestrian.tv/sport/eddie- mcguire-coronavirus-misinformation-fox-footy/

9

GERMANY

Between a patchwork and best-practice

Isabelle Borucki and Ulrike Klinger

Political context

Germany is a federal republic with 16 states, each with a constitution, government and parliament. German federalism is not just about the distribution of power, but also subsidiarity, i.e. some policy fields are exclusively matters for the federal government in Berlin (e.g. foreign policy). In contrast, other policy fields are affairs of the states (e.g. education policy). Hence, heated debates can occur about who should deal with some issues, states or federal governments, but also the federal government sometimes declares salient issues as executive priorities ('Chefsache'), taking them over from state legislation.

Germany is governed by a parliamentary government elected with a mixed voting system of list votes and personalised votes. The chancellor, Angela Merkel, coordinates the cabinet. Her party, the Christian Democratic Union (CDU), has been governing Germany in coalition with the Social Democrats or Liberals since 2005. Due to the emergence of the populist and increasingly radical-right party Alternative for Germany (AfD) in 2013, the German party system experienced polarisation and fragmentation of political discourse.

Both governing parties, SPD and CDU have recently experienced changes in party leadership. Angela Merkel stepped down from the CDU party leadership in 2018. As a consequence, the party is currently experiencing fierce competition among potential candidates for party leadership and hopefuls for the chancellor-candidacy for 2021. Some of the potential candidates held key positions during the COVID-19 crisis, so the looming election impacts how politicians and government members position themselves in the crisis.[1]

Chronology

See Table 9.1.

DOI: 10.4324/9781003120254-11

TABLE 9.1 Germany chronology

Date		Diffusion of COVID-19	Key official actions	Key communication events
January	27	First case in Germany (Bavaria).		
	29			Statement by the Federal Minister of Health Jens Spahn regarding the coronavirus.
February	1		Around 100 people returned from Wuhan. As a precautionary measure, they were isolated in a shelter for 12 to 15 days.	
	12			After meeting of the Health Committee on February 12, 2020, Health Minister Jens Spahn speaks on the current situation regarding the coronavirus and how to proceed.
	15	Super-spreading event during carnival party in Heinsberg district (North Rhine-Westphalia).	Germany implements the EU Health Council's recommendations. Travellers from China are asked about contact with infected persons and stays in infected areas.	
	21	First confirmed Italian Covid-19 death, 15 infected.		
	27		The federal government's newly established crisis team meets for the first time.	
March	2/3		The export of medical protective equipment (breathing masks, gloves, protective suits) abroad is prohibited. The Ministry of Health is responsible for the central procurement of personal protective equipment (PPE) for doctor's offices, hospitals and federal authorities.	Federal press conference on the coronavirus.

4		Government statement by Jens Spahn in Bundestag.
10	Infections in every German federal state.	The federal crisis team recommends the cancellation of all major events with more than 1,000 expected participants.
12		Chancellor Angela Merkel highlights importance to act in socially responsible manner. President Steinmeier calls the pandemic a huge test for societal cohesion.
13		Federal and state governments agree on hospitals recruiting additional staff, extending the number of ICUs and postponing scheduled surgeries and procedures.
16	Death toll reaches 10.	Schools and day-care centres closed in most states. Government imposes comprehensive border controls and entry bans.
17		No entry for third-country nationals, worldwide travel warning, restriction of non-essential travel within EU, closure of numerous shops.
18		Chancellor Merkel broadcasts a television speech – the first in her 15 years of office (except for annual New Year's speeches).
22		Contact restrictions established: only two people allowed to walk together in public at the same time (exceptions for core family). A minimum distance of 1.5–2 metres must be maintained. All restaurants, hair salons, most non-food stores and all establishments requiring closer contact are closed.

(Continued)

TABLE 9.1 (Continued)

Date	Diffusion of COVID-19	Key official actions	Key communication events
23	Death toll exceeds 100.	The federal government announces economic aid package amounting to 156 billion euros. Contact restrictions are extended until April 19.	
April 1			
2	The infection rate within a single day reached its peak (+6,536).		
3	Death toll exceeds 1,000.		
10		14-day quarantine obligation for returnees from abroad.	
12	Number recovered within one day exceeds new infections on same day for first time.		
15		Federal-state agreement: contact restrictions in place to at least May 3, schools to be opened gradually from May 4, shops under 800 m² open from April 20 (or later), no major events until August 31, everyday masks highly recommended.	
20		Some states start to relax restrictions, allowing shopping in stores up to 800 sq. metres. Berlin, Brandenburg and Saxony schools gradually reopened. Saxony first to make wearing of face masks in stores and on public transport compulsory.	Chancellor Angela Merkel warns against reopening too quickly and individual solutions in the states. Spahn: presentation of a 10-point plan to strengthen the public health service.
22	2,237 new infections. 4,200 recoveries.	Daily testing capacity rose from 31,000 to 136,000. Number of tests per week more than tripled from 125,000 to 400,000. Overall mortality rate is 8% higher than previous four years.	

26	Until April 26, companies filed for short-time working[a] for 10.1 million employees to avoid unemployment, the highest number of short-time working in German history.[b]
27	Face masks now compulsory, mostly for supermarkets as well as on buses and trains, sometimes only on public transport.
30	Federal and state governments agree on further easing of restrictions, plan to reopen playgrounds, museums, zoos and religious institutions.
	Starting in April 2020, smaller and larger protests against the anti-corona measures took place, Stuttgart (5,000 participants) Munich (3,000 protesters), among them radical and extreme right activists and conspiracy 'theorists.'
	Government approves contagion tracking app: voluntary, anonymous and no geolocation.
May 6	Merkel announces further easing of restrictions after meeting state prime ministers. Nationwide, people from 2 households allowed to meet in public places. People in nursing homes may receive visits from 'permanent contact person.'
9	New infections below 1,000 cases for tenth day in a row. Some states (Mecklenburg-Western Pomerania, Saxony, Thuringia) report 1–10 new infections.

(*Continued*)

TABLE 9.1 (Continued)

Date		Diffusion of COVID-19	Key official actions	Key communication events
	11		Thuringia reopens schools for most students.	
	18		After a compulsory eight-week corona break, regular operation of the day-care centres in Saxony and Thuringia start. Primary schools are also opening in Saxony.	
	25		The state prime minister of Thuringia, Bodo Ramelow, faces public criticism due to his plans to terminate the general corona restrictions as of June 6.	
June	2	689 in intensive care.		Contagions tracking app available on App Store and Google Play.
	3	Total cases: 195,758. Infected: 198,786. Death toll: 9,222.	After outbreak in Göttingen, several schools and day-care centres are closed, mass test is ordered. In Magdeburg, several schools, a day-care and a youth centre are closed because of rising infection rates.	
	23	Lockdown in Gütersloh and Warendorf (North Rhine–Westphalia) after infections at the Tönnies meat factory.	Plans to reopen schools and child-care on a regular basis, starting in August, are developed.	

[a] https://en.wikipedia.org/wiki/Short-time_working (July 8, 2020).

[b] www.tagesschau.de/wirtschaft/corona-kurzarbeit-arbeitslosigkeit-101.html (July 8, 2020).

The coronavirus pandemic drew attention to various social challenges: The need for office and home schooling highlighted social and gender inequalities and revealed massive digitalisation challenges, mostly concerning the lack of infrastructure. Only about 12% of households in Germany are connected via fibreoptic networks, making Germany one of the last among EU countries in this regard. Particularly in rural areas, up to 30% of households have no access to high-speed internet.[2] Many essential workers are underpaid, e.g. caregivers, cleaners, delivery workers and retail employees. Agriculture is highly dependent on low-income foreign workers for harvesting of produce, so harvesting Germans' favourite springtime vegetable asparagus turned into a public drama. The meat industry became a super-spreading hotspot; many meat-packing factories had to close, workers were sent into quarantine and the precariousness of work conditions were debated. Meanwhile, conspiracy theories have become very widespread and visible.

Analysis

When Chancellor Merkel delivered her televised address to the citizens, the severity of the situation was clear. This made the threat clear, as well as the language she used; talking of a dire situation, 'a historical task,' and set the tone for government communication: 'It is serious. Do take this seriously. Not since the day of German reunification, no, not since the Second World War, has our country seen a challenge that so severely depends on all of us acting together in solidarity.' She addressed aspects of democratic governance and executive actions:

> I address you today in this unusual way because I want to tell you what guides me as Chancellor and all my colleagues in the Federal Government in this situation. It is part of an open democracy: that we also make political decisions transparent and explain them. That we justify and communicate our actions as well as possible so that they are comprehensible.

With a background in academic research (Merkel holds a PhD in physics), she pointed at the emergent character of the situation:

> This is a dynamic situation, and we will remain capable of learning so that we can always rethink and react... I therefore ask you not to believe any rumours, but only the official communications, which we always have translated into many languages.

The speech was published online in several languages (English, Turkish, Russian, Arabic, Sign Language).[3] An empirical study showed that Merkel's TV speech indeed had a measurable effect on the population, an apparent reduction of stress and anxiety related to the coronavirus situation (Teufel et al., 2020).

Besides press conferences (usually, representatives of the German Government are invited three times a week by the Federal Press Conference, a unique institution hosted by a journalistic association[4]), the chancellor's TV speech, extensive information provided on government websites, a governmental information portal (zusammengegencorona.de) and various social media channels, the federal government published a series of podcasts. While podcasts are increasingly popular in Germany (24% of internet users listen to podcasts at least once per month, 54%among the 18–24 year-old population), this is a channel that hardly ever reaches the older population (13% among 55 years and older), who are particularly vulnerable to COVID-19 (all data from Hölig & Hasebrink, 2020: 50).

Was the expert guidance used consistently and clearly?

Government communication was clearly and explicitly guided by scientific expertise – to such an extent that prominent scientists became the target of public criticism about e.g. the closing of kindergartens, and had to repeatedly point out that it is not they who decide. In the early phase of the crisis, expert consultations were more or less focused on epidemiology and virology. In particular, the government was consulted by Christian Drosten, an internationally renowned expert on emergent viruses, one of the discoverers of the SARS-associated coronavirus in 2003 and who had developed the COVID-19 diagnostic test in January 2020 that was later used by the WHO.[5] To explain the scientific perspective to a broad audience, Drosten published a podcast, first daily and then every few days, starting February 25 (*Corona Update with Christian Drosten*). This podcast became the most popular information source during the crisis in Germany, with 41 million downloads by May 8, and a large international following in 60 countries.[6] Drosten soon became 'the country's real face of the coronavirus crisis.'[7]

The intense focus on virological expertise drew criticism, as the lockdown's social, psychological and economic consequences became salient. The government reacted declaring that potential relaxations of measures would be based on interdisciplinary expertise by the Leopoldina German National Academy. Published on April 13, this expertise drew much public criticism, too. For instance, the expert group suggested keeping kindergartens closed for further months – only two of the 26 experts were women.[8]

In cooperation with the Robert Koch Institute, a German federal government agency and research institute responsible for disease control and prevention, the German government developed an app to trace infection chains (Corona-Warn-App), published on June 16. By early July, around 15 million smartphone users had downloaded the app, roughly 25% of smartphone users in Germany. This is quite remarkable, as Germans are infamously sceptical when it comes to data privacy, and this is an app developed by the government that traces encounters with other smartphones running the app. In contrast to initial plans involving large tech companies such as Google and a central collection of trace data, the app does not share data, works on an anonymous basis with data remaining on the smartphone. However, again the older population benefitted least from this app. Based on state-of-the-art bluetooth interfaces, the app does not work on older phones or operating systems – technology that is prevalent predominantly among the elderly.

Who were the main actors?

Crises are the time of the executive, and Germany is no exception to this pattern. The federal government and state governments were key actors in both deciding and communicating measures to contain the pandemic. The government was also crucial in alleviating the economic fallout by issuing numerous support payment programmes, economic recovery programmes, lowering taxes, issuing a new national budget and, most importantly funding short-time working as a measure to counter unemployment. During the pandemic, government popularity skyrocketed: on June 26, 82% agreed Merkel was doing her job well (69% in January 2020), and 40% reported they would vote for CDU (27% in January).[9]

Most importantly, journalists and traditional mass media played a key role in explaining and classifying the measures taken. While 'the internet' and social media have overtaken TV as the primary news source among all German age groups under 55 years (Hölig & Hasebrink, 2019), traditional news consumption and the use of TV grew during the pandemic.

In hybrid media systems (Chadwick, 2017), information travels across platforms. To find out which news sources dominated on social media, we analysed the most popular (i.e. most shared) URLs on Twitter during the pandemic. Between January 27 (first case in Germany) and May 15, we analysed the ten most shared URLs per day in German-language tweets that contained the terms 'corona' and/or 'COVID' (data retrieved via Crimson Hexagon/Brandwatch, 110 days, N=1,100, three coders, Holsti 0.86).

The results clearly show that almost two-thirds (63.4%) of the most shared URLs on Twitter link to traditional mass media coverage. However, the second most popular source (8.5%) originated from German hyper-partisan right-wing media sites, among them notorious spreaders of disinformation and conspiracy theories which may have fuelled the protests against the anti-corona measures. Only 1.3% (N=13) of these most-shared URLs link to government communication. However, this indicates that government information, e.g. the government information portal zusammengegencorona.de, was among the most shared URLs on Twitter, which can be interpreted as an indicator of relevance. Other prominent government URLs include a corona-hackathon initiated by the federal government (wirvsvirushackathon.de), links to the Ministry of Health, the Foreign Ministry, the Federal Employment Agency and state government sites from North Rhine-Westphalia and Bavaria.

Throughout the pandemic, science and academic actors (scholars and academies) have been in the public limelight like never before. Science communication was very prominent, explaining statistics, exponential growths, reproduction rates, aerosols and other medical and statistical data. While only 0.5% of URLs are expert sources, the single most shared URL in our dataset is a YouTube video by the famous German scientist and science blogger Mai Thi Nguyen-Kim titled 'Corona is just getting started' from April 1.[10] On the other hand, the political conflict over the question of when to reopen and exit from anti-corona measures led to an instrumentalisation of science and the widespread impression that scientists frequently changed their opinion and could not agree on anything. Surveys show that trust in and reputation of science increased, but only a minority of Germans understand what science is about and how it works (Petersen, 2020). Distrust of science and experts is particularly common among AfD voters (76% vs 45% in the general population, Petersen, 2020). Like other countries, Germany was affected by the 'infodemic,' as the WHO[11] called it, a surge of disinformation, conspiracy theories and pseudo-expertise (Boberg et al., 2020). A study by the fact-checking organisation Correctiv.org found that Germans were most likely to encounter fake news about the pandemic on WhatsApp, but the source of information was YouTube.[12]

Did official sources contradict one another?

Official information was not directly contradictory, although recommendations changed as the pandemic evolved and research intensified, e.g. changes in recommendations on wearing face masks. However, a conflict between the federal government and some state governments arose over the exit strategy from (the comparatively soft and short) lockdown. While actors within the federal government cautioned against early relaxation of measures, some state prime ministers issued a reopening-race by unilaterally ordering early re-opening and ending the obligation to wear masks. This race to reopen was obviously linked to inter-party competition for CDU party leadership and chancellor-candidacy in 2021. The election of a new party leader had to be postponed from April 2020 to December 2020, giving all declared and potential candidates, among them the prime ministers of Bavaria and North Rhine-Westphalia and the Federal Health Minister, plenty of opportunity to compete for popularity and to develop a profile as successful crisis managers. Using this crisis as a platform to show leadership and efficient crisis management led to conflicting messages between the federal government (pursuing a cautious strategy not to reopen too soon) and some states' pressuring for a quick reopening. In frustration, Merkel denounced such 'opening discussion orgies' ('Öffnungsdiskussionsorgien') on April 20, but finally transferred the authority of decision-making about reopening to the states on May 6. This debate was on one dimension about centralised rules and measures for all Germany versus a so-called 'patchwork rug' of different rules and measures in the 16 states, on a second dimension about long-term measures (prioritising the epidemiologist's perspective) versus short-time measures (prioritising the economic and social collateral effects). The third dimension in this discourse stressed the benefits of having 16 'laboratories' – the states and their heterogenic structure to test best-practice measures.

Despite some protests and surging disinformation, public support for the federal government's measures to contain the pandemic remained very high. By May 15, two-thirds of respondents in a representative survey said the counter-measures were precisely right (17% said overdone, 16% said they were not enough).[13] Interestingly, those who thought measures were overdone were predominantly supporters of the radical-right populist party AfD. This party lost support during the pandemic (about −5%) and did not find a clear political position, attacking the government for not doing enough in the early phase of the pandemic, later attacking the government for regulating too much.

Conclusion

Overall, we conclude the government measures to contain the coronavirus were widely accepted and satisfaction with the government and communication was comparatively high. This rather positive picture is slightly spoiled by the counter-actions of the radical right and the demonstrations against reasonable measures, e.g. against wearing a mask. The German government acted quickly enough to prevent the spread of COVID-19, following scientific expertise. On a critical note, this expertise was very much focused on virology and epidemiology, while the economy, social science, psychology and other fields were given less prominent roles. German federalism and the internal leadership competition within the CDU ended centralised measures, resulting in a patchwork of different rules and counter-measures.

Notes

1 The sympathy towards Merkel, the coalition and their management of the crisis was about 50% in March and even grew until July to 71% (www.infratest-dimap.de/um fragen-analysen/bundesweit/ard-deutschlandtrend/2020/maerz/, www.infratest-d imap.de/umfragen-analysen/bundesweit/ard-deutschlandtrend/2020/juli/)
2 www.br.de/nachrichten/netzwelt/warum-der-glasfaser-ausbau-in-deutschland-nur -zaeh-vorangeht,S6J4d6F
3 www.bundesregierung.de/resource/blob/975232/1732182/d4af29ba76f62f61f1 320c32d39a7383/fernsehansprache-von-bundeskanzlerin-angela-merkel-data.pdf? download=1 (July 9, 2020)
4 www.bundespressekonferenz.de/information-in-english (July 9, 2020)
5 https://en.wikipedia.org/wiki/Christian_Drosten (July 9, 2020)
6 https://de.wikipedia.org/wiki/Coronavirus-Update
7 www.theguardian.com/world/2020/mar/22/coronavirus-meet-the-scientists-who -are-now-household-names (July 9, 2020)
8 www.zeit.de/2020/23/corona-studie-leopoldina-pandemie-akademie-wissenschaft (July 10, 2020)
9 www.forschungsgruppe.de/Umfragen/Politbarometer/Langzeitentwicklung_-_ Themen_im_Ueberblick/Politik_II/ (July 10, 2020)

10 www.youtube.com/watch?v=3z0gnXgK8Do&feature=youtu.be (July 10, 2020)
11 www.who.int/docs/default-source/coronaviruse/situation-reports/20200202-sit
    rep-13-ncov-v3.pdf (July 10, 2020)
12 https://correctiv.org/faktencheck/hintergrund/2020/05/12/datenanalyse-nutzer
    -finden-fragwuerdige-corona-informationen-vor-allem-auf-youtube-und-verbre
    iten-sie-ueber-whatsapp (July 10, 2020).
13 www.forschungsgruppe.de/Aktuelles/Politbarometer/ (May 15, 2020).

References

Boberg, S., Quandt, T., Schatto-Eckrodt, T., Frischlich, L. (2020). Pandemic Populism: Facebook Pages of Alternative News Media and the Corona Crisis – A Computational Content Analysis. *ArXiv*: 2004.02566 [Cs.SI], http://arxiv.org/abs/2004.02566.

Chadwick, A. (2017). *The Hybrid Media System: Politics and Power*. Oxford University Press.

Hölig, S., & Hasebrink, U. (2019). *Reuters Institute Digital News Report 2019 – Ergebnisse für Deutschland*. Verlag Hans-Bredow-Institut (Arbeitspapiere des HBI Nr. 47), https://hans-bredow-institut.de/uploads/media/default/cms/media/x52wfy2_AP47_RDNR19_Deutschland.pdf

Hölig, S., & Hasebrink, U. (2020). *Reuters Institute Digital News Report 2020 – Ergebnisse für Deutschland*. Verlag Hans-Bredow-Institut (Arbeitspapiere des HBI Nr. 50), https://www.hans-bredow-institut.de/uploads/media/default/cms/media/66q2yde_AP50_RIDNR20_Deutschland.pdf

Petersen, T. (2020). Die Stunde der Wissenschaft. *Frankfurter Allgemeine Zeitung*. 8, https://fazarchiv.faz.net/document/FAZ__FD1202006186023158?offset=&all=

Teufel, M., Schweda, A., Dörrie, N., Musche, V., Hetkamp, M., Weismüller, B.,...Skoda, E. M. (2020). Not All World Leaders Use Twitter in Response to the COVID-19 Pandemic: Impact of the Way of Angela Merkel on Psychological Distress, Behaviour and Risk Perception. *Journal of Public Health*. https://doi.org/10.1093/pubmed/fdaa060

10

INDIA

A spectacle of mismanagement

Chindu Sreedharan

Political context

The largest democracy and second most-populous country in the world, India casts a dominant shadow on all its South Asian neighbours bar China (Tellis, 2020). Its population, topping 1.35 billion, is expected to overtake China's 1.4 billion by 2024. Its economy, which recorded $2.94 trillion in 2019, is the fifth largest in the world in terms of nominal GDP, having overtaken that of the United Kingdom (UK) and France (United Nations, 2019). Geopolitically, it is an economic powerhouse with nuclear armaments persistently courted by leaders of the West. These achievements notwithstanding, India is a nation riddled with developmental challenges: income disparity is on the rise, there is persistent gender inequality and India is exceptionally vulnerable to climate change and disasters.

Presiding over all this are the polarising politics of Prime Minister Narendra Modi. Considered by many to be responsible for the spread of Hindu nationalism that has divided the country, Modi first came to power in 2014, and in 2019, though many of his campaign promises had not been met (BBC, 2020a), was returned with an even better majority – a feat made possible largely by his exceptionally well-organised election machinery that saturated India's news and social media networks with the image of Modi as 'the protector of the nation' (Verniers, 2019). His successive tenures have done much harm to India's secular fabric, stoking religious intolerance and undermining democratic institutions (Komireddi, 2019). Since 2018, India's economic growth has slowed down, and unemployment is at a 45-year high. There is a 'stark mood of despair,' particularly among the poorest (Basu, 2020).

DOI: 10.4324/9781003120254-12

Chronology

The first COVID-19 case in India was reported on January 30. By February 3, the number of infections rose to three. All were students who had returned from Wuhan, and all were in the south Indian state of Kerala, ruled by the Communist government of Chief Minister Pinarayi Vijayan, and known for its high literacy rate and investment in public health.

Kerala's response to the virus was admirably swift; it began ten days *before* its first patient tested positive. K. K. Shailaja, its health minister, started preparing Kerala for an epidemic soon after she learnt about the virus. Hence by January 27, the state had already adopted the World Health Organisation's (WHO's) test, trace, isolate and support protocol, and set up a Rapid Response Team (Spinney, 2020). On February 3, with confirmation of its third positive case, Kerala declared a state calamity, placing more than 2,239 travellers from affected countries in quarantine.

In the first week of March, around the time the patients in Kerala had all ended their quarantine, cases were identified in other Indian states. On March 3, the New Delhi-based *Hindustan Times* led with the headline 'Corona reaches Capital.' The same day, PM Modi, known for his sophisticated social media team and significant reach on @narendramodi, tweeted out an image, 'Basic Protective Measure For All,' together with a reassuring message to his millions of followers: 'There is no need to panic. We need to work together, take small yet important measures to ensure self protection.'[1] This was Modi's first direct communication on the virus. India also suspended visas issued to nationals of Italy, Iran, South Korea and Japan on March 3. By March 10, two days after the WHO announced 100,000 infections across 100 countries, India was beginning to see an increase in new cases. The nationwide total stood at 50, across ten states and the national capital region (Kumar, 2020).

On March 12, a day after WHO declared COVID-19 a pandemic, India reported its first death, in Karnataka (Wire, 2020a). The Government of India suspended tourist and student visas, as well as visa-free entry for persons of Indian origin, for a month beginning March 13. It also advised states and Union Territories to invoke the *Epidemic Disease Act, 1897* to enable them to enforce such measures as banning public gatherings, closure of schools and insistence on working from home where possible. While there was some criticism in the news media about the invocation of a colonial-era law to battle a modern-day pandemic (Kapur, 2020), analysts were quick to concede that, as Nanisetti wrote in *The Hindu* (2020), the Act served an immediate purpose in the absence of any new legislation. In any case, the government advice received little resistance from regional governments, with the states of Karnataka, Haryana and Goa, and the National Capital Territory of New Delhi invoking the Act in quick succession to declare an epidemic (Kapur, 2020).

By March 15, the total number of cases in India had reached 110. The death toll stood at two. The majority of cases were from Maharashtra in the west (32), followed by 22 in Kerala (south), 12 in Uttar Pradesh (north), and seven in the New Delhi region (north). Soon after, the Government of India issued an advisory to all states, urging social distancing measures till March 31. On March 21, in his first televised public address about the pandemic, Modi announced the formation of a task force to draw up measures to combat the economic effects of the pandemic. He also called for a 'Janta (People's) Curfew,' to be observed on March 22 between 7 am and 9 pm (*Economic Times*, 2020). The curfew will be 'a litmus test for us,' Modi said. 'This is also the time to see how prepared India is to fight off a global pandemic like the coronavirus.'

The call for the curfew was Modi's attempt at social mobilisation, to co-opt citizens into being responsible for their own well-being (Ninan, 2020). It was clear containment was critical to India; given its large population, highly crowded urban spaces and inadequate medical infrastructure, the country could easily be overrun if COVID-19 reached epidemic scales. Perhaps it was this awareness that brought the support the call received, cutting across political affiliations. The Indian National Congress, Modi's main opposition in the parliament, extended its support to the call. So did many of the state governments usually critical of Modi's leadership, including the Communist leadership in Kerala. The response to the curfew, hence, was overwhelming; millions stayed indoors on March 22, emerging at 5 pm briefly to show gratitude to health workers and essential service providers.

Parts of the nation, meanwhile, were beginning to submerge into complete or contained lockdowns. By the time the Janta Curfew ended, 82 districts in 23 of India's 29 states, among them, Rajasthan, Andhra Pradesh, Telangana, Punjab, Uttarakhand, and Jammu and Kashmir, were under lockdown (*Times of India*, 2020).

Tuesday, March 24, was particularly crucial. At 5:34 am, Modi's official Twitter account published a short tweet in Hindi and English: 'Will address the nation at 8 p.m. today, 24th March 2020, on vital aspects relating to the menace of COVID-19.'[2] After a day of suspense, including speculations the country might be headed for a state of emergency, Modi announced a three-week nationwide lockdown beginning at midnight, four hours after his address, applicable to 'every state, union territory, village and district' (Firstpost, 2020). Drawing on powers under the *National Disaster Management Act, 2005*, Modi said, 'If the situation is not controlled in 21 days, India could go 21 years behind' (*Economic Times*, 2020). Modi's televised speech acknowledged this would be an exceptionally difficult time for the poorest Indians, but stressed a nationwide lockdown was the only way to quell transmission.

The extreme measure, the 'most severe step taken anywhere' (Gettleman & Schultz, 2020) saw the world's largest and harshest pandemic measures implemented. Expectedly, it attracted a great deal of criticism. The rationale for the decision came under limited scrutiny, but the hastiness of the announcement, the lack of details on how essential goods would be made available, and the way lockdown was implemented presented significant concerns to the Indian public.

Across the nation, there was confusion, with the police adopting harsh measures to enforce the lockdown, including on essential service workers, doctors and journalists. In New Delhi, for instance, police were 'raining sticks' on pharmacists going to work (Gettleman & Schultz, 2020).

But the most visible and perhaps cruellest impact was on India's poor, many of them migrant workers. Suddenly jobless, millions of workers are believed to have moved back to their villages in a 'historic reverse-migration' to 'some of the poorest, least prepared places' (Roy & Agarwal, 2020). With limited resources and the public transport system shut down, tens of thousands of people left cities to walk hundreds of miles, some more than 500, in the immediate days after Modi's announcement. Nearly 200 migrants died on the road (Wallen, 2020). Though India announced a $22.5-billion stimulus package for the poor on March 26, this was too little to provide 'free staple grains for about 800 million' low-income citizens (Roy & Bellman, 2020).

By April 14, as the initial lockdown came to an end, the number of confirmed infections had climbed to 10,363 (Chowdhury, 2020), from the pre-lockdown figure of 500. And while the death toll, at 336, was significantly low comparatively, the twin vulnerabilities of high population density and weak healthcare system meant the nation was far from safe. India's test rate, too, was exceedingly low – barely 4,000 per day in early April. Against this background, Modi extended the lockdown to May 3. But the number of infections continued to rise over the next weeks, each day recording more than 1,000 new cases.

This trend was to continue into the next months. In May, Modi extended the lockdown twice, placing the nation under restrictions till May 31. By May 16, India recorded 85,940 cases, overtaking China. Three days later, it exceeded 100,000 infections. By June 1, India was the seventh most-infected country in the world, with 194,504 cases.

The June–September period is particularly noteworthy in India's COVID-19 response timeline. Uniquely, when infections were rising in record numbers, India began to reopen. Thus, on June 8, when India registered 9,983 cases in a single day to become the fifth most-affected nation in the world, the government initiated 'Unlock 1.0' (Singh, 2020). On June 11, India overtook the UK, with 298,283 cases, to become the fourth most-affected country. But Modi's address to the nation on June 30 framed this situation as a 'better position compared to many countries,' and that the government's decisions have saved 'lakhs of lives' (*Hindustan Times*, 2020). The next day, with infections exceeding 600,000 and the death toll at 17,495 and climbing, India entered 'Unlock 2.0.' On July 6, India overtook Russia to be the world's third most-affected nation, with 697,413 cases and 19,693 deaths. The government, however, continued with the third phase of reopening from August 1, arguably seeing this as an economic necessity as figures were to soon reveal, India's GDP had fallen by a spectacular 24% (Nahata, 2020), the worst in decades. On September 7, as the nation began 'Unlock 4.0,' India recorded 90,000 cases overnight, 4.2 million infections, and 71,642 deaths. It was now the second most-infected nation in the world.

Analysis

India awoke to the COVID-19 crisis late. In this, it followed the pattern of most nations, misjudging the threat level and misspending the lead time that news of the Wuhan outbreak offered. While Kerala, which recorded India's first case, was impressively proactive with its preparation, there was little evidence of crisis planning at the national level.

This oversight, to a significant extent, is attributable to the political events that preoccupied the Modi government, indeed most national politicians, in the pre-crisis and initial phases of the outbreak. Elections to the prestigious Delhi Assembly, the legislative body that governs the national capital region, were scheduled for February 8. The fallout of that election, which Modi's Hindu nationalist Bharatiya Janata Party lost, was 'the worst religious conflict that engulfed the Indian capital in decades' (Ellis-Petersen and Rahman, 2020a), when Hindu mobs attacked Muslims with tacit and explicit support from Delhi Police (Gettleman et al., 2020). This was followed by US President Donald Trump's visit in the last week of February and a political crisis in the state of Madhya Pradesh, which saw the BJP gaining control of the state government (Noronha, 2020). All of this commanded significant political attention, particularly from the prime minister.

It is unsurprising, then, that Modi's first tweet about coronavirus came on March 3, more than a month after India recorded its first case. Modi was not alone in this belatedness. An analysis of 23,115 tweets posted by 20 Indian politicians between January 30 and May 30 shows that there was very little discourse, barely an acknowledgement of the threat in fact, on social media: just 1% of the coronavirus-related tweets of politicians from January to May came in February (Live Mint, 2020). This included a tweet from Congress politician Rahul Gandhi on February 12, which said 'the government is not taking this threat seriously.' In all, of the 20 politicians, 14 were silent about the virus all through January and February (Live Mint, 2020).

It was only in March, after the infection reached New Delhi, that COVID-19 entered political discourses in a significant way. Till then, the virus was largely seen as a regional problem that concerned Kerala or the world outside, but of limited consequence to the Indian state. Once the national capital recorded its first case, this narrative began to change, albeit slowly. Into mid- and late-March, communications about the virus began to dominate public discourse, both on traditional and social media. This trend continued into April as lockdown was extended, with politicians devoting 45% of their tweets to COVID-19 (Live Mint, 2020).

An exceptionally powerful social media influencer[3] who routinely makes key announcements on Twitter, Modi's tweets in Hindi and English formed the basis of India's national crisis communication. Many of his social media communications struck the 'right' note and are categorisable as 'good' crisis communications. His tweets in March, for instance, advocated for calm and disseminated preventive measures adhering to crisis and emergency risk communication principles (Reynolds & Seeger, 2005). There were also efforts to involve society, with tweets calling for solidarity against the virus, framing the crisis as an 'us' versus 'it' situation. On March 22, going into the Janta Curfew, he tweeted, 'The people of India have decided, we are in this together. We will fight the menace of COVID-19 together.'[4] After the surprise lockdown, Modi devoted an entire episode of *Mann Ki Baat*, a monthly radio programme he hosts, to COVID-19, entreating listeners to respect the lockdown, and apologising to all his 'countrymen,' particularly his 'underprivileged brothers and sisters' for the hardships placed on them (PMIndia, 2020).

Though in line with Crisis and Emergency Risk Communication (CERC) principles, a closer look reveals several deep-seated issues with Modi's public messaging. The government was, as noted earlier, belated in its initial responsiveness, wasting much of the pre-crisis phase on other matters. In the initial phase, while Modi's tweets appear to show empathy and provided emergency courses of action, there was inadequate state support to enable civil society to implement the measures in any meaningful or timely manner. His communication, it would appear, was aimed at signalling the government was actively putting in place a coordinated national strategy. But there was little evidence of a crisis plan, or of coordination with states, when India entered its surprise lockdown, putting millions of her poorest into extreme hardship. The lockdown, arguably, was needed. However, its ill-planned nature, particularly its suddenness, appears to have been designed more to bolster Modi's image as 'protector of the nation' than to help the situation. It created a media spectacle as Roy & Agarwal (2020) put it, 'the mother of all spectacles.'

As lockdown was extended, Modi's popularity soared (Gettleman & Yasir, 2020b). Criticism was largely muted. While that in itself is not surprising, national crises often effect rallies around the flag (Chatagnier, 2012), Modi's public messaging did little to alleviate the framing of coronavirus as a 'Muslim disease' by Hindu nationalists (Ellis-Petersen & Rahman, 2020b). Nor was there an attempt to combat the xenophobia and social media trolling that emerged against Chinese citizens. Kohli and Dhawan (2020) suggest this was a deliberate political strategy to shore up Hindu nationalist support during the crisis framed as a catastrophic danger to the Indian society if 'left unrestrained.'

A corollary of this strategy that prioritised words over action, perhaps, was the fact that the government misspent the time it bought by the lockdown. The lockdown would have been 'effective had this period been used for improving the healthcare infrastructure or at least boosting the public health budget' (Harikrishnan & Chakraborty, 2020). But India's COVID-19 stimulus package has been identified at approximately 1% of the GDP, falling too short of what is required. There is little evidence, too, of an intergovernmental framework, crucial for policy coordination and fiscal transfers to deal with a pandemic (Harikrishnan & Chakraborty, 2020), particularly in a nation of India's complexity. Nor was there evidence of a strategy to alleviate the humanitarian crisis triggered by the surprise lockdown. As India began to open up, paradoxically with her death toll mounting and infections surging, COVID-19 dropped further down India's public communication agenda. Modi's Twitter feed, for instance, paid little attention to COVID-19 in July and August. The consequences of his ad hoc approach to the crisis, however, are starkly evident: at the time of writing, India's GDP has contracted a spectacular 24% and her surging infection rate is second only to the United States.

Notes

1 https://twitter.com/narendramodi/status/1234762662413660165
2 https://twitter.com/narendramodi/status/1242323791436320768?lang=en
3 Modi has 62.2 million Twitter followers, as of September 12, 2020.
4 https://twitter.com/narendramodi/status/1241603438036713472?lang=en

References

Basu, K. (2020). India's economic troubles are rooted in politics. *Foreign Policy*.

BBC (2020a). *India election 2019: Has India's BJP government kept its promises?* www.bbc.co.uk/news/world-asia-india-47771192

Chatagnier, J. T. (2012). The effect of trust in government on rallies round the flag. *Journal of Peace Research*, *49*(5), 631–645.

Choudhury, S. R. (2020). India extends coronavirus lockdown until May 3. *CNBC.com*. www.cnbc.com/2020/04/14/india-extends-coronavirus-lockdown-till-may-3.html

Economic Times (2020). *PM Narendra Modi forms economic response task force, calls for 'Janata Curfew.'* https://economictimes.indiatimes.com/news/politics-and-nation/pm-narendra-modi-forms-economic-response-task-force-calls-for-janata-curfew/articleshow/74715013.cms?utm_source=contentofinterest&utm_medium=text&utm_campaign=cppst%0A

Ellis-Petersen, H., & Rahman, S. A. (2020a). Delhi's muslims despair of justice after police implicated in riots. *The Guardian*. www.theguardian.com/world/2020/mar/16/delhis-muslims-despair-justice-police-implicated-hindu-riots

Ellis-Petersen, H., & Rahman, S. A. (2020b). Coronavirus conspiracy theories targeting muslims spread in India. *The Guardian*. www.theguardian.com/world/2020/apr/13/coronavirus-conspiracy-theories-targeting-muslims-spread-in-india

Firstpost (2020). *PM Narendra Modi announces a national lockdown for 21 days starting midnight of 24–25 March*. www.firstpost.com/health/pm-narendra-modi-announces-a-national-lockdown-for-21-days-starting-midnight-of-24-25-march-8185961.html

Gettleman, J., & Schultz, K. (2020). Modi orders 3-week total lockdown for all 1.3 billion Indians. *The New York Times*. www.nytimes.com/2020/03/24/world/asia/india-coronavirus-lockdown.html

Gettleman, J., Yasir, S., Raj, S. and Kumar, H. (2020) How Delhi police turned against muslims. *The New York Times*. www.nytimes.com/2020/03/12/world/asia/india-police-muslims.html

Harikrishnan, S., & Chakraborty, L. (2020). COVID-19 crisis: Lockdown, as a strategy to control the pandemic, has proven to be neither good nor bad. *Financial Express*. www.financialexpress.com/opinion/covid-19-crisis-lockdown-as-a-strategy-to-control-the-pandemic-has-proven-to-be-neither-good-nor-bad/1986615/

Hindu (2020). *Battling COVID-19 with a colonial-era law.* www.thehindu.com/news/cit ies/Hyderabad/battling-covid-19-with-a-colonial-era-law/article31195144.ece

Hindustan Times (2020). *PM Modi's address to the nation. Complete text.* www.hindustanti mes.com/india-news/pm-modi-s-address-to-the-nation-complete-text/story-pWz8 lPwjANttEsMd47YDZI.html

Kapur, M. (2020). A 123-year-old law, once used to imprison freedom fighters, is India's primary weapon against coronavirus. *Quartz India.* https://qz.com/india/1820143/i ndia-battles-coronavirus-with-british-era-epidemic-diseases-act/

Kohli, P., & Dhawan, P. (2020). *Dissection the Hindu Chauvinism in India's COVID-19 response, oxpol.* https://blog.politics.ox.ac.uk/dissecting-the-hindu-chauvinism-in -indias-covid-19-response

Komireddi, K. (2019). *Five more years of Narendra Modi will take India to a dark place.* www .theguardian.com/commentisfree/2019/may/21/five-more-years-narendra-modi -india-dark-place.

Kumar, D. (2020). Half a million COVID-19 cases in India: How we got to where we are. *Wire.* https://thewire.in/covid-19-india-timeline

Mint, L. (2020). *How top politicians tweeted about #coronavirus.* www.livemint.com/news/ india/how-top-politicians-tweeted-about-coronavirus-11591368662484.html.

Nahata, P. (2020). India GDP contracts a record 23.9% in April-June quarter. *Bloomberg Quint.* www.bloombergquint.com/business/india-gdp-contracts-a-record-239-in -april-june-quarter

Ninan, T. N. (2020). Janata curfew is Modi's 2nd stab at social mobilisation, but it can be a double-edged sword. *Print.* https://theprint.in/opinion/janata-curfew-is-modis-2nd-stab-at-social-mobilisation-but-it-can-be-a-double-edged-sword/38 5040/

Noronha, R. (2020). BJP's Shivraj Singh Chouhan sworn in as Madhya Pradesh CM for fourth time. *India Today.* www.indiatoday.in/india/story/bjp-s-shivraj-singh-chouh an-sworn-in-as-madhya-pradesh-cm-for-fourth-time-1658867-2020-03-23%0A

PMINDIA (2020). *PM's address in the 10th episode of 'Mann Ki Baat 2.0.'* https://ww w.pmindia.gov.in/en/news_updates/pms-address-in-the-10th-episode-of-mann-ki -baat-2-0/

Reynolds, B., & Seeger, M. W. (2005). Crisis and emergency risk communication as an integrative model. *Journal of Health Communication, 10*(1), 43–55.

Roy, R., & Agarwal, V. (2020). Millions of Indians are fleeing cities, raising fears of a Coronavirus 'Land Mine' in villages. *The Wall Street Journal.* www.wsj.com/articles /indias-migrants-head-home-as-lockdown-eases-prompting-fears-of-coronavirus -spread-11590579072

Roy, R., & Bellman, E. (2020). *India to spend $22.5 billion to help poor survive Coronavirus shutdown.* www.wsj.com/articles/india-to-spend-22-5-billion-to-help-poor-sur vive-coronavirus-shutdown-11585223446

Singh, S. G. (2020). *COVID-19: Here's a timeline of events since lockdown was imposed in India, business standard.* www.business-standard.com/article/current-affairs/here-s-a -timeline-of-events-since-lockdown-was-imposed-in-india-120070201413_1.html

Spinney, L. (2020). The coronavirus slayer! How Kerala's rock star health minister helped save it from COVID-19. *The Guardian.* www.theguardian.com/world/2020/may/14 /the-coronavirus-slayer-how-keralas-rock-star-health-minister-helped-save-it-from -covid-19.

Tellis, A. J. (2020). *Between Washington and Beijing: India's geopolitical challenges, carnegie endowment for international peace.* https://carnegieendowment.org/2020/05/18/betw een-washington-and-beijing-india-s-geopolitical-challenges-pub-81824.

Times of India (2020) *Coronavirus: Officially or unofficially, India in lockdown, restrictions put in place in 82 districts.* http://timesoia.indiatimes.com/articleshow/74765462.cms?utm_source=contentofinterest&utm_medium=text&utm_campaign=cppst

United Nations (2019). *World population prospects 2019.* www.ncbi.nlm.nih.gov/pubmed/12283219.

Verniers, G. (2019). *Modi's success in India's elections: Five factors, yale global online.* https://yaleglobal.yale.edu/content/modis-success-indias-elections-five-factors

Wallen, J. (2020). Warning over Indian road safety as almost 200 migrants killed in crashes. *The Telegraph.* www.telegraph.co.uk/global-health/science-and-disease/warning-indian-road-safety-200-migrants-killed-crashes

Wire (2020a). *Half a million COVID-19 cases in India: How did we get here?* https://thewire.in/covid-19-india-timeline

11

ITALY

The frontrunner of the Western countries in an unexpected crisis

Edoardo Novelli

Political context

After 20 years characterised by a bipolar political system, with conflict between a centre-right and a centre-left coalition, which took turns in government, the 2013 and in particular the 2018 political elections marked the emergence of new political forces and an unstable tripolar political scenario.

The COVID-19 crisis in Italy coincided with this period of political instability and conflict. The coalition government that tackled the pandemic, led by Prime Minister Giuseppe Conte, was composed of the centre-left Partito Democratico (Democratic Party), the Movimento Cinque Stelle (Five Stars Movement), plus some minor left and centre-left formations. This coalition, called yellow-red, was elected on September 5, 2019. From June 1, 2018 to August 2019, Conte had led a centre-right majority, 'yellow-green' coalition, composed of the Five Star Movement and La Lega (The League), a far-right-wing populist party. In addition to changes in economic and social policies, the new coalition assumed a more pro-European position, in contrast with previous Euro-critical and Eurosceptic administrations. As a lawyer and university professor, Conte became involved in politics only in 2018, becoming Prime Minister without having ever taken part in the elections and having never been elected to Parliament. The change of coalition from centre-right to centre-left, combined with Conte's lack of political experience, gave rise to a weak image of the leader and doubts about his leadership qualities, also within the new coalition, which produced an immediately divided and quarrelsome group.

As a consequence, in the first months of 2020 the Italian political system was characterised by conflict and the government was weak. At the same time, the popularity of the far-right opposition parties La Lega and Fratelli d'Italia (Brothers of Italy) continued to grow in the polls. In the weeks preceding the

DOI: 10.4324/9781003120254-13

discovery of the pandemic's spread in Italy (February 21), the public debate and mainstream media were focused on internal politics and local elections. The news coverage of COVID-19 was poor, mainly concentrated on the situation in China. The risks of contagion were underestimated, even by experts and the scientific community.

Chronology

See Table 11.1.

Analysis

Before the pandemic: an unprepared system

The Italian chronology of COVID-19 shows some important decisions were taken well before the discovery of infection cases on February 21 – first and foremost the six-month state of emergency declaration on January 31. However, the fact that the National Plan for Preparedness and Response to an Influenza Pandemic (Ministry of Health, 2007) – foreshadowed by article 13 of the International Health Regulations, issued in 2005 by the World Health Organisation (WHO) (WHO, 2005) – but not updated since 2007, mitigated the effects of these decisions. This delay, which cannot be attributed to the incumbent institutions, had consequences both on the medical and operational level and communication management. The main medical and operational consequences were a delay in monitoring and response to the pandemic; the absence of clear guidelines in the protocols for testing, hospitalisations and isolation of positive cases; a lack of testing kits, intensive care beds and pulmonary respirators; insufficient personal protection equipment for operators and finally, scarcity of medical masks for the population.

With regards to communication, the 2007 plan defined it as a 'skill and a resource of the Health Organization, essential for the management of public health events' (Ministry of Health, 2007). The plan also indicated in detail the main communication objectives that had to be achieved. Among the main ones were the preparation of national, regional and local organisational structures to establish collaborative relationships between institutions; the selection of spokespersons at the national and local level; the construction of a communication process that guarantees clarity, transparency, timeliness, uniformity and reliability of information and reinforcing the credibility of the institutions and finally, the development of a collaborative relationship with media through the constant and clear communication of information. Therefore, despite their clear identification, these goals remained on paper and were never accomplished.

Other events aggravated the weakened credibility in dealing with the pandemic. Firstly, some decisions dictated by the emergency, such as the circular issued by the Ministry of Health on January 27. Following WHO guidelines,

TABLE 11.1 Italy chronology

Date		Diffusion of COVID-19	Key official actions	Key communication events
January	1	Unofficial infection starts.		
	22		Minister of Health (MH) chairs first Coronavirus Task Force, 2019-nCov; plans for testing set out.	
	27		Following WHO guidelines, MH reduces cases calling for medical swabs.	
	30	2 Chinese tourists test positive in Rome.	Flights to and from China banned.	
	31		Government declares a 6-month state of health emergency.	Head of Italian Civil Protection appointed Extraordinary Commissioner and Coordinator of the COVID-19 Operating Committee.
February	3		Technical Scientific Committee established.	
	6	1 Italian from Wuhan positive.		
	21	First confirmed Italian COVID-19 death, 15 infected.	Government quarantines 2 small municipalities in Lombardy and Veneto.	
	22		Prime Minister Decree (DPCM) 14-day **lockdown in 11 northern municipalities.**	
	23		Lombardy closes schools, universities and public places, closes cafes and bars after 6 pm.	Start of the Civil Protection daily press conference.
	24		MH announces that only those who are symptomatic will be tested.	Conte on 5 main Italian Sunday talk shows: 'Everything is under control. Don't panic.' Milan stock exchange loses 5.43 points. The regions contest the government measures.

Month	Day	Death toll	Events	Media/Communication
	25	Death toll reaches 11.	DPCM extends restrictions to inter-regional movements, retail stores and public events to 6 additional regions.	
	26		Opposition parties call for an emergency government.	Politicians and mayors promote counter-campaigns against restrictions.
March	4	Death toll exceeds 100.	**Start Phase 1**. DPCM extends restrictions on inter-regional movements, retail stores, public events. All schools, universities closed.	Milan Cathedral and La Scala Theatre reopen. Conte announces DPCM on official Facebook page of the Presidency of the Council.
	5			President of the Italian Republic, Sergio Mattarella's televised speech.
	7		DPCM restrictions added to prevent travel within Italy, retail stores closed, public events banned in 6 regions. **Northern Italy lockdown.**	Televised nightly press conference of Conte at 2:30 am.
	9			MH launches campaign #iorestoacasa (I stay at home) on social networks. 'Everything is going to be okay' becomes the slogan against COVID-19.
	10		DPCM 'I stay home' extends restrictions until April 13. **Lockdown throughout Italy.** Government appoints a task force to organise logistics, healthcare.	Conte announces DPCM on his personal Facebook page. 'Let's stay apart today to hug each other stronger tomorrow.'
	12	Death toll exceeds 1,000.		Note from the President of the Republic to Europe: 'Italy needs solidarity, not obstacles.'

(Continued)

TABLE 11.1 (Continued)

Date	Diffusion of COVID-19	Key official actions	Key communication events
15		Some regions issue ordinances to close regional borders.	
18		'Cure Italy' law decree allocates 25 billion for economic aid.	
19	3,451 deaths – world highest.		
20		MH closes public parks for walking, sports activities.	
22		DPCM extends quarantine to all production activities. **Italy in hard lockdown.**	National Civil Aviation Authority authorises the use of drones for control.
23	Infected exceeds 50,000.		Conte's first report to Parliament.
25			
26		Fourth version of the self-certification form allowing citizens to circulate.	
27	Death toll exceeds 10,000.		President's second televised speech.
29			A Civil Protection call for 500 nurses receives 9,400 responses in 48 hours.
April 1		DPCM extends hard lockdown until April 13.	
4		MH presents 5-point strategic plan to exit crisis.	
5			Journalistic investigation reports deaths of extensive elderly residents in nursing homes where COVID-19 patients had been hospitalised.
7			Commissioner Arcuri guarantees availability of 20 million protective masks per week.

Date			
9	Death toll among doctors and nurses exceeds 100.		
10		DPCM extends total lockdown until May 4.	
11	Death toll exceeds 20,000, total infected 100,000, total cases 150,000.	DPCM establishes task force of economic and social experts.	
13		Minister of Education announces lessons will not be resumed. School year declared over.	
14			International Monetary Fund estimates for Italy: 9.1% drop in GDP, deficit at 8.3%, unemployment at 12.7%.
21	Second day of slowdown in spread of infection.		
26		Government sets surgical mask sales price at 50 cents.	Conte announces the 5 points of phase two in Parliament.
27			The surgical masks remain unavailable for weeks.
29		Government approves contagion tracking app: voluntary, anonymous and no geolocation.	Civil protection daily press conference at 8 pm ends.
May 4		**Start phase 2 – first step.** DPCM removes the strictest lockdown restrictions. Travel within regional borders allowed.	
8	Total cases: 200,000. Deaths: 30,000+. Number of infected drops to 90,000.		

(Continued)

TABLE 11.1 (Continued)

Date		Diffusion of COVID-19	Key official actions	Key communication events
	13		'Relaunch Italy' decree allocates 55 billion economic aid to companies and workers.	
	18		**Phase 2 – second step.** DPCM removes most of remaining restrictions in retail, production activities. Inter-regional travel allowed.	
	28	Number of patients in intensive care – below 500.		Contagions tracking app available on App Store and Google Play.
June	3	Death toll: 33,530. Infected: below 40,000. Total cases: 233,515.	**Start phase 3:** Government suspends remaining restrictions. Only a few minor limits remaining. **End of Lockdown.**	
July	14		DPCM extends the remaining restrictions on public activities and meetings until July 31.	
	16	Death toll exceeds 35,000. Infected drop to 12,443. Total cases: 243,736. Total medical swabs: 6,103,492.		
	29		Government extends the emergency state to October 15.	

this circular reduced cases calling for testing to all those with symptoms, who had come into contact with those who had tested positive, or had returned from China. A change that slowed down the discovery of the contagion. Secondly, in March it was discovered and made public that COVID-19 had been present in Italy since early January.

The Italian media were also caught off guard and underestimated COVID-19 until cases exploded. On February 21, the start of infections in Italy, the news that a group of Italians had returned from Wuhan was reported on page 23 of *la Repubblica*, one of the most important Italian newspapers. The next day, COVID-19 climbed to the top of the media agenda, discussed with emotional, emphatic and alarming tones. This attitude was partially motivated by the partisanship of certain media outlets but mainly related to the innate tendency for sensationalism of information by Italian media. Prime Minister Conte took a central role from the beginning of the crisis, managing the key moments of communication, institutional appointments and political decisions first-hand. While holding important roles, the Ministers of Health and Economy adopted lower profiles. Conte was joined by two technicians appointed for the operational management of the crisis: the head of Civil Protection, Angelo Borrelli, and the COVID-19 emergency commissioner, Domenico Arcuri. The President of the Republic played an essential institutional and communicative role, issuing messages, notes and declarations at crucial moments during the crisis.

The government's response: personalisation and communication

One sign of Conte's leadership was the extensive use of Prime Ministerial Decrees. The 17 Prime Minister Decrees (DPCMs) approved from February 22 to June 3 indicate the exceptional and urgent nature of the situation and the centrality of the Prime Minister.

Before the real threat from COVID-19 was understood, Conte had already appeared on the main television talk shows and news programmes, reassuring the population that everything was under control. When the situation worsened at the beginning of March, Conte communicated almost exclusively through institutional and official statements dedicated to COVID-19.

Conte's frequent TV press conferences, speeches to the nation and videos on Facebook – a total of 20 between January 31 and June 3 – were central, solemn moments for providing information. Conte announced all the most important measures and various phases of lockdown directly to the Italian people. In his speeches, he showed an understanding of the difficulties and suffering, highlighted the exceptionality and seriousness of the moment, emphasised community spirit, national pride and his commitment. His communications were more empathetic and emotional than they were pragmatic and authoritative. 'It is not the first time our country has faced national emergencies. But we are a strong country, a country that does not give up: it is in our DNA,'[1] or 'let's stay distant today to embrace each other with more warmth and to run faster tomorrow,'[2] are examples of the rhetoric that characterised Conte's speeches. In short, Conte adopted a leadership style that was better suited to a father of the nation than to a commander-in-chief.

The prevailing trend was to deliver monologic, disintermediated speech without the presence of journalists, who were often not invited. The diffusion of official announcements through Conte's personal Facebook page or the official Facebook page of the Presidency of the Council further accentuated this communication style. This tendency annoyed both Italian and international press,[3] which criticised Conte and the institutions for their uncertain management of the emergency and inadequate communication of the crisis. Some of the main problems highlighted by the media included the practice of announcing measures before their approval, the absence of opportunities for questions, the lack of clarity and precision and the lack of punctuality in television events (Alfonso & Comin, 2020). Conte and the government in turn criticised journalists and the mass media for leaking and precociously spreading information, which risked jeopardising the measures' effectiveness. One such example is March 7 when the media anticipated a measure which led thousands of Italians to return to their regions just before the lockdown.

The 'collaborative relationship with the media, through the constant and clear communication of information' (Ministry of Health, 2007) that was hoped for in the 2007 plan was not achieved. On the contrary, the government and media engaged in a competition and conflict that a more effective governmental media and information management strategy could have reduced (McNair, 2017).

Many actors, many conflicts

The power delegated to the regions to implement the government's emergency rules caused confusion within the command hierarchies. Especially in the early days of the pandemic, the lack of coordination between national and local institutions slowed the health response. Various actors were involved in the management and communication of the emergency: the government, ministries, Civil Protection, the Higher Institute of Health, the regions; everyone issued decrees, devices, ordinances, regulations.

The government appointed commissioners and task forces on specific topics: the app for tracing the infection, the fight against fake news on the internet, the analysis of social-healthcare and economic data, schools and many others. The result was more than 300 people involved at national level, thereby affecting the efficiency and speed of the reaction.

The health emergency did not reduce excessive bureaucracy, a historic defect in Italian legislative and administrative systems. From January 1 to June 3, the national authorities issued 291 provisions on COVID-19, almost all of them very complicated and inaccessible. The Coordinated text of the ordinances on COVID-19 released on March 24 by Civil Protection (Presidenza Consiglio dei

Ministri, Dipartimento Protezione Civile, 2020) was 295 pages with 123,000 words.

The management and communication of the crisis highlighted conflicts between authorities, powers and institutions, first and foremost those between national Government and the Regions, which often contested the national provisions. With their own autonomy in the healthcare sector, the latter issued conflicting and uncoordinated ordinances.

In the days following the fall of the Milan stock exchange on February 2, key institutional and political figures – including the secretaries of the Democratic Party and La Lega and the mayors of Milan and Bergamo – promoted counterinformation campaigns against the government's regulations for closures. Public events were organised, and videos were released to support tourism and commerce,[4] creating a short circuit in institutional communication.

The institutional conflict that occurred with the European institutions and their leaders had an opposite, positive effect, for example the President of the European Central Bank (ECB) Christine Lagarde and the President of the European Commission, Ursula Von Der Leyen, with which the government repeatedly argued about European economic aid and anti-COVID-19 measures (see Chapter 6 on the European Union (EU)). The firm stance towards so-called European selfishness – also supported by the President of the Republic[5] and even the Pope[6] – and the progressive granting of aids – up to the 172 billion foreseen by Recovery Fund for Italy – strengthened the internal consensus towards the government against an external enemy, led by the 'frugal four countries': Austria, Denmark, the Netherlands and Sweden.

Experts played an essential role in the disease management and emergency communication. This category included scientists, mainly engaged in research, and communicators, with the task of providing concise and easily understandable explanations. Although some experts had initially underestimated COVID-19, with the explosion of the crisis virologists, biologists, infectious disease specialists, as well as statisticians and physicists, became its main communicators.

On the one hand, communication regarding COVID-19 was an opportunity to reaffirm the value of expert knowledge, in contrast to the death of expertise (Nichols, 2017) and the delegitimisation of intermediaries, driven by the emergence of various populist parties and ideas (Taggart, 2004; Di Cesare, 2020). On the other hand, experts became newsworthy (Chadwick, 2013) and the dynamics of the current hybrid media system, the goal of which is to win audiences by producing controversial talk shows and mobilising opposing fans and communities on social networks, shifted.

The internet and especially social networks helped to communicate the crisis, manage the emergency and share segregated sociality. Among the initiatives proposed by the institutions, the #iorestoacasa campaign promoted at the beginning of March by the Ministry of Health to convince Italians to stay home was supported by dozens of famous personalities and celebrities.

Museums, libraries, archives and cultural institutions proposed online initiatives such as events and virtual itineraries. The daily Civil Protection Press Conference launched in early March on Facebook became a popular event, a sort of collective ritual.

Many individual user initiatives went viral. The most famous one, promoted on Facebook in mid-March, brought thousands of Italians to their balconies to play and sing every day at 6 pm.[7] 'Italy on the balcony' became a national participatory phenomenon, a sign of the will to resist: an event known worldwide,[8] defined by Conte as 'an ideal collective hug.'[9] COVID-19 and the lockdown also gave rise to an extensive production of pages, memes, videos and posts with a strong participatory, creative and ironic component. However, there was no lack of fake news and controversial uses of social networks, in particular concerning possible medical treatments or the infection's origins. However, these cases were limited overall.

Conclusion

In Italy, the COVID-19 infodemia (Rothkopf, 2003) was fuelled by three sectors of public communication. First, the communication of institutions and politics, aimed at the public good and managing the emergency, but weakened by operational delays and many conflicts. Second, the communication of the media, which in addition to a public function, also met its own criteria of 'newsworthiness, relevance, audience,' sometimes in contrast with the general interest. Third, the communication of scientists and medical experts, characterised by high prestige and reliability, but based on long-term hypotheses and research, and not always able to provide absolute and immediate answers. It is, for example, the case of the questions: 'when will the contagion curve start to fall?' or 'when will a vaccine be available?' that were continually asked of experts and scientists by journalists and analysts who repeatedly answered that they were not yet able to respond.

In addition to the contrasts between national and local institutions, mentioned above, in the Italian case, the communication of these three actors – political institutions, media and scientific experts – was not always coordinated and convergent. Raising the question of who of these was most appropriate to manage communication during a pandemic.

Italy was the first Western and European country to deal with the COVID-19 emergency in mid-February 2020, the nation where the most drastic measures were adopted and maintained longer than in any other country. It was the nation where in the northern area the world's highest death toll was reached between February and April. Considering the above, the Italian Government and authorities did not have a reference point to help them tackle COVID-19's spread. China offered a precedent, but the policies adopted by this dictatorial regime could not be replicated in a modern Western democracy. The policies adopted by the Conte Government were on the one hand to exercise clear leadership in the management of the crisis, and on the other to proceed very gradually, introducing rules and limitations step by step, hand in hand with the worsening of the situation.

There were delays, errors and underestimations in the management of the health emergency and communications, which highlighted long-term defects of the Italian health system, focused more on caring for the sick than on protecting the healthy (De Maria, 2020). Nonetheless, the constant and consistent flow of communication aroused a sense of solidarity, community and sharing. The Italians accepted the emergency and the drastic containment measures: not an obvious response, given the weak civic culture and intolerance to respecting rules shown by Italians on other occasions.

Italians' approval of the prime minister and government grew, reaching 61% and 56% (Pagnoncelli, 2020). The so-called 'rally around the flag' phenomenon which has emerged in several countries involved in the pandemic has been particularly notable in Italy due to the low initial popularity of Conte and the government. An approval that, unlike other countries, persisted in the post-emergence phase (Diamanti, 2020).

In conclusion, it is widely believed that the Italian Government managed to cope with both health and emotional emergencies. An opinion strengthened by comparison with other European countries such as the United Kingdom (UK) and France. In this regard, the highest international recognition arrived from the WHO Director-General. Tedros Adhanom Ghebreyesus officially praised the response of Italy to the coronavirus emergency and the control of the epidemic highlighting 'a combination of leadership, humility, active participation by every member of society, and implementing a comprehensive approach.'[10]

A judgement confirmed by a survey carried out in July 2020, which revealed that over 40% of Italians believes that Conte is the world leader who best managed the COVID-19 crisis.[11]

Notes

1 Conte's speech, March 4, 2020, www.governo.it/it/articolo/conferenza-stampa-del
-presidente-conte/14294 (June 21, 2020).
2 Conte's speech, March 11, 2020, www.governo.it/it/articolo/conferenza-stampa-del
-presidente-conte/14294 (June 21, 2020).
3 www.nytimes.com/2020/03/21/world/europe/italy-coronavirus-center-lessons.ht
ml (June 21, 2020).
4 www.youtube.com/watch?v=650DSCkp_VY, https://www.youtube.com/watch?
v=_ZH9-Pvew_4 (June 21, 2020).
5 www.quirinale.it/elementi/46574 (June 21, 2020).
6 https://angelusnews.com/news/vatican/full-text-pope-francis-easter-urbi-et-orbi-
message-2020/ (June 21, 2020).
7 www.thelocal.it/20200317/here-are-italys-official-top-five-balcony-chart-hits
(June 21, 2020).
8 *The New Yorker*, www.youtube.com/watch?v=EBByYjjvNzs (June 21, 2020).
9 www.facebook.com/watch/?v=225656135146923 (June 21, 2020).
10 www.who.int/dg/speeches/detail/who-director-general-s-opening-remarks-at-the
-media-briefing-on-covid-19---1-july-2020.

11 www.affaritaliani.it/politica/conte-miglior-leader-mondiale-contro-la-pandemia-b
attuta-la-merkel-sondaggio-677104.html?refresh_ce (July 21, 2020).

References

Alfonso, L., & Comin, G. (2020). #*Zonarossa*. Guerini Associati, Milano.

Chadwick, A. (2013). *The Hybrid Media System*. Oxford University Press, Oxford.

De Maria, R. (2020). Caratteristiche ed errori della gestione sanitaria della pandemia
da COVID19 in Italia: una défaillance di sistema. *Rivista Trimestrale di Scienza
dell'Amministrazione*, 1, doi:10.32049/RTSA.2020.2.05 http://rtsa.eu/RTSA_2
_2020_de_Maria.pdf.

Diamanti, I.(2020). Conte, Leader rifugio di un Paese Impaurito. *La Repubblica*, June
29, p. 8. Accessed June 13, 2020: https://rep.repubblica.it/pwa/generale/2020/0
6/28/news/conte_leader_rifugio_di_un_paese_impaurito_il_piu_amato_e_an
cora_lui-260468262/. Research available at: www.demos.it/a01741.php accessed
13-6-2020.

Di Cesare, D. (2020). *Virus Sovrano*. Bollati Boringhieri, Torino.

McNair, B. (2017). *An Introduction to Political Communication*. Taylor & Francis, London.

Ministry of Health (2007). *National Plan for Preparedness and Response to an Influenza
Pandemic*. Roma. Accessed June 13, 2020: www.salute.gov.it/imgs/C_17_pubblic
azioni_501_ulterioriallegati_ulterioreallegato_0_alleg.pdf.

Nichols, T. N. (2017). *The Death of Expertise*. Oxford University Press, Oxford.

Pagnoncelli, N. (2020). Scenari. *Corriere della Sera*, April 26, p. 14. Accessed June 13,
2020: www.corriere.it/politica/20_aprile_26/effetto-coronavirus-meno-consensi
-lega-254percento-pd-4-punti-balzo-m5s-186percento-cf3b6f68-8727-11ea-9b77
-4fc0668b38e0.shtml.

Presidenza Consiglio dei Ministri, Dipartimento Protezione Civile (2020). Raccolta delle
disposizioni in materia di contenimento e gestione dell'emergenza epidemiologica da
COVID-19 e Testo coordinato delle ordinanze di protezione civile. Accessed May
13, 2020: www.upi.emilia-romagna.it/?option=com_fileman&view=file&routed
=1&name=TESTO%20UNICO%20COORDINATO%20COVID-19_24_3_2020
.pdf.pdf&folder=&container=fileman-files

Rothkopf, D. J. (2003, May 5). When the Buzz Bites Back. *The Washington Post*, p. B01,
Accessed June 10, 2020 www1.udel.edu/globalagenda/2004/student/readings/info
demic.html.

Taggart, P. (2004). Populism and Representative Politics in Contemporary Europe.
Journal of Political Ideologies, 3, 269–288.

WHO – World Health Organization (2005). *WHO Global Influenza Preparedness Plan.
The Role of WHO and Recommendations for National Measures before and during Pandemics*.
WHO, Geneva. Accessed June 13, 2020: www.who.int/csr/resources/publications/i
nfluenza/WHO_CDS_CSR_GIP_2005_5.pdf.

12

SPAIN

Managing the uncertain while facing economic collapse

Sergio Pérez Castaños and Alberto Mora Rodríguez

Political context

The COVID-19 outbreak in Spain took the newly created coalition government by surprise. For the first time in 40 years of modern democracy, Spain has a coalition government formed by the traditional labour party (PSOE) and the former communist party, now in an electoral coalition with a smaller party called United We Can (UP). This government came from the 2019 'year of elections' in which there were up to five different elections, two of them national. The first, held in April, led to a deadlock in government and voters were called again in November. This call depicted a quite similar Congress, but by the end of the year an agreement was achieved.

The government formed in January 2020, and the greatest number of members (17) in it, including the Prime Minister, Pedro Sánchez, are designated as PSOE. The parties govern Congress with no majority, leaving them to continuously negotiate within the political branches to get policy working. Summing up, from those elections, the coalition gets 155 seats from an overall of 350; 120 from PSOE and 35 from UP based on a vote of 40.8%, 28% for PSOE and 12.8% for UP.

Chronology

When this chapter was completed in early September 2020, there were around 283,000 official cases in Spain and up to 29,000 deaths from COVID-19.[1] To reduce the spread of the virus, there were several actions taken by the government. First, on March 14, the State of Alarm[2] was declared through Royal Decree 463/2020. This suspended some civil liberties such as the freedom of mobility, forcing citizens to stay inside their homes and to only go out for essential

DOI: 10.4324/9781003120254-14

activities such as work or grocery shopping. But, due to the rapidly increasing cases of COVID-19, the government decided two weeks later on what they called 'freezing of all non-essential activities' and the general confinement of any person not working in essential economic areas. This had a clear impact on the economy and unemployment levels increased to 9.3% during March alone.[3] To help the economic situation, the Commission for Reconstruction was created by Congress. Its aim is to develop certain lines of action to get the economy back on track, approving fund allocation, tax benefits or unemployment measures, among others.

This generated a new system that allowed entrepreneurs and business owners to close their offices and companies and temporarily fire workers with the compromise of hiring them back when everything goes back to normal. This is called the Temporary Work Regulation Expedient (ERTE) and led to thousands of people losing their income and job.[4] Hand in hand with this, the government created the so-called Minimum Vital Income. This is a guaranteed minimum income system that worked with other existing social benefits. These measures were passed by the government on May 29 and by Congress on June 10, counting on the support of almost all the political groups except the far-right political party, VOX, which abstained.

During all this process, there are several important dates to point out. The first one is the first appearance of the Director of the Centre for Coordination on Sanitary Alerts and Emergencies (CCAES), Dr Fernando Simón, on February 2, as the first case was detected in Spain on January 31 in the Canary Islands. When the cases 'jumped' into continental Spain, by February 24, the press conferences became more and more frequent, often held on a daily basis.

The next important media event was on March 13, when the government declared the 'State of Alarm' and the lockdown began. On this day, Prime Minister Sánchez (PSOE) spoke to the nation and explained the measures being put in place such as the reduction of mobility, the mobilisation of the military to help the police and the health services and the most novel one, the creation of four 'super ministries' in charge of the main areas of importance[5] during the pandemic. The plurality of profiles in the Crisis Cabinet responds to the need for establishing different communicative strategies as there are several actors with different strategic and operative needs in terms of communication (Frandsen & Johansen, 2020).

From that moment on, every week there was a joint press conference held by all those four ministries plus some of the main actors fighting the pandemic, such as the director of the National Health Institute or the General Director of the Police. Every Saturday, the Prime Minister would address the nation announcing new measures or modifications during the State of Alarm.

Of all the different challenges the government had to overcome, the most important was regarding the lack of sanitary materials for first responders. This, combined with press conferences in which there were no questions allowed, led to the development of a more aggressive opposition discourse. During the first weeks, almost all political factions supported the government measures but, since April, the discourse among the main opposition parties became more and more belligerent. This led to several civil society initiatives such as popular demonstrations against the government and its 'suspension of civil rights.'[6]

Despite this, every day since the lockdown began, at 8 pm citizens spontaneously came to their windows to clap. These so-called 'sanitary claps' had the objective to highlight the job that first responders were doing. This happened since March 14 up to late May, when the severe restrictions were lifted. See Table 12.1.

Analysis

How did the government manage the crisis?

When facing a sanitary crisis, preparation is essential, and this has been the main topic for political and media confrontation in Spain. Despite Spain being structured internally into 17 regions, each with competences about Public Health, it seemed clear none of them or Central Government were ready for the situation that unfolded. The main issue to underline here is that at the beginning of the crisis the situation was being downplayed during the speeches, mostly in an attempt to limit social alarm, which caused a negative readiness to face the incoming situation throughout the system. This only changed after March 12, when the Prime Minister stated that 'The Government, in Coordination with the Regions, will take whatever measure needs, when and where it is needed' foreshadowing the State of Alarm.

The following period of management was characterised by a periodical and constant feed of information from the government to the media. Each actor had a clear purpose: from the ministers in announcing new measures, to the technicians providing daily information. From March 16, the most relevant measures and a weekly summary was reserved for the Prime Minister, who every Saturday addressed the media. The strategy of naming technical speakers in crisis situations is quite usual. Thanks to the legitimacy and neutrality that they provide, it limits the rejection from citizens. In this sense, Dr Fernando Simón was a key speaker. Nevertheless, his knowledge, pedagogic skills and calm when addressing the media did not make him immune to criticism from the political opposition, mostly focused on his minimising of the risk in January.

The communication strategy of the government aimed to demonstrate all measures were supported by science, constantly referring to both national and international epidemiological and health experts. But social unity was encouraged by the warlike language used by the Prime Minister, including elements such as 'war,' 'battle,' 'frontline,' 'common enemy,' 'weapons' or metaphorical rhetoric such as 'The enemy is not awaiting, it went through our defences long time ago. Now the wall to contain it is in everything that we have built as a country and community,' 'Every one of us have a specific mission in this battle' or 'We are deep in a vital stage in the battle against the virus.' These messages

TABLE 12.1 Spain chronology

Date		Diffusion of COVID-19	Key official actions	Key communication events
January	1	Unofficial infection starts.		
	24		The Ministry of Health (MH) defines the criteria to be tested for COVID-19.	
	31	First positive case.		The director of the CCAES during a press conference states, 'There will be a couple of cases.'
February	25	Five new positive cases.	MH decided to get tests for every sick person with pneumonia symptoms.	The president of the Spanish Epidemiology Society states, 'There will be no held up hospitals in Spain.'
	26		MH changes the risk level from 'low' to 'moderate.'	The director of the CCAES begins to address the nation and media every day.
March	2	Infected toll exceeds 100.		
	3	First person dead and tested for COVID-19.	MH recommends celebrating every sport event with no public attendance.	
	7			When asked about March 8 demonstration, the director of the CCAES says that 'it does not seem to be a risk element.'
	9	Infected toll exceeds 1,000.		
	10	Infected toll exceeds 1,500.	Spanish Government cancels every event for more than 100 people.	
	11	Infected toll exceeds 2,500.	World Health Organisation (WHO) declares global pandemic.	
	12		Schools are closed in every Spanish region.	President Sánchez announces an economy plan holding a more dramatic attitude.

14	Death toll exceeds 100.	The State of Alarm is declared for 15 days by royal decree.	
15	Infected toll exceeds 5,000.	National quarantine begins.	President Sánchez announces that there would be 5 super ministries in charge of managing the crisis.
16		All borders are closed.	Weekly briefings by the Prime Minister commence.
18			The King addresses the nation followed by anti-Monarchy demonstrations.
27	Death toll exceeds 5,000. Infected toll exceeds 56,000.	Government forbids by royal decree to fire employees under Temporary employment regulations (ERTE). A second State of Alarm is declared.	
30	Death toll exceeds 7,000. Infected toll exceeds 85,000.	Every non-essential activity remains closed for 7 days.	
April 9	Death toll exceeds 15,000. Infected toll exceeds 152,000.	Congress approves the extension of the State of Alarm until April 26. Economic activity is activated again.	
12			President Sánchez states the implementation of a 'Minimum Vital Income to help families in distress.
17	Death toll exceeds 20,000.	The government changes how to count deaths.	Government officials declare data is not 'real' since every region counts cases and the deceased differently.
22		Congress approves new State of Alarm from April 26.	President Sánchez declares that sanitary material such as mask will have a government-controlled price.

(Continued)

TABLE 12.1 (Continued)

Date		Diffusion of COVID-19	Key official actions	Key communication events
	26	Death toll exceeds 23,000. Infected toll exceeds 200,000.	Children under 14 years-old can go out for one hour.	First of the 14 conferences with regional prime ministers. All of them held online.
May	2		Government prepares 4 different phases in the post-lockdown process.	
	4		Phase 0 begins. Many businesses can open up again.	
	6		A new State of Alarm is passed.	
	8	Death toll exceeds 26,000. Infected toll exceeds 223,000.	Phase 1 begins in some parts of the country.	
	14		Commission for Reconstruction begins to work in Congress.	
	18		Masks become compulsory on public transport and in indoor public spaces.	
	20			President Sánchez publicly asks for forgiveness if any mistakes have been made.
	22		Phase 2 begins in half of the country.	
June	3		Congress approves last State of Alarm.	
	8		Phase 3 begins. Almost everything back to normal.	
	10		The Minimum Vital Income is approved.	
	21	Death toll exceeds 28,000.	The State of Alarm ends. The country begins the so-called 'New Normality.' Masks compulsory in any public area.	Last of the 14 conferences with regional prime ministers held.

aimed to reinforce the exceptionality of the situation and appeal to the political and public opinion unity to earn legitimacy and social support. The seriousness transmitted with the warlike rhetoric was matched by the measures adopted, mobilising almost 20% of GDP in economic measures. The main objective was to face the health, economic and social crisis, elements that were emphasised in all the speeches and that would take form in the measures published in the 17 royal decrees approved from March to June.

The other dimension emphasised in speeches was the international scope of the problem, a strategy of minimising the guilt and sharing the burden with other organisations and governments. In this sense, the Prime Minister stated that 'the world is facing a war against a common enemy to every citizen wherever they live'; adding pressure on the European institutions and looking at them and their compromise to solve the situation: 'Europe cannot and would not fail, it has to be up to the challenge.'[7]

In terms of communication management, there were a significant number of pro-government communicators who, in prime time, were called on to speak about the measures. Likewise, the government created the hashtag #Estevirusloparamosunidos (#WeStopThisVirusTogether), which was widely used across online communities.

From an accountability point of view, the Prime Minister appeared 14 times in Congress and celebrated 14 conferences with the regional prime ministers. The Minister of Health appeared 13 times before the Parliamentary Commission. As stated before, the Commission for the Reconstruction was created. Likewise, between March 12 and June 21 the government held a total of 187 press conferences[8] and up to 47 meetings with societal agencies.

The government response was not free of mistakes both in the technical dimension and in the communication area. In addition to the lack of anticipation and the delay in the acquisition of medical elements, several mistakes were made which provided the political opposition with ammunition to attack the government management of the crisis. This, combined with social media agitation, provoked several demonstrations, but they were small and biased by social class. Among the most important mistakes were the constant modifications to the measures, such as the definition of which workers are catalogued as essential, or the use of masks to avoid the spread of the virus. Another well-criticised issue was the very small amount of time between new measures being approved and when they came into effect, with almost no time for the affected economic sectors to adapt themselves.

In the technical area, changes in how statistics regarding new cases and deaths were reported created fear and insecurity, even more when adding up all the data provided by regions did not result in the same numbers stated by the government. Likewise, a longstanding problem was the purchase of medical supplies that were against medical standards.

During the first weeks there were also several speakers that provoked some confusion on who was leading on measures. This, combined with the quite long press conferences and the enormous amount of questions asked, increased the probability of making mistakes. One clear example is a statement given by the Chief of the Civil Guard, who affirmed that the police force was fighting fake news to minimise opposition to the government. This was interpreted by the opposition to mean the government was using the police to pursue their own political interests.

There were also delays in addressing the media, calling the media to be present at a certain hour and appearing much later, and the selection of questions made by the Press Secretary meant that several media outlets decided not to cover those press conferences for a while. Additionally, there were mistakes in coordination and cooperation across levels of government. The clearest example is that every Sunday there were meetings with all the regional prime ministers, but all the measures that were supposed to be discussed had already been announced during Saturday's press conference. There were also divergences among the parties in the government coalition, which gave the impression there was no internal cohesion and that there was no leadership and coordination among ministries.

The other actors in play

Political opposition has not been homogeneous nor supportive of governmental measures or their consistency during the most critical stages. Thus, while regional and the left-wing parties have supported the government, the right-wing parties (the conservatives (PP) and VOX) have been critical of the government's management of the crisis. The opposition's main argument was to depict the government as clumsy and incompetent. One of the key discursive frameworks used by these parties was to try to connect the mobilisations held in Madrid during Women's Day, March 8, with the fact that this city and region was, by far, the most affected by the virus. Likewise, there were references to the lack of democratic guarantees. This face-off between the two major political parties, PSOE and PP, saw the regions become the major battlefield as conservative-ruled regional governments attacked central government over the lack of funds, sanitary materials and the responsibility for elderly residences, one of the most affected groups. There was such an aggressive tone in Congress that the President of the Chamber had to call order and threaten to suspend the session several times and publicly denounce the behaviour of representatives. The media was also polarised and aligned with one or another party.

Despite this, we have to point out two outstanding phenomena: the first one is the clear position of several well-known television commentators who were the most critical of the government; the second is the inclusion of clear fake stories in well-established media platforms' news bulletins. The uncertainty of the moment and the context of growing political polarisation created the perfect environment for fake news to flourish. This fake information is powered by political news flows (Flores-Vivar, 2020) as the main objective is to disseminate misinformation for political advantage (Amorós-García, 2018: 35). In this sense, while normally, fake news spreads within pseudo-media outlets with no rules or editorial process at all, this content also appeared in trusted mainstream media bulletins. But this forced media to also publicly refute this information, as well as public institutions. In this sense, the so-called 'verifiers' have increased their visibility as fact-checkers and have helped in denouncing fake news and facilitating real data or information (Paniagua-Rojano et al., 2020).[9] The Centre for Sociological Research, which polls public opinion monthly, found 66.7% of the population believe that information and news should be controlled by establishing just one official source.[10]

Conclusion

Communication management in Spain took on a choral structure with a strong presence of government members reinforced by the work of technical experts. There has been a continuous flow of information emphasising measures were justified by the legitimacy of science and the internationalisation of the crisis. The government also appealed to a national effort of collaboration and solidarity. Despite the missteps and errors, the exceptionality of the moment which tends to reinforce the position of government, known as the 'rally a round the flag' effect (Mueller, 1970: 21), the activation of strong economic measures and the difficulties held by the opposition in generating a solid contra-argument made the government's approval ratings quite stable. On the other hand, there has been a growing political, social and media polarisation which combined with the upcoming economic and social crisis foretells increasing levels of institutional disaffection in the upcoming years.

Notes

1 Data from Ministry of Health: www.mscbs.gob.es/profesionales/saludPublica/ccayes /alertasActual/nCov-China/home.htm
2 This exceptional regime is included in the Spanish Constitution article 116.2 and when activated, several basic rights can be suspended such as mobility, occupation of private sector companies or public prices fixation, among others. The first time it is declared, it can be done by the government and only for 15 days. From that moment on, it is necessary to count on the support of the majority of the Congress.
3 This 9.3% of increase in March is added to the 7.9% increase in unemployment during April and 0.7% during May.
4 The exact number affected by these measures can be found at: www.mitramiss.gob .es/estadisticas/reg/welcome.htm
5 These were Transportations and Communications, Health, Interior and Defence. All of them ruled by PSOE.
6 Examples of these demonstrations were those that took place in mid-May in the conservative Salamanca district (Madrid), or the one against masks, held on August 16 also in Madrid.
7 Both sentences are included in the speech given by the Spanish Prime Minister on April 28, video available at: www.lamoncloa.gob.es/consejodeministros/resumenes/ paginas/2020/280420-consejo_ministros.aspx

8 Twenty of them made by the Prime Minister, 80 by ministers, 43 by technical members of the government and 44 by experts.
9 Two major examples have been Maldita (https://maldita.es) and Newtral (www
   .newtral.es).
10 These related to question number 6 (Pregunta 6) in the poll: www.cis.es/cis/export
   /sites/default/-Archivos/Marginales/3260_3279/3279/es3279mar.html

References

Amorós-García, M. (2018). *Fake News. La verdad de las noticias falsas*. Plataforma Actual.

Flores-Vivar, J. M. (2020). Datos masivos, algoritmización y nuevos medios frente a desinformación y fake news. Bots para minimizar el impacto en las organizaciones. *Comunicación y Hombre*, 16, 101–114. https://doi.org/10.26441/rc17.2-2018-a12

Frandsen, F., & Johansen, W. (2020). Public Sector Communication: Risk and Crisis Communication. In V. Luoma-aho & M. Canel. *The Handbook of Public Crisis Communication*. Wiley. https://doi.org/10.1002/9781119263203.ch15

Mueller, J. E. (1970). Presidential Popularity from Truman to Johnson. *American Political Science Review*, 64(1), 18–34. https://doi.org/10.2307/1955610

Paniagua-Rojano, F., Seoane-Pérez, F., & Magallón-Rosa, R. (2020). Anatomía del bulo electoral: la desinformación política durante la campaña del 28-A en España. *Revista CIDOB d'Afers Internacionals*, 124, 123–145. https://doi.org/10.24241/rcai. 2020.124.1.123

13

SWEDEN

Lone hero or stubborn outlier?

Bengt Johansson and Orla Vigsø

Political context

Sweden is governed by a coalition between the Social Democratic party and the Green Party (28% and 4% in the 2018 general election), led by Prime Minister (PM) Stefan Löfven (Social Democrats). The minority government is dependent on support from two small centre parties (Liberal Party and Centre Party) and the Left Party. The support from the centre parties was formalised after the longest period (18 weeks) of attempts to form a government in Swedish modern history. In February 2020, the support for the government was at an all-time low, with only 23% support for the Social Democrats and 4–5% for the Green Party.

During recent years, the political debate has been dominated by migration, and all other issues have more or less been viewed through a 'migration frame,' where (organised) crime and deficits in the welfare system or the general development of the Swedish society have been related to the proportion of immigrants in Swedish society. The Sweden Democrats, who built their political capital on a critical approach to immigration, have won increasing voter support. From winning their first mandates in parliament in 2010, they became the biggest party in the opinion polls by early 2020. For the first time, the party was larger than the Social Democrats.

This changed dramatically during the months to follow. Sweden – as many other countries – experienced a 'rally around the flag' opinion swing, with the Social Democrats increasing their support to more than 30%. Government agencies in general and in particular the ones responsible for managing the crisis also experienced increased support, especially during the initial phase of the crisis (Esaiasson et al., 2020; Kantar/Sifo, 2020). However, the support for government and authorities has to some extent declined during the later phases of the pandemic, when the Swedish strategy has been criticised (Novus, 2020).

DOI: 10.4324/9781003120254-15

Chronology

The news media coverage and public debate about the pandemic contains a number of general themes:

(1) Crisis management (measures taken, and problems accomplishing them).
(2) Consequences of the pandemic, in different parts of society (business, tourism, restaurants, sports, culture etc.).
(3) Living and dying with corona (stories of how people deal with the pandemic, both in terms of victims/survivors and coping with social distancing).
(4) Sweden abroad (how Sweden is portrayed in foreign news media, but also how other nations evaluate the Swedish strategy and their decisions regarding open or closed borders with Sweden).
(5) COVID-19 in different countries (news stories about the crisis in different countries, especially countries with large outbreaks like Brazil, China, the United States etc., but also countries which limited the spread of the virus like Germany, Austria and New Zealand.

Even if the political debate was limited, some political discussions arose related to problems of crisis preparedness (supplies of medical equipment), the rather low intensive care capacity, problems of testing for COVID-19, and the quality of elderly care (especially working conditions in retirement homes). Another area where political aspects have been prevalent is the role of the state in saving businesses from bankruptcy, and the long-term consequences. See Table 13.1.

Daily broadcasted televised press conferences were a central part of the government's and the authorities' crisis communication, while public debate took place on Twitter, Facebook and other social media during the whole phase. It is hard to estimate the effects of this at the present stage, but what is clear is that the public debate on social forums has been agitated, both in favour of and in opposition to the official policy.

When PM Löfven gave a televised speech to the nation on March 22, this was the first time a PM used the opportunity to address the nation. The tone was sombre and serious, and the speech contained few specific points. It was mostly a call for collective efforts.

Analysis

When analysing the communication in Sweden regarding COVID-19, there are some basic facts that need to be taken into consideration. First, Sweden has for centuries had highly autonomous agencies, and the locus of expertise, resources and work force lies in the agencies rather than in central government offices. The government rules by instructions, budgets and informal contacts, but the government cannot directly command agencies how to act in a specific situation. Secondly, the Swedish political system is highly decentralised, with 21 regions in charge of the health care system, having the power to allocate taxes. Elderly

TABLE 13.1 Sweden chronology

Date		Diffusion of COVID-19	Key official actions	Key communication events*
February	1			
	23		COVID-19 is classified as a dangerous disease.	The Public Health Agency (PHA) is criticised by medical doctors for playing down the risk of community transmission and dissemination of inaccurate information about crisis preparedness.
	26	First Swedish infected case.		
	30	14 confirmed cases in Sweden.		
March	1			Media discussion about PHA recommendation to let children returning home from holidays (in Italy) to return to school.
	6			Daily (weekdays) press conferences from PHA and other authorities broadcast on public service TV at 2 pm (continues until June 10).
	10		COVID-19 is announced to be in the phase of community transmission in Sweden.	
			Public gatherings limited to max. 500 participants.	
	11	First Swedish death from COVID-19		
	13		The Public Health Agency abandons its earlier strategy of testing all persons that have symptoms after travelling abroad.	Stock market falls amid media talk of an economic recession. News stories about hoarding and empty shelves in the stores.
	15		Citizens to avoid unnecessary visits to hospitals/care homes and non-essential travel abroad.	

(Continued)

TABLE 13.1 (Continued)

Date	Diffusion of COVID -19	Key official actions	Key communication events*
16		The government presents a large crisis package to support business. Short-term layoffs are introduced.	
17		The government, in line with European Commission recommendations, stops all non-essential travel from outside Europe. PHA recommends remote learning to all upper secondary schools, adult education schools and universities. People over the age of 70 are advised to avoid unnecessary social contact.	
19		Citizens to avoid non-essential domestic travel.	PM Stefan Löfven gives speech to the nation.
22			Debate about the high death tolls in immigrant-dense Stockholm suburbs.
23			Public debate on companies receiving support from the state and giving dividends to shareholders.
24		PHA establishes new rules for bars and restaurants to avoid crowding.	
27		The government restricts public gatherings to maximum 50 participants.	
26			News stories begin to criticise shortages of medical supplies.
31	4,835 confirmed cases, 332 deaths.	National ban on visiting care homes. PHA presents more detailed information on how to achieve social distancing in different parts of society (business, restaurants, personal responsibility etc.).	

April	1		Editor of the prestige newspaper *Dagens Nyheter* criticises the government's COVID-19 strategy.
	2		First media reports about COVID-19 outbreaks in care homes.
	3	The Ministry for Foreign Affairs advises against travel to all countries up to June 15, 2020.	
	4	The government proposes temporary law changes to be able to take quicker measures against COVID-19.	
	5		King Carl XVI Gustav addresses the nation.
	13	The Swedish National Agency for Education assesses that traditional student graduation will be possible.	A large number of news stories are covering local decisions and reactions from students.
	14		22 researchers claim the strategy has failed, leading to intense debate.
	15		The well-known Swedish television and radio host Adam Alsing dies from COVID-19, aged 51.
	16		Reports about fear of increased spread when people gather to celebrate Walpurgis night.
	20	Minister of Finance Magdalena Andersson estimates the cost for short-term layoffs being 5 billion Euro.	Companies cheating to receive support is heavily criticised.
	22		Reports of people not paying attention to social distancing in outdoor seating at restaurants leads to temporary closure if regulations not followed.
	30	21,715 cases, 876 deaths.	

(Continued)

TABLE 13.1 (Continued)

Date		Diffusion of COVID-19	Key official actions	Key communication events*
May	4			Critical reports about prioritising among patients with COVID-19 symptoms (some elderly not receiving intensive care).
	5			Lena Hallengren, Minister of Health, urges regions to speed up testing of COVID-19.
	7			PHA clarifies position on wearing masks to protect from COVID-19. No recommendation for use by private citizens in public spaces.
	13		Domestic travel restrictions are changed. Recommendations allow non-essential journeys one or two hours by car from home residence.	
	21			Sweden reported having the highest average death toll in last seven days.
	24			Reactions to Swedes being banned from entering other countries when borders are opened.
	26			Less than 10% of the Stockholm population have COVID-19 antibodies, much lower than expected.
	28			Former chief epidemiologist Ann Linde admits she has concerns about the Swedish strategy.

29	PHA presents new recommendations to allow sporting events and matches to take place from June 14	
31	38,849 cases, 4,622 deaths.	
June 5	The government seeks to secure large-scale testing.	Party leader of Sweden Democrats demands the resignation of chief epidemiologist Anders Tegnell.
7		Party leaders debate on public service TV, government is attacked for shortcomings.
10		COVID-19 party leaders debate in Parliament.
11		Reactions to decisions in Denmark, Finland and Norway to keep the borders to Sweden closed.
13	Travel restrictions for domestic travel are removed.	
14		First day without any COVID-19 related deaths since mid-March.
15		Massive local outbreak of COVID-19 in Gällivare, in the north of Sweden.
17	The Ministry for Foreign Affairs removes travel restrictions on a number of EU countries, but prolonged restrictions outside of Europe until August 31.	
29	67,667 cases, 5,310 deaths.	

Note: ★ = data is collected from when the issue was covered on the public service website SVT Online for the first time.

care and care homes are the responsibility of 250 municipalities. This means that crisis management takes place in a highly decentralised system where coordination and information are central parts, which slows down crisis response. In addition to this, the government can only declare a state of emergency in order to centralise authority during wartime, not during other crises (Pierre, 2020).

Another important prerequisite is the high trust Swedes have in public authorities, which played an important role for the choice of crisis management strategy. Using 'nudges' rather than prohibition, i.e. recommendations of behaviour rather than legal restrictions, was considered a more effective and, most importantly, a sustainable way to manage the pandemic.

From the very beginning, the government made it clear that the response to this epidemic would be according to the same procedures used in earlier pandemics: the Public Health Authority (PHA) was put in charge and expected to issue recommendations for regions, municipalities and citizens, based on scientific evidence (Giritli Nygren & Olofsson, 2020). Dealing with the virus was a question of collecting facts, analysing them in a scientific way and suggesting measures based on the conclusions. This strategy was from the beginning (March and April) widely applauded by all political parties and media, and chief epidemiologist Anders Tegnell was given a key role as he presented daily analyses and recommendations by the PHA. He also gained the status of a popular icon for his calm communicative style and his steady appeal to react according to 'what we know in the scientific community.' No recommendations were presented until there was what the PHA deemed as solid scientific proof to back them up.

Even if some experts criticised the chosen strategy, the general media frame portrayed Tegnell and the PHA as a sensible, calm, scientific representative of the Swedish way. Swedish media reported how governments in neighbouring countries acted contrary to the advice of their own scientific expertise when deciding on a lockdown, and reports of other countries' criticism were generally framed as a lack of understanding of how things ought to be done.

The Swedish strategy was never to stop the disease, but instead to contain the spread of the virus in order to avoid overloading hospitals with patients, the famous 'flattening the curve' approach. The virus was not seen as a mortal threat to people who did not belong to the high-risk groups (the elderly, those with underlying illnesses), and it was believed that a lockdown would cause more severe problems for the whole population. Therefore, only people with symptoms were asked to stay home and isolate themselves, while schools, restaurants, shops and factories remained open.

The PHA issued recommendations regarding the distance between people and the maximum number of people in one room. In general, the system relied on individual responsibility and sound judgement about self-protection. The PHA underlined that restrictions would become more severe if people did not follow the recommendations issued.

With the protection of the elderly and sick as a top priority, this also entailed a transfer of responsibilities to the regional and local levels, due to the structure of the Swedish health care system. Making sure that care homes, hospitals etc. had the equipment to secure both staff and patients or occupants became a task for regional/local authorities, and this proved to be highly problematic. During the deregulation of the last 20 years or so, the central authority securing a stock of medicine and protective wear had been cancelled, and everything had been reduced to a just-in-time basis, meaning that supplies were kept at an absolute minimum. When suddenly the whole world was demanding medicine, rubber gloves, facial masks etc., supply could not keep up with demand. Other short-comings related to the conditions in the elderly care, such as high levels of staff turnover, limited training and limited knowledge of Swedish language among the staff has been pointed out as factors worsening the situation. This led to care homes becoming hot spots of the disease, with high death tolls among the weak and elderly. The curve may have been flattened, but the main goal of the action had been missed.

While support for the government's way of handling the situation by leaving it in the hands of PHA had been unanimous, criticism was by the end of May being voiced as the number of deaths kept rising. A contributing factor might have been the rather cool way the deaths were presented at the daily press conferences, where chief epidemiologist Tegnell kept assuring the press and the public that the path chosen was the right one, and that Sweden was moving in the right direction. Critics found this a somewhat offensive framing for the news that 100 more people had died since yesterday. Where Swedes had been safe in the knowledge that their country was the only one which did the right thing, an 'outlier' in the positive sense, it now became clear that Sweden may be an outlier in a negative sense. Sweden was no longer admired by others as the courageous, rational agent.

Until late May, criticism of the strategy had mainly been presented by other researchers and experts. One observation is that experts to a large extent replaced politicians as central actors in the media logic of news covering COVID-19. The fight over how to interpret the COVID-19 strategy became an expert discourse (as well as a layman's discussion on social media).

In June, the critique of leadership and choice of strategy increased, notably from other politicians, criticising the slow testing capacity and the high death tolls in care homes; a critique which to some extent backfired when the regions and municipalities with the most severe problems turned out to be led by these parties. The lack of leadership was also questioned, with some arguing that the government had been a backseat driver letting the PHA and other authorities take the lead in managing the pandemic. This critique was expressed during previous crises and reflects what has been seen as a general critique of Swedish crisis management (Pierre, 2020).

The sharp line between government and expert authorities and the decentralised political system complicates strong political leadership during a crisis. Experts play a very important role, and a great deal of government work is about coordinating crisis management. This is perhaps symbolically made visible by the fact that the government and authorities to a large extent had separate press briefings during the early phases of the pandemic. Even if PM Stefan Löfven held a speech to the nation and was visible, it was chief epidemiologist Anders Tegnell who was regarded as the commander in chief fighting the COVID-19 in Sweden.

By the end of June, Swedes are still prohibited from travelling to many countries in Europe. As testing increases, the number of COVID-19 cases increases, but the number of patients needing intense care is declining, as is the death toll (from a rather high level). Sports events are taking place – without an audience – but most amusement parks are closed, and big events are postponed or cancelled. Still, life goes on almost as usual, not many wear face masks (not recommended but debated) and social distancing is – more or less – performed in public spaces. The general feeling is that the pandemic is far from over.

References

Esaiasson, P., Sohlberg, J., Ghersetti, M., & Johansson, B. (2020, April 30). How the coronavirus crisis affects citizen trust in government institutions and in unknown others – Evidence from 'the Swedish Experiment.' https://doi.org/10.31235/osf.io/6yw9r

Giritli Nygren, K., & Olofsson, A. (2020). Managing the COVID-19 pandemic through individual responsibility: The consequences of a world risk society and enhanced ethopolitics. *Journal of Risk Research*, doi:10.1080/13669877.2020.1756382.

Kantar/Sifo. (2020). *Rapport om förtroende, oro och beteende under coronakrisen 21 mars–15 juni Rapport till MSB*. Stockholm: Kantar/Sifo.

Novus. (2020). *Väljarbarometer*. https://novus.se/valjarbarometer-arkiv/

Pierre, J. (2020). Nudges against pandemics: Sweden's COVID-19 containment strategy in perspective. *Policy and Society*, doi:10.1080/14494035.2020.178378.

14

THE UK

From consensus to confusion

Ruth Garland and Darren Lilleker

Political context

The UK government entered the COVID-19 crisis with a legacy of ten years of austerity and a country divided by nearly four years of Brexit. Boris Johnson started his premiership in July 2019 as one of the least trusted leaders in recent history (Grieve, 2019). In the lead up to the general election six months later, a litany of mishaps appeared to undermine his reputation further. His decision to prorogue (close) Parliament was ruled unlawful by the Supreme Court, 21 senior Conservatives were expelled from his party, and the government lost 12 parliamentary divisions (votes).

However, Johnson could rely on three sources of political capital when the crisis hit. He had vanquished his opponents to win the most decisive general election victory in ten years, he fulfilled his promise to 'Get Brexit Done' when the new parliament ratified the EU Withdrawal Bill, and as a consistent supporter of the National Health Service (NHS) he had distanced himself from his party's austerity agenda by promising more money for hospitals, schools and the police in the 2019 Conservative party manifesto.

Full of confidence following election victory, he started to marginalise the media. Journalists were excluded from political briefings, and ministerial appearances were limited. Johnson's controversial senior adviser Dominic Cummings exceeded his powers by sacking a political adviser and was accused of threatening to 'whack' the BBC (Shipman, 2020). Disagreements with the three devolved nations, not least over Brexit, threatened consensus within the Union. Hence the context is of a leader with a semi-authoritarian approach to governance with significant strength in parliament, but not necessarily commanding the support of the whole country.

DOI: 10.4324/9781003120254-16

Chronology

Communication moments and media events

The Health Secretary chaired the first government emergency (COBRA) meeting to discuss the virus on January 24, informing reporters the threat to the UK was 'low' (ITV News, 2020a). The next day, the Foreign Office advised against all travel to China's affected Hubei province. The prime minister (PM) missed four further COBRA meetings, chairing his first on March 2 (Calvert et al., 2020a). At a televised press briefing on March 3, Johnson spoke positively about shaking hands with hospitalised coronavirus patients, on the same day that a sub-group of SAGE, the government's scientific advisory group, advised against 'handshakes.' On March 16, he led the first daily press briefing. These 60–90-minute sessions were broadcast by the BBC, establishing a format that placed government scientists alongside ministers. Deploying short, memorable slogans and distinctive 'emergency' graphics that were widely disseminated on hoardings, the www.gov.uk website, newspapers and social media, the briefings provided the focal point for public communication. See Table 14.1.

Four key media moments challenged the government's narrative: the response to Johnson's sickness absence from March 27 to April 27, the rising criticism of government delays (Calvert et al., 2020b), Johnson's widely criticised launch of the 'roadmap' to easing lockdown on May 10, and the government's response to the behaviour of Johnson's adviser Dominic Cummings in driving 264 miles to Durham on March 27, the day Johnson tested positive for coronavirus.

Political and social issues

Although the government had distanced itself from post-2010 austerity it could not avoid the damaging legacy of local public service cuts and a largely privatised 'inadequate, unfair and unsustainable' system of elderly care desperately in need of reform (Dilnot, 2011; LGA, 2018). Report recommendations were ignored although the 2019 Conservative Manifesto contained a commitment to bring plans for an integrated and sustainable social care system to parliament within a year (Conservative Party, 2019). A three-day pandemic planning event in October 2016, Exercise Cygnus, revealed flaws in Britain's Emergency Preparedness, Resilience and Response (EPRR) plan but the conclusions were never published (Nuki & Gardner, 2020).

Public trust in government was already low following a series of controversies dating back to the Iraq War of 2003 (Ipsos MORI, 2019) but there were three impartial public institutions that continued to unite the nation: the NHS, the BBC and the monarchy. Protecting the NHS became a key part of the message while the Queen and BBC amplified the government's message; the latter only being critical when there were clear inconsistencies between government announcements and evidence, particularly in relation to the supply of personal protective equipment (PPE) to frontline medical staff, the situation in care

TABLE 14.1 UK chronology

Date		Diffusion of COVID-19	Key official actions	Key communication events
January	24		Health Secretary Hancock chairs the first COBRA emergency meeting to discuss COVID-19.	Johnson quoted in media saying the threat to the UK was low.
	31	First case detected, a Chinese tourist in the city of York.		
February	6	Second case detected in Brighton, a UK man returning from France.		
	28	First case of local transmission in the UK.		
March	2			Johnson chairs first weekly emergency committee (COBRA) on COVID-19, saying the UK is 'very well prepared.'
	5	First confirmed COVID-19 death in hospital. Case numbers pass 100.		
	13	Confirmed cases rise from 208 to 798.	Government advises care homes close to visitors with symptoms. Premier League fixtures and London marathon postponed.	
	14	Cases rise to 1,140 and deaths to 21.		Government announces that UK has moved from 'contain' to 'delay', and ends community 'test and trace.'

(*Continued*)

TABLE 14.1 (Continued)

Date	Diffusion of COVID-19	Key official actions	Key communication events
16			PM leads the first daily COVID-19 televised press briefing on BBC1, 5 pm; these continue daily til June 23.
17		Chancellor announces largest package of emergency state support for business since the 2008 financial crash with £330bn loans, grants and tax cuts.	
23	Infections rise to more than 6,000.	Government begins lockdown, banning people from leaving home except for essential tasks or exercise. NHS contacts 1.5m clinically vulnerable telling them not to leave home.	
25		*Coronavirus Act 2020* gives government emergency powers.	
26			First 'Clap for Carers'; this would run to end of May.
27	Infections double every 3–4 days. Deaths total 759.	PM Johnson and Health Secretary Matt Hancock test positive and start isolating.	

April	2	Daily hospital admissions peak at 3,121.	Hancock declares target of 100k tests/day by the end of April.	
	5		Johnson admitted to hospital and later intensive care.	Televised broadcast by the Queen is watched by 23.5m.
	10	Daily hospital deaths peak at 980. Doubling time for cases is six days.	Crime falls by 21%. Police report issuing 1,084 fines for flouting lockdown in four weeks.	
	14		Office for Budget Responsibility (OBR) estimates that public sector borrowing will reach £273 billion (15% GDP).	
	21	Deaths up 828 to 17,337.	Parliament votes to agree a 'hybrid' virtual parliament.	
	27		Johnson returns to work.	
	29	Deaths in all settings recorded, reaching 26,097. Estimated 1/3 deaths found in care homes.		
	30		UK's testing capacity reaches 100k per day.	
	14			
	21			
	26			
	29			
May	5	At 29,427 deaths, the UK has the highest number in Europe.		
	10			Johnson launches widely criticised roadmap to lockdown.

(Continued)

TABLE 14.1 (Continued)

Date	Diffusion of COVID-19	Key official actions	Key communication events
11		Tax payers are now paying the wages of 7.5m people at a cost of £8bn a month.	Johnson briefs parliament on 'roadmap' for easing lockdown. Schools to reopen in England from June 1.
15		Transport for London negotiates £1.6bn bailout following 90% fall in public transport use.	
20			Slogan 'Stay Alert, Control the Virus, Save Lives' introduced to much criticism and satire.
23			Cummings' travel during lockdown revealed in press.
28	Deaths reach 37,460.		
31	People in hospital with COVID-19 falls 15% week-on-week. New admissions fall by 20%.	Health Protection (Coronavirus, Restrictions) (Amendment) 2020 removes many of the lockdown rules in England.	
June 2	Official report shows people from ethnic minority backgrounds twice as likely to die from COVID-19.	MPs vote to end hybrid parliament.	
9	129 further deaths recorded. Overall, 50,335 deaths by end June.		Education Secretary Williamson U-turns on schools fully opening.

homes and the ability to test for COVID-19 and develop a track and trace system for those with symptoms.

Social networks and the web

Social networks were polarised over Brexit into ideological camps, including a vociferous anti-Johnson and anti-government one. During the crisis, further ideologically diverse camps emerged, one in favour of lockdown and another that questioned strict social distancing, citing Sweden as more successful in protecting public health and the economy. The dominant group supported lockdown, evidenced by the public shaming of those flouting rules even before lockdown was fully introduced: the #covidiots hashtag went viral during the weekend of March 21–22 (O'Reilly, 2020). There was also extensive sharing of messages which reinforced the government's initial slogan: 'Stay home. Protect the NHS. Save lives.' Social media users promoted a weekly 'Clap for Carers,' mirroring the similar initiative in Italy, that ran from March 26 to the end of May. While conspiracy theories abounded regarding COVID-19 being caused by 5G networks, as well as whether Johnson's diagnosis was a hoax to gain public sympathy, these were spread by a minority and largely drowned out by messages of solidarity with key workers and the sharing of volunteering opportunities to support the most vulnerable.

The tenor changed with the introduction of a new slogan on May 20, alongside the easing of lockdown. 'Stay Alert, Control the Virus, Save Lives' was widely mocked with a meme generator (imgflp.com) allowing users to share subverted humorous versions. Critics of easing restrictions, the flocking of citizens to beauty spots during the hot May Bank Holiday weekend, U-turns over the full opening of schools and the enforced wearing of face masks from June 15 abounded. These, on the back of the scandal over Cummings' journey to Durham, and subsequent 60-mile round trip to Barnard Castle at the height of the pandemic, allegedly to test his ability to drive led to more widespread criticisms of the government's handling of the pandemic.

Hence, social media initially amplified the government's message and encouraged social norms to develop through shaming and supporting key workers, especially as health professionals turned to social media to plead with the public to obey the guidelines. However, it was also a platform for criticism, in particular, the sharing of alternative perspectives from non-British media sources (Dettmer, 2020). Anti-government voices also focused on the long-term record of post 2010 Conservative governments as well as the specific handling of the crisis, mirroring downward shifts in the polls.

Analysis

After a slow start, the UK lockdown began on March 23 and achieved high compliance largely through consent rather than enforcement (Nice, 2020). The government communications campaign focusing on the widely viewed televised daily briefings achieved high levels of political consensus, media cooperation and public engagement (Mayhew, 2020; Tobitt, 2020). Approval was 72%, according to YouGov, during the first week of lockdown and remained high despite Johnson's absence (Opinium, 2020), demonstrating the largely 'non-partisan status-quo bias' also seen on social media (Blais et al., 2020). This started to slide after May 10 when Johnson launched a widely criticised 'roadmap' for the easing of lockdown and worsened in response to the Cummings affair two weeks later. Approval dropped to 46% as lockdown was eased and the downward trajectory continued to 41% by May 29 (Walker, 2020a). By June 8, a YouGov international survey of 22 countries found that the UK government's net approval rating of −15 was joint lowest with Mexico (Armstrong, 2020). What changed in the intervening 11 weeks?

A 'part-time' prime minister?

As the pandemic took hold in China during January 2020, Johnson and his girlfriend Carrie Symonds returned to London after a week's holiday on the Caribbean island of Mustique. In mid-February, as floods threatened homes in the north, midlands and Wales, Johnson spent ten days at his country home. At weekly parliamentary questions to the prime minister on February 26, outgoing opposition Labour leader, Jeremy Corbyn, described him as 'a part-time Prime Minister,' calling on him to chair a COBRA meeting (Walker, 2020b). Three days later, and 11 days after a court approved Johnson's second divorce, Symonds announced their engagement and her pregnancy on Instagram, saying the baby would be born in the summer. Wilfred was born on April 29.

The intrusion of the prime minister's complicated private life, the use of vaguely inaccurate statements and an on-off approach to visible leadership continued to influence communication processes during the first months of the pandemic. The format for briefings was established at the first session at 5 pm on March 16, and deviated little thereafter: the elegant but neutral wood-panelled room, the three wooden lecterns facing the camera, with the prime minister at the centre flanked by the Chief Scientific Adviser and Chief Medical Officer and two Union Jack flags. The session began with a daily update on the statistics, followed by thankyous, announcements, a rundown on charts by the scientist of the day and finally, questions from the media, starting with the BBC, and later involving the public. The refrain throughout was 'This is an unprecedented global pandemic, and we have taken the right steps at the right time to combat it, guided at all times by the best scientific advice.'

Before his illness, Johnson chaired seven of the ten daily briefings. After his return on April 27, he chaired eight of the 50 (16%) remaining broadcasts until June 23. Given the campaign's focus on the daily briefings, this is a significant reduction in his public presence as leader of the UK Government's response to the crisis. This contrasts with that of Scotland's First Minister Nicola Sturgeon, who chaired 69 briefings during the same period, often taking advantage of her earlier 12:30 slot to subvert the agenda of the UK government. Johnson's place at the lectern was taken by a revolving cast of 11 senior ministers, of whom only one was female. Most prominent was the Health Secretary, Matt Hancock, with 24 appearances, followed by Dominic Raab, Foreign Secretary and Deputy during Johnson's illness, with 12.

Where the campaign went wrong

The *Coronavirus Act 2020* passed into law on March 25 giving the government wide-ranging emergency powers but why did it choose to draft a new bill when it could have invoked pre-existing emergency law, the *Civil Contingencies Act* (CCA)? It has been argued that in bypassing the CCA the government also avoided its in-built accountability, local funding imperatives and the principle of *subsidiarity* whereby decisions are taken at the lowest appropriate level and coordinated at the highest necessary level (Lent, 2020). This made consensus less sustainable over time as central government side-lined local authorities and public service providers.

A failure to deliver timely and accurate information to all stakeholders began to reassert itself, firstly in response to Johnson's illness. On April 6, Raab told the daily briefing Johnson 'continues to lead the government.' That evening, Johnson was admitted to intensive care. On April 3, Hancock described staying at home as an instruction 'not a request,' later saying 'you should "play your part. Do it for the people you love."' On April 11, the Home Secretary Priti Patel told viewers to 'play your part' or the police would be 'unafraid to act.' Speculation grew in early May that there were moves to ease lockdown when anonymous sources were cited in Conservative-supporting newspapers culminating in a detailed rundown of the 'roadmap' in the *Sunday Telegraph* on May 10, followed that night by Johnson's much-criticised broadcast (Malnick, 2020). MPs, the opposition, the devolved governments and the rest of the media had to wait until the following day for a full briefing. This was the moment when Wales, Scotland and Northern Ireland began to publicly diverge from the UK-wide timetable.

On May 23, two left-supporting newspapers published details of Cummings' journeys across the country over the Easter break. Downing Street[1] insisted that his actions were 'in line' with government advice, devoting 90 minutes of live TV to Cummings to defend himself personally. More than 180,000 constituents bombarded their MPs with complaints (Procter et al., 2020), 44 Conservative MPs and a petition of 1m people called on Cummings to resign (Mason, 2020) and social and mainstream media exploded with critique. A series of polls found that confidence in government advice fell following the controversy (Fletcher et al., 2020) while a national survey conducted immediately before and after the Cummings story broke found that the number saying they were prepared to break lockdown rules had doubled (Cartwright, 2020).

Then came the damaging U-turn. On June 9, the Education Secretary Gavin Williamson admitted what teachers had been saying for weeks, that opening primary schools to all children before the summer break as stated in the 'road-map' was not practical with social distancing. Attempts by ministers on May 16 and 17 to isolate the teaching unions and councils by upholding those still teaching as heroes, and those who questioned the plan as operating against the interests of children, had failed. Following the schools U-turn, political editor Nicholas Watt told the BBC's *Newsnight* programme that he had picked up 'lots of unease' among Conservative MPs, being told by 'a very senior Tory MP' that 'our leadership is pitiful. Boris Johnson needs to be honest.'

Conclusion

The UK entered lockdown relatively late but public, media and political cohesion and compliance remained high, despite the illness of the prime minister. The government moved quickly from its habitual side-lining of mainstream media to a bold attempt at accountability, with ministers and science advisers presenting a united front. The failure to build a national consensus, despite government claims to the contrary, and a return to anonymous briefing of favoured sources, undermined trust between the government, media and the public. This reached a climax over Johnson's support of a controversial senior aide widely believed to have broken lockdown rules at the height of the pandemic. The adviser survived but the reputation of the government and the prime minister fell dramatically, leaving the field increasingly open to critical voices. A series of policy U-turns bred confusion, eroding the simplicity of the government's message. However, the crisis proves it is possible even for divisive governments to instil a shared national purpose and a sense of equality by suspending partisan conflict but to be effective, this must be sustained.

Note

1 The official residence of the prime minister; when official statements are made by the office, but not from any named official, they are classified as having been made by 'Downing Street.'

References

Armstrong, M. (2020). The coronavirus and leader approval ratings. *Statista*, 21 April. Accessed 12 June at www.statista.com/chart/21437/coronavirus-and-leader-approval-ratings/

Blais, A., Bol, D., Giani, M., & Loewen, P. (2020). Covid 19 lockdowns have increased support for incumbent parties and trust in government. *LSE Blogs*, 8 May. Accessed 15 June at https://blogs.lse.ac.uk/politicsandpolicy/covid19-lockdowns-democracy/

Calvert, J., Arbuthnot, G., & Leake, J. (2020a). 38 days when Britain sleepwalked into disaster. *Sunday Times*, 19 April. Accessed 15 June 2020 at www.thetimes.co.uk/article/coronavirus-38-days-when-britain-sleepwalked-into-disaster-hq3b9tlgh

Calvert, J., Arbuthnot, G., Leake, J., & Gadher, D. (2020b). 22 days: how three weeks of dither and delay at no 10 cost thousands of British lives. *Sunday Times*, 24 May. Accessed May 24 2020 at www.thetimes.co.uk/article/three-weeks-of-dither-and-delay-on-coronavirus-that-cost-thousands-of-british-lives-05sjvwv7g

Cartwright, E. (2020). We asked people if they were breaking lockdown rules before and after the Dominic Cummings scandal – here's what they told us. *The Conversation*, 3 June. Accessed 15 June 2020 at https://theconversation.com/we-asked-people-if-they-were-breaking-lockdown-rules-before-and-after-the-dominic-cummings-scandal-heres-what-they-told-us-139994

Dettmer, J. (2020). Critics knock Britain's handling of COVID pandemic. *Voice of America*, 20 May. Accessed 11 June 2020 at www.voanews.com/europe/critics-knock-britains-handling-covid-pandemic

Dilnot, A. (2011). *Fair funding for all – the commission's recommendations to government.* (Dilnot Commission Report). London: Department for Health. 4 July. Accessed 15 June at https://webarchive.nationalarchives.gov.uk/20130221121529/https://www.wp.dh.gov.uk/carecommission/files/2011/07/Fairer-Care-Funding-Report.pdf

Fletcher, R., Kalogeropoulos, A., & Neilsen, R. K. (2020). Trust in UK government COVID-19 information down, concerns over misinformation from government and politicians up. *Reuters Institute*, 1 June. Accessed 4 June at https://reutersinstitute.politics.ox.ac.uk/trust-uk-government-and-news-media-covid-19-information-down-concerns-over-misinformation

Grieve, D. (2019). Former Attorney General interviewed on LBC Radio, cited in *The New European*, 14 November. Accessed 20 March at www.theneweuropean.co.uk/top-stories/dominic-grieve-who-would-he-vote-for-1-6375244

Ipsos MORI (2019). *Veracity index 2019: trust in professions.* London: Ipsos MORI. Accessed 15 June 2020 at www.ipsos.com/sites/default/files/ct/news/documents/2019-11/trust-in-professions-veracity-index-2019-slides.pdf

ITV News (2020a). Coronavirus timeline: how has the virus spread? *ITV Report*, 25 January. Accessed 15 June at www.itv.com/news/2020-01-25/coronavirus-timeline-how-has-the-virus-spread/

Lent, A. (2020). We have special legislation to cope with crises like Covid – so why didn't the government use it? *Civil Service World*, 5 June. Accessed 6 June 2020 at www.civilserviceworld.com/articles/opinion/we-have-special-legislation-cope-crises-covid-%E2%80%93-so-why-didn%E2%80%99t-government-use-it

Local Government Association (2018). *Local government funding: moving the conversation on.* 3 July. Accessed 15 June at https://local.gov.uk/sites/default/files/documents/5.40_01_Finance%20publication_WEB_0.pdf

Malnick, E. (2020). Stay alert: PM's new message to the nation. *Sunday Telegraph*, 10 May. Accessed 10 May at www.telegraph.co.uk/politics/2020/05/09/stay-alert-boris-johnsons-new-message-nation/

Mason, R. (2020). Tory anger at Dominic Cummings grows as 61 MPs defy Boris Johnson. *The Guardian*, 27 May. Accessed 28 May at www.theguardian.com/politics/2020/may/27/tory-anger-at-dominic-cummings-grows-as-dozens-of-mps-defy-boris-johnson

Mayhew, F. (2020). BBC faces £125m in lost income over COVID-19 as it reveals surging audience for news coverage. 20 May. Accessed 15 June at https://pressgazette.co.uk/bbc-faces-125m-in-lost-income-over-covid-19-as-it-reveals-digital-at-heart-of-news-plan/

Nice, A. (2020). *The government should stop avoiding parliamentary scrutiny of its coronavirus legislation.* London: Institute for Government. 2 June. Accessed 6 June at www.instit

uteforgovernment.org.uk/blog/government-stop-avoiding-parliamentary-scrutiny-coronavirus-legislation

Nuki, P., & Gardner, B. (2020). Exercise Cygnus uncovered: the pandemic warnings buried by the government. *Sunday Telegraph*, 28 March. Accessed 15 June 2020 at www.telegraph.co.uk/news/2020/03/28/exercise-cygnus-uncovered-pandemic-warnings-buried-government/

Opinium (2020). *The political report: from the opinium/observer polling series.* Opinium Research. 27 April. Accessed 15 June at www.opinium.co.uk/wp-content/uploads/2020/05/Opinium-Political-Report-27th-April.pdf

O'Reilly, L. (2020). #Covidiots trends on Twitter as people urge others to stay inside amid coronavirus outbreak. *Evening Standard*, 23 March. Accessed 11 June 2020 at www.standard.co.uk/news/health/covidiots-twitter-trend-social-distancing-self-isolation-a4394826.html

Procter, K., Murray, J., & Brooks, L. (2020). Constituents bombard MPs with thousands of emails over Dominic Cummings. *The Guardian*, 29 June. Accessed 15 June 2020 at www.theguardian.com/politics/2020/may/29/constituents-bombard-mps-with-180000-emails-about-dominic-cummings

Shipman, T. (2020). No 10 tells BBC licence fee will be scrapped. *The Times*, 16 February 2020. Accessed 15 June 2020 at www.thetimes.co.uk/article/no-10-tells-bbc-licence-fee-will-be-scrapped-hzwb9bzsx

Tobitt, C. (2020). 'Staggering demand' for trusted television news. *Press Gazette*, 17 March. Accessed 15 June at https://pressgazette.co.uk/coronavirus-leads-to-staggering-demand-for-trusted-tv-news/

Walker, B. (2020a). Polls show the UK has lost faith in the government's ability to handle the COVID-19 crisis. *New Statesman*, 9 June. Accessed 15 June 2020 at www.newstatesman.com/politics/health/2020/06/uk-government-coronavirus-response-boris-johnson-approval-poll

Walker, P. (2020b). 'Part-time PM': Corbyn criticizes Johnson's response to floods. *The Guardian*, 26 February. Accessed 8 June 2020 at www.theguardian.com/politics/2020/feb/26/part-time-prime-minister-jeremy-corbyn-criticises-boris-johnson-response-to-floods

15

EGYPT

Emotive speech masks a complicated reality

Dalia Elsheikh

Political context

The Egyptian public sphere is highly polarised due to the aftermath of the 2011 Arab Spring, President Mubarak's removal and subsequent 2012 presidential elections dividing Egyptians into two camps: Islamists and supporters of the Mubarak regime. Morsi's victory led to further division and his removal by the army, who cracked down on Morsi supporters during what is known as The Rab'a Massacre, prior to Al-Sisi being elected as president in 2014.

Conflict between supporters of the Al-Sisi and Muslim Brotherhood continues despite Muslim Brotherhood leaders being in prisons or exile in nations opposing the Al-Sisi regime such as Qatar and Turkey. Brotherhood members actively engage in Egyptian politics through media broadcasts, blogs and vlogs and astroturfed campaigns. Egyptian authorities try to limit access to independent media inside Egypt and buy channels in an attempt to monopolise media output. Hence the current media landscape is polarised between state-controlled domestic media and anti-regime media broadcasting into Egypt.

The current polarisation of opinion and media provided a space for misinformation and politicisation of the pandemic.

Chronology

See Table 15.1 .

Analysis

Government strategy followed four distinct phases. The first 'prevention phase,' saw the government attempt to prevent the virus from entering the country by deploying health officials in airports and ports, measuring

DOI: 10.4324/9781003120254-17

TABLE 15.1 Egypt chronology

		Diffusion of COVID-19	Official government milestones	Major communication events
February	1		Flights temporarily suspended between Egypt and China.	
	28			Rumours of large numbers of cases have to be denied by government.
March	2	2 foreign cases discovered.		
	5	First Egyptian diagnosed.		Ministry of Health's daily bulletins begins.
	7	45 infected on Nile River cruise ship.		
	14		Schools and universities closed. 100 billion Egyptian pounds pledged to combat the virus.	
	15			Minister of Supply and Internal Trade announces sufficient commodity stocks for 29 months.
	16		Church suspends prayers.	First televised briefing by Prime Minister. Announcing border closures dates & a decree to reduce the number of workers working in office in the public sector.
	17		Central Bank of Egypt announce economic support measures.	
	20		Border closure.	
	21		Mosque closures. President appoints Tag-Eldine new adviser for health affairs.	
	22			First public speech by Al-Sisi to mark Mother's Day.

24	Closure of cafes, restaurants and entertainment venues. Closure of shopping centres at weekends. Closure of governmental public service offices.	PM announces partial lock down, with curfew from 7 pm until 6 am.
		Televised briefing by Prime Minister.
April 2		
5	Total cases 1,173, total deaths 78, new cases 103.	
7	Al-Sisi inspected Armed Forces anti-COVID-19 equipment and teams assisting the state civil sector.	Public speech for Al-Sisi.
8		Televised briefing by Prime Minister.
9		Video of Al-Sisi reprimanding officials at a construction site for not providing workers with masks to protect them from COVID-19 released.
12	Announces grant of EGP 500 to irregular, seasonal workers.	
16	Closure of public transportation, parks and beaches on Easter.	Televised briefing by Prime Minister.
22		Public speech by Al-Sisi.
23	Curfew hours reduced to start from 9 pm ahead of Ramadan. Allowing restaurants and shops to work till 5 pm.	Televised briefing by Prime minister.
25	Parliament passes amendments to the *Law of Health Precautions against Infectious Diseases.* Among which, refusal to bury COVID-19 victims is punishable by imprisonment.	

(Continued)

TABLE 15.1 (Continued)

		Diffusion of COVID-19	Official government milestones	Major communication events
May	5	Total cases 7,201, total deaths 452, new cases 338.		
	7		Amendment of Emergency Law to tackle COVID-19 including requisition of premises to act as temporary field hospitals.	
	11		International Monetary Fund (IMF) approves request for emergency financial assistance of US$ 2.772 billion.	
	17		Banning Eid prayer and closing all public transportation, curfew times 5 pm to 6 am during Eid and 8 pm to 5 am after. Introducing wearing of facemasks from May 30, failure punishable by fine.	
	20		Deducting 1% from salaries for 12 months beginning on July 1 to offset economic repercussions.	
	21			Announcement of modelling system, infection rate and estimation of unregistered cases, and hospitals capabilities.
June	5	Total cases 31,115, total deaths 1,166, new cases 1,348.		
	15		Two field hospitals established.	
	23			PM lifts curfew, eases restrictions from June 27.

passengers' temperatures and installing thermal gates in some airports. The second, containment phase, when infections erupted in hotspots and the source of infection was known, the government tracked, traced and tested their contacts. The third, community spread, phase started when the number of cases reached thousands. Preparations for a fourth worst-case scenario phase included amending emergency laws temporarily nationalising private companies and converting them to field hospitals and deploying the army to help tackle the virus.

Prevention and containment phases

During the first two phases, the government was unable to control the agenda. Government initiatives were politicised by opposition forces – mainly Muslim Brotherhood and affiliated media organisations abroad, as well as astroturfing campaigns. Opposition forces claimed the government were not carrying out measures they announced, such as having medical staff at airports; they also used photos of nurses to claim they were purely performing for the media.

Egyptians learned about Al-Nagila Hospital's conversion into a quarantine hospital from social media, after some doctors revealed the Ministry of Health package of incentives to those agreeing to work there. The action was framed by a social media astroturfing campaign as Egypt hiding COVID-19 patients there, sending medical staff to death in return for 20K which pushed citizens living in Matrouh to protest in front of the hospital. The protest was broadcast by Aljazeera framing Egyptian government preparations through a politicised lens.

In late February and early March, some confirmed cases were reported abroad but no domestic cases were announced as these were only detected after sufferers showed symptoms. At this stage, the 14 days incubation period for the disease was not known yet. The government was thus accused of hiding cases, allegations which were denied in an official statement by the Cabinet with the help of further statements from the World Health Organisation (WHO).

Despite denials, the allegations were heavily politicised, affecting Egypt's economy and Egyptians working abroad. On March 1, Qatar banned all arrivals from Egypt, except Qatari nationals. In return, Egypt instituted a 'reciprocal' ban for Qataris on March 6. On the March 2, Kuwait asked for results of COVID-19 tests for any Egyptian entering its border resulting in rumours spreading that Egyptians workers in Kuwait were the source of the virus and demands for their deportation. On March 8, both Saudi Arabia and Bahrain asked those arriving from selected countries, including Egypt, to self-isolate for 14 days; the following day Saudi Arabia suspended travel between nine countries including Egypt.

During this period there were no televised speeches by the president. Affiliated opposition media abroad politicised the absence claiming the Egyptian president was in 14 days quarantine after contact with a top army personnel who died from the virus.

As the politicised critical reporting was proven to be wrong, the government communication was strengthened and strategy changed from mid-phase two: (a) the Prime Minister (PM) began a series of televised speeches abandoning the depersonalised press releases and providing visible technocratic leadership; (b) the President made appearances at official meetings followed by televised speeches; (c) a daily bulletin by the Ministry of Health released the number of cases.

Official messages and communication

On March 16, the PM gave his first televised speech, providing clear information describing what was known about the disease at each stage, its treatment and the efforts in place to contain and overcome the virus until a vaccine is discovered. The Cabinet Facebook page was used to expose and deny rumours. The public debates at this stage centred on the correctness and credibility of government information. Little discussion focused on the number of tests conducted or the resources available to the health system and its efficiency. At this stage, no one knew about or discussed the total number of critical care beds and ventilators in Egypt.

The mass media, mainly owned and controlled by the government, did not amplify government messages, instead playing a negative role by spreading false information. This included interviewing an actress undermining the threat from the virus, and a presenter claiming that India has no cases of COVID-19 because of spices used in their cooking which are high in chromium. Others claimed Egyptians have immunity against the disease, that drinking tea kills the virus in the throat before it reaches one's chest or suggesting Shallolu, an ancient Egyptian recipe, as the best way to fight the virus (Amin, 2020); one programme even consulted an astrologer (Adib, 2020).

Despite government efforts to control the spread of fake news either through legislation or through the Cabinet Facebook page or by designating phone numbers on WhatsApp for reporting coronavirus 'rumours,' it failed to tackle the misinformation being spread by its own media channels. ElGomhoria ElYoum website was blocked for six months after publishing an article suggesting the Public Health Ministry had found a treatment for coronavirus, yet the wider picture is of an irresponsible media. State-controlled media provided false information; independent outlets concentred more on highlighting government deficiencies. The pandemic was covered like any other news story: politicised, sensationalised and personalised with minimal information content.

During these first phases, stigmatisation and bullying were evident in many examples such as of patients not reporting symptoms, others escaping from the quarantine hospitals, refusing to bury the deceased, bullying doctors and incidents of attacks on a Chinese citizen on Cairo's streets. Yet neither government nor media communication were able to protect and empower the vulnerable. The police had to fire tear gas on protesters banning the burial of a deceased female in their village. The government strategy failed to tackle stigma in advance.

Credibility

On March 15, the UK *Guardian* claimed Egypt had more than 19,000 cases triggering Egyptian authorities to ask the journalist to leave the country, which undermined Egypt internationally (Safi, 2020). But surprisingly, it acted in Egypt's favour at a domestic level. The article was refuted scientifically by some academics (Ibrahim, 2020), but more importantly it was also refuted by some prominent Egyptian journalists abroad who opposed the Al-Sisi regime (Aboelgheit, 2020). This gave credibility to government figures in the eyes of many Egyptians and moved the debate from 'hiding cases' to the differences between confirmed and real cases caused by minimal testing capacity or the absence of people with symptoms. Debates also centred on quarantining whole villages when cases erupt, the lower number of elderly people in comparison to European countries which affects the numbers and a failure by Egyptians to report symptoms. A research paper (Hassany et al., 2020) on estimating cases was published by Egyptian scientists, including the Health Minister. However, the article was directed to foreign audiences and so gained no coverage in Egyptian media.

Official messages

Egyptian officials expressed significant empathy during the early phases. Al-Sisi used emotional rhetoric to recommend containment measures and was careful to speak in a way that did not spread panic. He promised to offer masks for half price or for free if needed. He also called on the private sector to avoid laying off employees and cutting salaries and gave orders to return Egyptians stranded abroad even when borders were closed.

Al-Sisi, who often appeared wearing a mask, also appeared in a video reprimanding an official at a construction site for not providing workers with protective facemasks. Government messages at the beginning of the pandemic were also used to reassure Egyptians that food and essential goods would last for 29 months, after panic buying broke out in supermarkets. Al-Sisi also appeared inspecting the army's infrastructure dedicated to help fighting the pandemic. He also appointed well-known and experienced Tag El-Deen as his adviser for health affairs. An action that was welcomed by ordinary citizens who disliked the current health minister.

The first phases witnessed personal phone calls from ministers to ordinary citizens. After villagers demonstrated against the burial of a doctor, the Prime Minster called her husband and apologised on behalf of the Egyptian people. This period also witnessed several calls from the Minister of Egyptians Abroad who had posted videos speaking about their situation. The actions raised the expectations of some as posting videos on social media became the main method of gaining both media and official attention, and they expected officials to respond.

Zakat, the systematic giving of 2.5% of one's wealth each year to benefit the poor, was allowed to be paid early to help those affected economically by the crisis. Egypt's Al-Azhar Grand Imam described the refusal of burying COVID-19 victims as a far cry from morality, humanity, religion (Al-Tayeb, 2020).

Egypt's empathy was expressed internationally as well. The Egyptian state sent personal protective equipment (PPE) donations to China, Italy and for the first time in history, Egypt sent donations to the United States. Egypt reverted the same slogan it used to receive donations from the USAID saying, 'from the Egyptian people to the American people' a symbolic message only Egyptians might understand. The US ambassador in Cairo replied via video thanking the Egyptian people (US Embassy, 2020). After Egypt exported shipments to help the United Kingdom (UK) amid its shortage of PPE, the UK minister of trade thanked Egypt in a tweet (Hands, 2020). Actions Egyptians are not used to.

These charitable actions sparked debate among Egyptians. They saw their country as an ethical player helping wealthy countries in the crisis despite others fighting over cargos. The debate extended to what Egypt can take in return from these countries in the future when a vaccine or a cure is found. Yet fears that the state might be doing this irrespective of domestic needs were also voiced. Ex ambassador Elashmawy (2020) argued the truth will not be known until the disease hits Egypt hard. This evidences weak trust, which the state was trying to restore. Others argued Egypt over-reacted during the H1N1 pandemic and this resulted in a huge amount of PPE being stored and unused: Egypt had 30 million n95 masks and one tonne of Tamiflu raw materials all in storage unused (Kamel, 2020).

Officials' actions

In comparison to other European countries, Egypt acted early enough (Kaldas, 2020) in taking tougher measures such as shutting schools, banning gatherings, closing borders and applying a partial curfew in an attempt to ban unnecessary socialising in a country that is known to be open 24 hours. Yet containment measures were undermined by citizens crowding during the day, in addition to politically motivated events in Alexandria, protest against the virus and a later March call for opening mosques. The corporate sector also called for businesses to open, calls the government bowed to by reducing the Ramadan curfew hours from 9 pm instead of 8 pm lasting till 6 am on April 23 for the sake of communal Iftar gatherings and the economy with 26% of workers having lost their jobs (Nosaed, 2020). The government also announced preparations to 'open the economy' and restore normal life[1] even when cases were still rising and without reaching the peak.

These announcements left Egyptians divided between two conflicting ideas. The first is the government changing its strategy into a herd immunity strategy. The second is that Egyptians are immune to the disease. By the end of Ramadan, the total number of cases was 17,265, and total deaths 764. By the end of Eid, the hospitals became full and Egyptians called for help and shared their experiences on social media outlets, in what was known as the 'Ramadan gatherings effect.'

Community spread

Throughout May the number of registered cases increased. Meanwhile Egyptians were self-isolating at home or deteriorating without registering symptoms. The Ministry of Health hotline was always busy. Yet the government were relaxing the lockdown measures and preparing for opening the economy.

Private hospitals were charging a huge amount of money. They refused to abide by prices suggested by the Ministry of Health and threatened to close, raising questions about government authority over a private health sector partially funded by foreign investments, and why the amended emergency law was not applied to the private sector (Saleh, 2020).

New businesses erupted such as brokers to find patients spare beds in hospitals, and there was a black market for selling medicines used in critical care units. What is known as the treatment protocol used by the health ministry was leaked on Facebook, and so was followed by ordinary citizens. Egypt was participating in a convalescent plasma trial, asking recovered patients to donate their bloods. Yet, it was transferred to another business. Recovered patients were selling their blood for thousands of Egyptian pounds. Rich people converting their homes to intensive care (IC) units (ElHawary, 2020). New private drive-through COVID-19 testing centres were also opened.

There were calls to fully implement the emergency law and for the army to intervene. By mid-June, without prior announcements, two field hospitals were built. The first by Ain Shams University on 4,500 m2. The second by the army with a capacity of 3,000 beds, on 40,000 m2. These sudden announcements were consistent with Al-Sisi's traditional 'forces of evil' rhetoric, where projects are announced only after completion in fear it could be attacked by 'forces of evil.'

This phase exposed the defects in the Egyptian health system, which is different from many other countries. Not all hospitals fall under the direct control of the Ministry of Health. It also exposed the important role some NGOs were playing, two women-led organisations either rented beds in private hospitals, transferring those in need to them or dedicated their buildings to COVID-19 patients. Egyptian women launched groups on Facebook offering free healthy cooked meals for patients in neighbourhood areas.

The computer modelling used by the government to calculate infection rates was unknown in Egypt until a televised event attended by the President on May 21. The event saw the Minister of Scientific Research reveal for the first time collaboration with Egyptian experts abroad on a modelling system. In addition to announcing for the first time the 5.5% rate of growth, adding that the estimate numbers of non-registered cases were five times the numbers of registered cases. This announcement indicated that containment strategies had failed.

Conclusion

During the early phases of the pandemic, there was a sense of equality among Egyptians. For the first time in recent history, officials were unable to travel abroad for treatment. All Egyptians, independent of status, had to undergo treatment within the Egyptian health system. Yet when numbers increased and the Ministry resorted to other hospitals, discrepancies appeared mainly because of the private hospital crisis and state failure to contain the virus. The feeling of equality was displaced with fears that money was the keyword.

The dramatic change in the government's message easing lockdown measures despite not reaching the peak led to mixed reactions from ordinary citizens. There were several entities dealing with crisis and not a united single committee. There was the presidency, the armed forces, Ministry of Health, Ministry of Higher Education and Scientific Research, private hospitals, doctors on Facebook and a committee established and known as the Higher Committee for Novel Coronavirus Crisis Management. Yet, there was no direct communication with citizens except through daily diagrams, the social media pages of organisations, officials speaking on talk shows programmes and prime ministerial speeches which announced new rules and curfew times, and presidential televised speeches which were usually piggybacking on another event.

Yet, despite fluctuations in government performance, it managed to adopt an empathetic tone and cut through the polarised and politicised information environment. It also succeeded in presenting a new technocratic civilian leadership, in contrast to the single leadership and security apparatus Egyptians are used to. However, while it gained important experience throughout the crisis, which may pave the way for changes in future crisis management methods, it failed to learn from other nations and remains in a parlous position dealing with COVID-19.

Note

1 On April 23, PM announced that economy will be opened in June. On June 23, he announced the details of reopening starting from June 27.

References

Aboelgheit, M., 2020. Comment on Guardian report on Egypt's cases. *Facebook* [online]. 16 March. Available from: www.facebook.com/mohamed.aboelgheit/posts/101 58003690338674

Adib, A., 2020. Interview in Elhekayyia programme [video, online]. *YouTube*. Available from: www.youtube.com/watch?v=se4tp3J2ESs [Accessed 22 June 2020].

Al-Tayeb, A., 2020. Comment on refusal of burying COVID-19 victims. *Facebook* [online]. 11 April. Available from: www.facebook.com/GrandImam/posts/1245715 75853485?__tn__=-R

Amin, S., 2020. Egypt battles COVID-19 amid flood of misinformation, conspiracy theories. *Al-Monitor*. 31 March. Available from: www.al-monitor.com/pulse/origi nals/2020/03/egyptian-superstitions-jokes-on-coronavirus.html#ixzz6Q6LW8AP0 [Accessed 15 June 2020].

Elashmawy, F., 2020. On PPE Egyptian donations. *Facebook* [online]. 21 April. Available from: www.facebook.com/fawzy.elashmawy/posts/2816406855074659

ElHawary, D., 2020. The rich establishing IC units in their homes. *Alyoum7*. 16 June. Available from: www.youm7.com/4828093 [Accessed 22 June 2020].

Hands, G., 2020. Twitter [online]. 13 April. Available from: https://twitter.com/GregH ands/status/1249742429160439812

Hassany, M., Abdel-Razek, W., Asem, N., Abdallah, M., & Zaid, H., 2020. Estimation of COVID-19 burden in Egypt. *The Lancet* [online]. 27 April. Available from: https://doi.org/10.1016/S1473-3099(20)30319-4 [Accessed 22 June 2020].

Ibrahim, H., 2020. How did the Guardian miss professionalism in its report about cases in Egypt? *Future Centre for Advanced Research and Studies*. 17 March. Available from: https://futureuae.com/ar/Mainpage/Item/5370 [Accessed 22 June 2020].

Kaldas, T., 2020. Egypt's disdain for transparency will backfire in this coronavirus crisis. *The Guardian* [online]. 31 March. Available from: www.theguardian.com/comme ntisfree/2020/mar/31/egypt-coronavirus-transparency-sisi-crackdown [Accessed 15 June 2020].

Kamel, A., 2020. Personal interview with Ahmed Kamel, ex spokesman, ministry of health. June.

Nosaed, 2020. ONS: 26% of employee lost their jobs because of coronavirus. *Nosaed*. 20 June. Available from: https://www.nosaed.com/2020/06/20 [Accessed 22 June 2020].

Safi, M., 2020. Egypt forces Guardian journalist to leave after coronavirus story. *The Guardian* [online]. 26 March. Available from: www.theguardian.com/world/2020/ mar/26/egypt-forces-guardian-journalist-leave-coronavirus-story-ruth-michaelson [Accessed 22 June 2020].

Saleh, M., 2020. Enriching pirates. *Al-Masry Al-youm*. 13 June. Available from: www.a lmasryalyoum.com/news/details/1987474 [Accessed 22 June 2020].

US Embassy Cairo, 2020. US ambassador thanking Egypt. *Facebook* [online]. 21 April. Available from: www.facebook.com/watch/?v=2561292964138646

16

RUSSIA

A glass wall

Svetlana S. Bodrunova

Political context

After 30 years of political transformation, Russia in 2020 is a state witnessing deep social fragmentation accompanied by a rise in authoritarian leadership and rigid power structures. The Russian President Vladimir Putin has been in power for over 20 years (in 1999–2000 and 2008–2012 as Prime Minister). Half of the upper chamber of parliament (The Federal Council) consists of regional governors directly appointed by the president. The lower chamber (The State Duma) has seen the same three 'systemic oppositional' parties for five electoral cycles in a row, with unchanged leaders and without posing substantial challenges to 'United Russia,' the biggest party that officially supports the president.

Public life in the country is affected by two major divisions. The first is a division between the populace and *sistema* ('the system,' Ledeneva, 2013) – a complex of formal and informal governance institutions and practices based on clientelist connections and involving all the three branches of power, the military and security services, police and organisations around these. Second, there is a stable and unequal values-based division between a dominant traditionalist majority and a politically disadvantaged minority with a mostly liberal-oppositional stance, reproduced in media consumption (Bodrunova & Litvinenko, 2016). These divisions are linked to different levels of public trust in institutions in Russia where support for the leader is high within the majority (FOM, 2020), while wider trust in institutions and media is much lower than in the other 29 world countries assessed in the report by Edelman agency (Edelman, 2020).

At the same time, a substantial share of public discussion on the Russian Internet, or Runet, has been conducted by what Toepfl (2020) has identified as 'leadership-critical publics,' in contrast to uncritical and policy-critical ones. In this respect, a range of major Runet discussion platforms were in a sharp contrast

DOI: 10.4324/9781003120254-18

to the federal TV channels and major tabloids. These factors all shaped how the state actions were perceived during the pandemic.

Chronology

See Table 16.1.

Analysis

Maximum presence, maximum calm, maximum spin

The communicative strategy of the Russian authorities during COVID-19 has been two-layer. The first layer was, contrary to expectations, oriented to maximum openness and equanimity, perhaps to prevent panic. Governmental measures that ensured openness included the following. First, establishment of stopcoronavirus.rf and other important data portals which, at least partly, became a reference point for those who sought basic instructions and explanations of the state policy on COVID-19. Second, adding more options to gosuslugi.ru ('stateservices.ru'), the main portal for state-provided social security and administration services. Third, streaming of Putin's direct lines and meetings with various officials; ministerial briefings; gatherings of the Operative Staff etc. Fourth, presence of ministries and their projects on social networks and Telegram (despite its official blockage), as well as collaboration with Yandex, the local Google competitor. Yandex established a map tracker of the spread of contagion, infection/death statistics widgets, news channels and the page with Johns Hopkins University data reworked. These services became points of reference for millions of Russians. Also, a notable example of explanatory and antipanic discourse was the late-evening *Doc talk* show on Channel One that was completely dedicated to COVID-19 during March to May. At the same time, the regional level of openness was much lower; this was especially true when it came to evidence on statistical fraud.

Perhaps, continuous governmental action was most visible thanks to nearly everyday televised online meetings of Vladimir Putin and Prime Minister Mikhail Mishustin with ministers, governors, mayors, NGOs, volunteers, business representatives etc. However, Putin and Mishustin contributed to openness quite differently. The latter was shown mostly 'in third person,' in the process of decision-making. The former has exploited direct forms of communication like multiple TV addresses on COVID-19, Victory Day and the constitutional referendum, critically raising the level of personalisation of crisis communication – even if pre-pandemic televised political communication had already been predominantly fixed on the figure of the Russian president as a part of a continuous strategy of his portrayal as a long-term national leader. Often, his speeches combined with distant conferencing with his subordinates, staged for declarations rather than for discussions, and his direct 'appeals to Russians' had fatherly

TABLE 16.1 Russia chronology

Date		Diffusion of COVID-19	Key official actions	Key communication events
January	19		Creation of COVID-19 polymerise chain reaction (PCR) tests starts.	
	24		Chief Medical Officer of the Russian Federation introduces measures to prevent the spread of COVID-19.	
	29		Operational Staff Board for prevention of COVID-19 is created. It is chaired by Tatiana Golikova, Deputy Prime Minister, and includes ministers, deputy ministers and senior health experts	
	31	First COVID-19 cases (Chinese citizens) in Tyumen and Chita.	National plan against COVID-19 is approved China-Russia border closes.	
February	1		Emergency situation declared in two China-Russia border districts.	
	20		Chinese citizens are prohibited from entering Russia.	
March	2	First case confirmed in Moscow.		
	3		Medical controls (temperature tests and visual checks) introduced for flights from South Korea, Iran and Italy.	
	5		Moscow placed on high alert.	Announcement that XXIV St. Petersburg International Economic Forum is cancelled.
	10		Moscow prohibits public events of 5,000+ visitors.	

12	Daily production of PCR tests reaches 100,000; actual testing figures still unavailable.		Prime-time talk show *Doc talk* switches focus to coronavirus-related topics стопкоронавирус.рф (stopcoronavirus.rf) opens.
16		The government announces national help action and allocation of 300 bln roubles to support the economy. Borders with Belarus close, most international air travel stops.	St. Petersburg government publishes a list of 20 local public polyclinics where testing is to take place. They are found not to be ready.
18		Entrance of foreigners is barred. Federal Agency on Consumer Rights and Wellbeing (Rospotrebnadzor) urges regions to introduce prevention measures (locally implemented halfway, at best).	Federal Communication Agency publishes a warning for COVID-19 fake news disseminators.
20			*Echo of Moscow* is warned after publishing claims by an independent expert that authorities are hiding real statistics.
21			#мывместе (#wearetogether) all-Russian volunteer action starts.
24		St. Petersburg bans pre-planned hospitalisation, patient reception and vaccination till June 23.	Putin visits Kommunarka, the first Moscow COVID-19 hospital.
25	The first two official COVID-19 deaths in Moscow.	The **first short lockdown**: March 30 to April 5 are 'days off'. Russia sends 15th batch of aid to Italy.	Putin's first TV address announces 'days off', postponement of the constitutional referendum, and additional economic measures.
26		Moscow introduces 'self-isolation regime' for 65+ and chronically ill.	Defence Minister announces construction of 16 modular hospitals.

(Continued)

TABLE 16.1 (Continued)

Date	Diffusion of COVID-19	Key official actions	Key communication events
27	Infection toll exceeds 1,000.		
28		Moscow closes non-essential businesses and parks.	
30		Russia fully closes borders. Full self-isolation in Moscow and St. Petersburg, with five exceptions, provoking criticism and latent disobedience.	Yandex.ru creates self-isolation index of cities. Putin's online meetings become regularly televised.
31		26 regions introduce self-isolation. Russia sells an aircraft of medical supplies to the USA.	
April 1		160,000 tourists arrive by special charter flights.	
2		'Days-off' prolonged until April 30. 45 of 85 regions prolong restrictions; in others, policies vary.	On TV, Putin announces region-by-region policy on self-isolation.
3			Moscow implements the 'Social monitoring' app. Rocketing surveillance suspicions follow.
4		Eight regions ban alcohol retail in order to prevent excessive home drinking and the rise of drinking-related crimes during the lockdown.	
5		Borders with Chechnya close.	
7		Putin approves one-time payouts to families with children.	Kommersant publishes poll data on high dissatisfaction and stress among doctors.

8			Putin announces extra payouts for medical workers, later postponed and cut by regional authorities.
9	Infection toll reaches 10,000.	The first Moscow fines for breaking self-isolation.	
13		Moscow introduces digital transport passes.	Rospotrebnadzor claims 55% of 74 infection hotbeds are hospitals.
14		1,000,000+ passes are cancelled due to wrong user data, to outrage of Muscovites.	
16	Infections confirmed in all regions.		
18			*Kommersant* publishes a leaked report on lack of personal protective equipment (PPE) and artificial lung ventilators (ALVs) in 28 regions.
19			Televised Easter service without worshippers.
20		In North Ossetia, special troops dispersed a large anti-isolation riot.	St. Petersburg announces extra payments to health workers; the money is delayed and controversially distributed by Yandex. Maps-based online protest rallies spread to nine cities including Moscow.
22	Infection toll reaches 50,000.	St. Petersburg bans funerals for COVID-19 victims.	
27			'Immortal battalion online' starts. 2.3m+ veterans' pictures are uploaded by May 9, becoming, arguably, the world's biggest pandemic-induced participatory action.

(Continued)

TABLE 16.1 (Continued)

Date	Diffusion of COVID-19	Key official actions	Key communication events
May			
1		Nizhny Novgorod region closes for non-residents.	
6		Rospotrebnadzor suggests a three-step renormalisation plan for regions.	
7	Russia becomes #5 globally for infections.	In Moscow, self-isolation is prolonged till May 31. Many cities follow.	
9		Victory Day. The airborne part of military parade takes place.	Putin, alone, lays flowers to the Tomb of Unknown Soldier. Nationwide flashmob – singing the 'Victory Day' song at balconies.
10	Infection toll reaches 200,000.		
11	Peak of the first wave: 11,656 infections in one day. Russia becomes #3 globally for infections.	End of the all-Russian lockdown. Restrictions remain for 65+ people. Most limitations remain in Moscow and St. Petersburg.	On TV, Putin claims the lockdown helped the medical system cope with the crisis. The *New York Times* and the *Financial Times* claim Moscow has 1,700 extra deaths; Russia demands apologies.
12	Russia becomes #2 globally for infections.	St. Petersburg bans all funeral ceremonies, regardless of diagnosis.	The Moscow Healthcare Department refutes death toll lowering.
13	In St. Petersburg, community-based pneumonia toll is 5.5 times and the death toll 10 times higher than in May 2019.		
19			*Mediazona* publishes the medical workers' death toll as 16 times higher than in most countries.

20	Infection toll 300,000. Infection index <1.0 Russia is #1 by testing volumes.	Compulsory mask wearing implemented in 82 Russian regions.	
22		St. Petersburg allows 10-min. funerals.	
23	100,000 recovered.		
27		St. Petersburg lifts the ban on COVID-19 burials.	
28			A poll reveals 30% do not believe in the pandemic.
30	Infection toll 400,000 (up 15%) Russia's hospital beds re-profiled for COVID-19. St. Petersburg leads in mortality rates outperforming Moscow by three times.		
June 01	Death toll 5,000.	Moscow allows non-essential retail and introduces 'scheduled walks,' which are widely ridiculed by people.	
02			Rospotrebnadzor announces Russia has passed 'the acute phase.'
08		Ban on travel abroad is lifted for work, study, medical treatment and caretaking.	
09		Moscow abandons self-isolation, digital passes and scheduled walks. Many public services reopen.	
10	50% of the infected recover.		
11	Infection toll 500,000.	School graduation exams non-compulsory.	
16		Moscow reopens museums, zoos and limited sports.	
20	Death toll 8,000.		

(Continued)

TABLE 16.1 (Continued)

Date		Diffusion of COVID-19	Key official actions	Key communication events
	23		Moscow reopens restaurants/cafés and kindergartens.	
	24		St. Petersburg reopens planned hospitalisation. The Victory Day military parade takes place in Moscow, evoking criticism for wasting money and risk to veterans.	
	25		Start of seven-day constitutional referendum.	Federal TV reports the referendum as safe. Popular criticism of the referendum is partly linked to COVID-19.
July	01		Hotels in Crimea open for Russians, with dangerous number of tourists arriving.	Putin's press secretary calls the referendum results 'triumphal.'
	08	Infections reach 700,000. Moscow death toll 4,000.		
	11		Putin institutes a medal for #wearetogether.	#wearetogether gathers 110 mln roubles of donations.
	12	Clinical trials on the world's first vaccine (second trial stage) are declared successful.		
	14	St. Petersburg mortality rates reach a 10-year high, jobless toll 100,000.		
	15		For incoming foreigners, 14-day quarantine is lifted.	

intonations. TV shows like *Russia, Kremlin, Putin* (a 20-interview project with or about Putin), several interviews to TASS he gave during the pandemic and opening a World War II memorial in Rzhev were also part of a maximally personalised communication strategy.

Putin's role was the glue between the first and the second layer of the communication strategy mentioned above – and the second layer was based on unequivocally values-laden discourse. The largely illiberal and sometimes openly anti-Western values were, most of all, voiced on federal TV channels. In particular, they showed up in news reporting and daytime and late-evening 'battle discussion' shows on Channel One (*Time will show* and *Big game*) and Russia 1 (*60 minutes* and *Evening with Vladimir Solovyov*). Rather than raising real issues, these shows, by imitating multi-sided discussion, were putting the COVID-related realities into the previously formed frameworks of dangerous cosmopolitanism, a weak and disunited Europe and a cynical global chessboard.

The most extreme form of this discourse was found in the series of adverts, mostly billboards and TV ads, that promoted the constitutional referendum. The plebiscite was to introduce over 200 changes to the Constitution; among them, 'zeroisation' of presidential incumbency, priority of the Russian legal system against international law, a further widening of presidential power, and protection of traditional values like defining marriage as the union of man and woman only. The advertising campaign, formally, called for participation, but the commercials explained the importance of voting in relation to traditionalist values: 'Let's preserve our native culture and language,' 'Let's protect the memory of our ancestors' (with visual references to the World War II), 'We will not give away an inch of homeland,' etc. Non-cancellation of the referendum during the pandemic (only two regions could vote online) was criticised on social networks but went virtually unnoticed by the World Health Organisation (WHO) and international human rights watchdogs.

Disregarding the Leviathan: people's reaction to information on COVID-19

The pandemic has put Russians in a paradoxical situation when *sistema* stood on the side of good. Researchers on the Soviet relations between the state and people described practices of disregard and indirect disobedience that, under the ideological rule, lead to 'normalisation' of private life and consumption (Schopflin, 1995; Pertsev, 2013). Similar to this, during the pandemic, mistrust of authorities manifested itself in massive breaches of self-isolation, disbelief in the pandemic among as much as 30% of the population (Kepinski, 2020) and inherent mistrust in official statistics. These factors contributed to a belated loosening of restrictions by the government when everyone was already on the streets. This time, collaboration with the Leviathan of the state would be reasonable, and solidarity expected; despite this, mistrust in both the state and media widened the gap between COVID-denialists and COVID-paranoids.

To our viewpoint, there were three major popular concerns beyond immediate safety. These were national and local statistics on the disease, the appropriateness of the containment measures, and surveillance. They cut across age and political differences. While these factors were highly salient to the public, economic depression and the rapid drop of living standards were discussed much more on VK.com, the most popular Russian-speaking social network, and on Yandex.District, a new service for local discussions, than on Facebook where users, in general, are more economically self-dependent. This 'platform bubble effect' had previously been described in the field of political and values-based polarisation (Bodrunova & Litvinenko, 2016); the pandemic showed that this division also has an economic dimension. Interestingly, fake news, bots and trolls, or conspiracy theories were of minor concern for people, perhaps because the very fabric of information on COVID-19 was flawed enough; rather, fears manifested themselves via Rabelais-reminiscent ridiculing and denial.

Of the three issues, the rise of surveillance was, perhaps, the most telling. Thus, introduction of the 'Social monitoring' mobile app for tracking of the quarantined was perceived negatively, as both highly inefficient and highly suspicious in its goals (data collection instead of social care). If NGOs were, indeed, concerned about the six types of COVID-related surveillance they have detected (Gainutdinov, 2020), for people, both inefficiency and non-transparency of tracking were a reason for additional distrust that only supported the previous wariness towards the state.

The 'glass wall': the state, media, and people in a triangle of mistrust

On the media side, low trust in media and audience fragmentation have led to an interesting phenomenon of 'informationalist' reporting. Seeking to both raise trust, avoid anxious reporting and not to challenge the official picture too much, textual media have *en masse* introduced statistical widgets and inverted-pyramid news sections on COVID-19. However, top-down editorial gatekeeping and sterile objectivity were a trap: they hardly matched audience agendas and under-represented public concerns. Such reporting failed to address issues that were voiced on social networks and did not help in creating more cohesion in the social reaction to the challenge of self-isolation. Few exceptions from this strategy included business dailies and a few oppositional and activist outlets; but their single investigative publications were unable to break the general 'informationalist' picture.

Another lack was that of proper contextualisation. Despite the rocketing growth of medical expertise in media and hundreds of explanatory 'how-to' publications, for the general reader, it was hard to understand the trends in the development of the pandemic itself and the pandemic-hit economies from the overwhelming amount of news that, at the same time, mostly lacked depth and contextualised interpretation. Thus, the audiences that neither trusted the official optimistic line nor had access to independent analysis were left having to rely on personal evaluations of risk. This is how the 'glass wall' between the authorities and the people formed and worked: federal and local governments were producing strategic decisions, creating rules and informing the population, with media trying to better convey the details, while people distrusted the paternalist tone and statistics which did not reflect the evidence from personal experience and the medical community. Unable to access data they could believe, they followed highly individualised perceptions and the habit of tacit disobedience.

Positive grassroots: search for trustworthiness and contributive action

The positive side of the situation was that it has also led to the rise of active information seeking and defining trustworthy sources for oneself. A small pilot poll conducted by the author in July 2020 among 65 respondents on Facebook and VK.com exploring sources of information on COVID-19 has shown that trustworthiness might also be affected by participation in 'platform bubbles.' Thus, VK.com users tended to name Channel One and stopcoronavirus.rf, while 'Facebookers' named international media, statistical sources like Yandex widgets and individual social media accounts. The high trust given to analytical doctor-controlled Telegram channels and 'anchor' Facebook experts needs to be underlined.

Also, connective action (Bennett & Segerberg, 2013) turned into contributive action. Users uploaded 2.3+ mln pictures of soldiers to the 'online rally' of the 'Immortal battalion' during celebrations of the 75th anniversary of the World War II victory, contributed to online protests by posting on Yandex.Maps and reproduced hundreds of world-renowned paintings by improvised materials in the Facebook's 'Izoizolyacia' ('Fine-art isolation') community. These activities, each in its own way, were linked to coping and a renormalisation of memory, political and cultural experiences amid the crisis.

Overall, COVID-19 in Russia has demonstrated that long-term immersion of state communication into values-laden framing that intensifies during a crisis and is opposed only by a politically minor and predominantly online-based counter-public produces an environment of distrust and non-compliance. Moreover, it showed deep alertness of citizens towards state paternalism and a rejection of media who stuck to formal objectivity instead of breaking the 'glass wall' between the authorities and people. However, social solidarity and responsiveness was evident in contributive action, volunteer activities and active search for trustworthy analytics.

References

Bennett, W. L., & Segerberg, A. (2013). *The logic of connective action: digital media and the personalization of contentious politics.* Cambridge University Press.

Bodrunova, S., & Litvinenko, A. (2016). Fragmentation of society and media hybridisation in today's Russia: how Facebook voices collective demands. *Journal of Social Policy Research, 14*(1), 113–124.

Edelman (2020). *2020 Edelman trust barometer.* www.edelman.com/trustbarometer.

FOM (2020). *Vladimir Putin: otsenki raboty, otnoshenie [Vladimor Putin: evaluation of work, attitudes].* Public Opinion Foundation (FOM), July. https://fom.ru/politika/10946.

Gainutdinov (2020). Pandemia slezhki [Surveillancedemic]. *AGORA website.* https://spy.runet.report/assets/files/Пандемия_слежки.pdf.

Kepinski, O. (2020). Tret' rossiyan ne verit v pandemiyu koronavirusa [One third of Russians do not believe into the coronavirus pandemic]. *Euronews.* May 28. https://ru.euronews.com/2020/05/28/ru-russians-dont-believe-in-pandemic.

Ledeneva, A. V. (2013). *Can Russia modernise? Sistema, power networks and informal governance.* Cambridge University Press.

Pertsev (2013). Neuchtennye dohody naselenia RSFSR i bor'ba s nimi v 1970–1980-e gody [Unrecorded popular revenues and countering them in the 1970s and 1980s]. *Bulletin of Voronezh State University, Series 'History. Politology. Sociology,' 2,* 149–152.

Schöpflin, G. (1995). Post-communism: a profile. *Javnost – The Public, 2*(1), 63–74.

Toepfl, F. (2020). Comparing authoritarian publics: the benefits and risks of three types of publics for autocrats. *Communication Theory, 30*(2), 105–125.

17

AUSTRIA

A ski resort as the virus slingshot of Europe

Katie Bates and Lore Hayek

Political context

2019 had been a politically turbulent year in Austria. The emergence of the infamous 'Ibiza'-video, which showed the head of the right-wing Freedom Party, Heinz-Christian Strache, discussing potential business opportunities in return for government favours with an alleged Russian oligarch in a holiday finca on the Spanish island (Al-Serori et al., 2019), led to the collapse of the centre-right government and snap elections in September. Extensive talks eventually resulted in the first ever coalition between the conservative ÖVP and the Green Party. The coalition took office on January 7, 2020 with Werner Kogler of the Green Party becoming Vice Chancellor to Chancellor Sebastian Kurz. While the ÖVP has the largest proportion of ministers, Health Minister Rudolf Anschober of the Green Party rapidly became one of the main players in the government as the first COVID-19 cases were confirmed in late February. Surveys about trust in government members found the highest levels of trust ever in Austria during the peak of the crisis (DiePresse.com, 2020).

Chronology

Compared to other European countries, Austria managed to reduce the impact of COVID-19 with an 'aggressive' and 'early' response, despite the ski resort of Ischgl once considered the superspreader of Europe (Gibney, 2020). On March 5, just under 100,000 COVID-19 cases had been reported worldwide and the World Health Organisation (WHO) Director-General appealed to all countries to pursue 'aggressive preparedness' (WHO, 2020a). The same day, the Icelandic Directorate of Health officially identified the Austrian ski resort of Ischgl a COVID-19 risk area. The previous day, Iceland had reported to the Early

DOI: 10.4324/9781003120254-19

Warning and Response System (EWRS) that 15 people returning to Iceland on a flight from Munich tested positive for COVID-19, 14 of which had been skiing in Ischgl (Spiegel International, 2020). Despite this, on the same day, WHO listed Austria as having 37 'imported cases only' (WHO, 2020b).

On March 7, a bar worker at the 'Kitzloch' Après Ski bar in Ischgl tested positive for COVID-19 (Spiegel International, 2020). On the same day, the WHO updated the transmission classification in Austria to 'local transmission' (WHO, 2020c), with 104 cases reported in Austria. However, tourism businesses were reluctant to agree to any measures as the winter season in the Alps was in full swing – bars, clubs, restaurants and hotels remained full.

By mid-March, Ischgl was considered the location of a significant super-spreading event in Europe, labelled the 'Virenschleuder Europas' (Europe's virus slingshot), with skiers taking the virus home to Germany and many Nordic countries. In March, infections across Germany were higher in areas closer to Ischgl (Felbermayr et al., 2020). The superspreading not only fuelled transmission internationally: by the end of April, 'Cluster S' (Ischgl and surrounds), just one of 141 clusters in Austria, was identified by the Austrian Agency for Health and Food Safety as the source of 41% of infections in Austria.

The first death from COVID-19 in Austria was reported on March 12 (WHO, 2020c). The *COVID-19 Measures Act* (COVID-19 Maßnahmengesetz, 2020) came into force on March 16, 12 am, one week after Italy and one week before Germany. The Act supplemented the existing *Austrian Epidemics Act 1950* and made provisions for restrictions on movement by prohibiting access to certain business premises and public places. Fines were imposed for any infringement, alongside employment, tax and financial measures. As a result of the act and its measures, the population were only allowed to leave the house for four specific reasons: to aid other people, particularly those at high risk, for everyday basic needs (such as grocery shopping), for work and to walk the dog or look after other animals. After ongoing public confusion, this last provision was clarified to also allow taking exercise. The province of Tyrol introduced additional measures, limiting people to their own municipality (Bote für Tirol, 2020); the Paznaun valley (where Ischgl is located) was put under full lockdown by the health authority for more than four weeks (Verkehrsbeschränkende Maßnahmen, 2020).

The peak in infections occurred on March 26, with 1,065 new cases and 78 deaths reported (BMSGPK, 2020). Measures were tightened on March 30 to include obligatory use of face masks when grocery shopping and enforced working from home or leave of absence (with government pay where required) for people that fell into medically high-risk categories. A week later, the government extended the requirement to wearing face masks whilst shopping and on public transport, whilst also outlining plans for the incremental lifting of certain measures with a view to reopening the economy and public life in Austria. A clear caveat was made, measures would be re-imposed if new cases rose significantly. Peak prevalence occurred on April 3 with 9,069 active cases, at that time 158 deaths had been reported (BMSGPK, 2020).

The prospect of Easter family celebrations led to some confusion in both communication and legislation. The government issued an 'Easter decree' limiting the number of people at private festivities to five. However, this contradicted the COVID-19 law as 'paying someone a visit' was not one of the four permitted reasons to leave the house (Grüll, 2020). A few days later, the Easter decree was subsequently renounced. This U-turn undermined government communication from then on.

New regulations eased the COVID-19 measures from April 14, four weeks after lockdown began, with non-essential, smaller stores opening. Restaurants and hotels opened their doors in mid-May with servers required to wear masks, only four people per table and tables to be 2 metres apart. From mid-June, face masks were only mandatory on public transport, in health facilities including pharmacies and other places where social distancing is difficult, including hairdressers. Obligatory masks in grocery shops and services like post offices and banks were re-introduced on July 24. See Table 17.1.

Analysis

Crises call for intense communication. Political leaders are expected to reduce public uncertainties caused by the crisis and provide 'meaning making' (Boin et al., 2005; Drennan & McConnell, 2007). One of the most trustworthy forms of political communication is the live press conference; press conferences are considered a strong and effective way to convey key political messages (Eshbaugh-Soha, 2013), as they require politicians and journalists to be in the same room at the same time and are therefore only employed for matters of great importance. Press conferences broadcast live on national television are quite unusual in most countries and are only held on rare occasions such as government formation/dissolution etc. Further, they circumvent the gatekeeping function of the media by letting politicians address the public directly, without a media filter.

During the COVID-19 crisis, many such press conferences were held in European countries. Politicians used press conferences to share general information about the current COVID-19 situation (number of new cases/hospitalisations/deaths etc.), to communicate concrete rules and measure, and to frame the national and international situation for their citizens.

In this chapter, we analyse the Austrian government's televised press conferences as the main channel of communication during the COVID-19 crisis. Our dataset includes all televised national press conferences, taking place almost daily, including weekends, from their start on March 10 until the last press conference on May 27 (n = 64). Within these 64 press conferences, 187 statements were made by 47 different actors. The content of each statement was coded, focusing on the proximity level of the threat(s) communicated (from a threat to the self to a threat to the world) and the main issues discussed. These were analysed by the characteristics of the actors in each press conference (sex, political party or organisation), the use of 'facts' and the timing of the press conference (by month) at both the press conference and statement level. Additionally, press conferences

TABLE 17.1 Austria chronology

Date		Diffusion of COVID-19	Key official actions	Key communication events
February	24		Installation of a panel of experts to advise the Minister of Health about COVID-19.	
	25	First two confirmed cases in a hotel in Innsbruck, Tyrol.		
March	5		Iceland classifies the ski resort Ischgl (Tyrol) as a high-risk area.	
	7	Barkeeper in Ischgl tests positive, followed by the identification of Ischgl as one of the first 'clusters.'		
	10		Travel restrictions apply.	Start of (almost) daily televised government press conferences.
	11	COVID-19 declared a pandemic by WHO.	Museums, tourist attractions etc. closed.	
	12	First COVID-death in Vienna.	Schools and universities switch to distance learning.	
	15		Military are deployed.	
	16		COVID-19 measures law comes into force. Restrictions on leaving the house, restaurants, bars and non-essential shops and services are closed. Tyrol goes into full lockdown for two weeks.	
	18		Chaos at Austro–Hungarian border due to travel restrictions.	

	28		'It is not a sprint, it is a marathon' (Nehammer).
	30		'Soon, we will all know somebody who will have died of Corona' (Chancellor Kurz).
April	1	Number of infected >10,000.	
	4	Number of recovered exceeds infected for the first time.	
	6	Compulsory face masks in shops, on public transport and in public buildings.	
	13		Presentation of the prevalence study: 0.33% of the population are infected.
	14	After Easter: non-essential shops reopen, small family gatherings are allowed.	
	21		'We are now able to slowly, carefully set steps towards reopening' (Health Minister Anschober). 'We have to get used to a new normality' (Chancellor Kurz).
	30	>500,000 people unemployed (+60% compared to 2019), >1.2 million employees on short time.	
May	1	Shops, hairdressers etc. reopen.	
	4	Pupils return to schools in shift operation.	

(Continued)

TABLE 17.1 (Continued)

Date		Diffusion of COVID-19	Key official actions	Key communication events
	15		Restaurants and bars reopen: Max. 4 guests at a table, staff must wear masks, curfew at 11 PM.	Chancellor Kurz invites German tourists to spend their summer in Austria rather than in Italy.
	21	No additional deaths for 24 hours.		
	25		Start of modified *Matura* (nationwide school leaving examination) – oral examinations are cancelled.	
June	15		Masks only compulsory on public transport.	
July	14		Constitutional court rules parts of the early COVID-19 measures (denial of access to public places) unconstitutional.	
	24		Re-introduction of compulsory masks in grocery shops and most public buildings.	
	31	21,000 infected, 718 deaths, 1,654 active cases.		

were categorised as implementing or relaxing social protection measures (or otherwise); these categories were then analysed using the threats and issues discussed alongside key actor characteristics and the use of 'facts.'

Press conferences varied considerably in their style (presentation format, frequency, actors (politicians/scientists/others; gender balance), settings, duration, admission of journalists' questions etc.). Of 187 statements, 152 (81.3%) were delivered by government politicians. Of these, 91 were by ÖVP politicians, Chancellor Kurz delivered the majority (21%, n = 19). The Green Party delivered just over a third of the politician-led statements (n = 58), Rudolf Anschober, the Health Minister delivered the majority (53.4%, n = 31). Indeed, Anschober delivered the most politician-led statements between March and May, even more than the Chancellor. Only ten statements (5.4%) were delivered by experts from the health care and research sectors. Other organisations, including telecommunications and unions, got their say in the remaining 25 statements (13.4%). Women spoke in just under one third of all statements (n = 51).

At press conferences, government politicians spoke at 63 of the 64, with 45 of press conferences (70.3%) only featuring politicians. The ÖVP was represented in 78.1% (n = 50) and the Green Party at 61.0% (n = 39). Health specialists spoke at six. Practitioners from other fields spoke at 15 (23.4%). Of all press conferences, 42.2% (n = 27) involved male actors only, 45.3% (n = 29) had both male and female actors and just 12.5% involved female actors only. The largest press conference was held on March 11, the day the WHO declared a pandemic, which contained eight actors, (seven male, one female), when measures for the closure of schools and kindergartens were introduced. The composition of the press conferences changed dramatically over time. In both March and April, 25 press conferences occurred. During May, only 14 press conferences were broadcast and only politicians were present.

Health Minister Anschober was the dominant presence, with this dominance increasing over time – Anschober spoke in 50% of press conferences in March, 54.6% in April and 62.5% in May. Anschober was also the main communicator of the facts and figures that supported government's decisions; almost all his press statements began with an overview of the numbers of infected, hospitalised and deceased people. Only 44 of all statements contained statistics directly related to the COVID-19, 27 of these were delivered by Anschober.

The issues discussed in the press conferences were quite obviously dominated by health care, which was the central concern in over a quarter of the statements. However, the analysis of issues shows the extent of the COVID-19 crisis, as measures had to be taken (and communicated) in almost all sectors of public life: the economy, civil protection and the military, kindergarten and schools, law and justice, transport and culture were each addressed in more than ten statements. Many statements also acted as appeals for national unity and cohesion:

> We achieved a great deal as a republic and a bouquet of flowers goes to all
> our citizens, who enabled this success. We did apply the right measures at

the right time – but it was the people who implemented them. Nothing would have been possible without the people.

(Rudolf Anschober, April 28,2020 [translated by authors])

Health was the dominant issue at press conferences, addressed in 29 of 64, followed by the *economy* (n = 22). Health was most commonly discussed in multi-issue press conferences which addressed two or three main issues, highlighting the challenging, intersectional nature of the effects of COVID-19. The *economy*, in contrast, was most commonly addressed in single issue press conferences (n = 11). Most issues were consistently raised across the months of March, April and May. The exceptions were *education* and *infrastructure* – reference to these issues declined over time. As restrictions eased in May, *leisure* became a more important theme.

One feature of effective crisis communication is employing messages that seek to induce behavioural change by presenting a threat (Reynolds & Seeger, 2005). The press conferences extensively discussed the threat that the virus posed on different levels, which we coded on a scale based on proximity to an individual from 1 (threat to the world as a whole) to 10 (threat to your own self). Almost 60% of the press statements discussed at least one kind of threat.

In over 40% of the statements, Austria was identified as under threat, which is in line with the government's strategy to frame COVID-19 as a national crisis and reinforced the call for national unity. Indeed, at the press conference level, 85% of press conferences identified at least one threat and Austria as under threat. In press conferences identifying one sole threat (n = 17), the threat to Austria dominated (n = 13), reinforcing the framing of the pandemic as a national crisis. Very frequently, older people, as the at high-risk population, were mentioned, with appeals by the chancellor and ministers not to visit older family members.

Under no circumstances should you take your children to their grandparents, as they are the people we need to protect the most

(Sebastian Kurz, March 11, 2020 [translated by authors]).

The Minister of the Interior, Karl Nehammer, used the most drastic words when he called people who would not adhere to the social distancing rules 'Lebensgefährder' (endangerers of lives, as opposed to 'Lebensretter' – life-savers).

Social protection measures were introduced in 11 press conferences, ten of which were in March. Press conferences differed when social protection measures were being introduced, in all but one on March 11, only politicians were present. In the 20 press conferences where measures were relaxed, politicians were always present with other actors involved in five. Threats to Austria were raised in every single press conference where a measure was introduced, eight raised the threat to Europe, seven a threat to those at risk and six a threat to the Austrian health system. The use of COVID-19-related statistics was highest in press conferences introducing measures (70%) and lowest in press conferences introducing no measures (n = 31), just over half of these press conferences referred to statistics related to other issues.

In the first few weeks of the crisis, the public perceived the government's communication as consistent and trustworthy (Austrian Corona Panel Project, 2020). However, the government caused bewilderment when the so-called 'Easter decree' was published, further restricting private gatherings to a maximum of five people to prevent large family meetings over the Easter holidays. Constitutional lawyers, opposition parties and civil liberties activists protested this regulation, for restrictions that affect private households are not covered by the COVID-19 legislation (Negwer & Medlitz, 2020). In July, the Constitutional Court ruled it unlawful. Survey data shows while citizens perceived the government's measures as quite effective and adequate in the early weeks, this support, albeit remaining high, became less stable over the course of the crisis: a panel survey shows, on a 10-point scale, a decline in trust in the government of 1.7 points (Austrian Corona Panel Project, 2020).

Conclusion

As the governor of Tyrol stated in the midst of the crisis, it is easier to read the book from the end. After the initial strict but firm communication of measures, Easter brought a mix of conflicting decrees and messages, which led to a perception of 'management by chaos.' Whilst sometimes fractured and inconsistent, the rapid implementation of social distancing measures were able to interrupt transmission early within Austria, no doubt reducing the peak of COVID-19 infections and sharply reducing the burden of excess mortality other countries faced. This comparatively rapid response has meant Austria stands out as an example of a relatively successful strategy protecting its own population, although the argued failure to react in a timely manner to emerging evidence of an outbreak in Ischgl undermined the credibility of the Austrian government's response internationally.

References

Al-Serori, L., Das Gupta, O., Münch, P., Obermaier, F. & Obermayer, B. (2019). Caught in the Trap. https://projekte.sueddeutsche.de/artikel/politik/caught-in-the-trap-e675751/ abgerufen

Austrian Corona Panel Project (2020). *Austrian Corona Panel Data*. Vienna: University of Vienna.

BMSGPK (Bundesministerium für Soziales, Gesundheit, Pflege und Konsumentenschutz) (2020). Ein einfaches COVID-19 Dashboard für Österreich. www.data.gv.at/anwendungen/covid-hallofreunde/

Boin, A., t'Hart, P., Stern, E., & Sundelius, B. (2005). *The Politics of Crisis Management: Public Leadership under Pressure*. Cambridge: Cambridge University Press.

Bote für Tirol (2020). Bote für Tirol Stück 10c. www.tirol.gv.at/fileadmin/buergerse rvice/bote/downloads/2020/Bote_10c-2020.pdf

COVID-19 Maßnahmengesetz (2020). Bundesgesetz betreffend vorläufige Maßnahmen zur Verhinderung der Verbreitung von COVID-19. www.ris.bka.gv.at/GeltendeFass ung.wxe?Abfrage=Bundesnormen&Gesetzesnummer=20011073

DiePresse.com (2020). Umfrage: Rekordwerte für Regierung. www.diepresse.com/57 95128/umfrage-rekordwerte-fur-regierung

Drennan, L. T. & McConnell, A. (2007). *Risk and Crisis Management in the Public Sector*. New York: Routledge.

Eshbaugh-Soha, M. (2013). Presidential Influence of the News Media: The Case of the Press Conference. *Political Communication* 30(4), 548–564. https://doi.org/10.1080/1 0584609.2012.737438

Felbermayr, G., Hinz, J. & Chowdhry, S. (2020). Après-ski: The Spread of Coronavirus from Ischgl through Germany. www.ifw-kiel.de/fileadmin/Dateiverwaltung/IfW -Publications/Gabriel_Felbermayr/Apres-ski__The_Spread_of_Coronavirus_ from_Ischgl_through_Germany/coronavirus_from_ischgl.pdf

Gibney, E. (2020). Whose Coronavirus Strategy Worked Best? Scientists Hunt Most Effective Policies. *Nature* 581(7806), 15–16. https://doi.org/10.1038/d41586-020-01248-1

Grüll, P. (2020). Austria's Government Presents COVID-19 Exit Schedule. www.euract iv.com/section/coronavirus/news/austrias-government-presents-covid-19-exit-schedule/

Negwer, G. & Medlitz, H. (2020). Was die Betretungs-Verordnung wirklich verbietet und was nicht. www.diepresse.com/5798542/was-die-betretungs-verordnung-wirk lich-verbietet-und-was-nicht

Reynolds, B. & Seeger, M. W. (2005). Crisis and Emergency Risk Communication as an Integrative Model. *Journal of Health Communication* 10(1), 43–55.

Spiegel International (2020). Chronical of Failure – A Corona Hotspot in the Alps Spread Virus Across Europe. www.spiegel.de/international/world/ischgl-austria-a -corona-hotspot-in-the-alps-spread-virus-across-europe-a-32b17b76-14df-4f37-bfcf -39d2ceee92ec last accessed 22.06.2020

Verkehrsbeschränkende Maßnahmen (2020). Gemeinden im Paznauntal und Gemeinde St. Anton a. A.; Verkehrsbeschränkende Maßnahmen nach dem Epidemiegesetz 1950. www.tirol.gv.at/fileadmin/buergerservice/kundmachungen/bh-landeck/Jan-Jun_2020/EPI-57-9.pdf

WHO (2020a). WHO Director-General's Opening Remarks at the Media Briefing on COVID-19 – 5. March. www.who.int/dg/speeches/detail/who-director-general-s-o pening-remarks-at-the-media-briefing-on-covid-19---5-march-2020

WHO (2020b). Situation Report 45. www.who.int/docs/default-source/coronaviruse/ situation-reports/20200305-sitrep-45-covid-19.pdf?sfvrsn=ed2ba78b_4

WHO (2020c). Situation Report 48. www.who.int/docs/default-source/coronaviruse/ situation-reports/20200308-sitrep-48-covid-19.pdf?sfvrsn=16f7ccef_4

18

IRAN

Disciplinary strategies and governmental campaigning

Azra Ghandeharion and Josef Kraus

Political context

Due to heavy international pressure caused by many unilateral and multilateral sanctions, Iran has a special place in global politics. It seems that Iranian governments, like all, are under the spotlight not only during elections but always since we are in a state of permanent campaigning in this new media environment (Lilleker, 2014: 4). Since the Islamic Revolution (1979), the country is ruled by *velayat-e faqih*, Guardianship of the Islamic Jurist. It is based on ideas of Muslim Shia political thought developed by the mastermind and the leader of the Revolution – Ayatollah Ruhollah Khomeini (1979–1989). The highest authority in the state is the Supreme Leader, nowadays Ayatollah Sayyed Ali Khamenei (1989–present), who controls, disciplines and supervises Iranian politics, its orientation and main actors. There are three pillars of power in the state: first, a president and his cabinet as executive power responsible for internal and international affairs; second, the body of parliament as the legislative power; third, the judicial system headed by Chief Justice. A security system also protects the state, the political administration and the Islamic Revolution legacy.[1]

Chronology

Iran has been one of the most affected countries by COVID-19, experiencing rapid growth before the pandemic touched Europe or the United States. Iran reported its first case of infections (two deaths, February 19, 2020) in the holy city of Qom, the centre of religion and politics of the country and important pilgrimage destination for Muslim Shiites. Saeed Namaki, the Minister of Health and Medical Education (MHME) said that one of the casualties from the virus was a merchant who regularly shuttled between Iran and China using indirect

DOI: 10.4324/9781003120254-20

flights after Iran stopped direct passenger flights to China. Though Qom transportation was partially suspended by MHME (Radio Farda, February 23, 2020),
just a few days after the news, coronavirus infections were reported in 24 of the
31 Iranian provinces. The rapid growth had been combined with an extremely
high mortality rate (20+%). Suddenly, Iran became one of the global epicentres
of the COVID-19 pandemic (Wright, 2020).

By the end of February, there were almost 600 cases in the country. The
number increased to nearly 6,000 (March 1–7). At the end of the month, around
44,000 cases were reported. The peak of daily new cases can be identified in
the last days of March with 3,000 infections a day and 30,000 active cases
(Worldometers.info).[2] It is possible to identify three milestones of the spread
from the beginning of February until the end of March. First, commemorat-
ing the anniversary of the Islamic Revolution (February 11), the overthrow of
Shah Mohammad Reza Pahlavi (1979) by the masses with a crucial contribu-
tion from the clergy (i.e. based in Qom). Second, the parliamentary elections
(February 21) at which participation was encouraged and campaigned for by
state representatives. The Supreme Leader, who on the Election Day proclaimed
voting was 'a religious duty,' blamed the low turnout on the 'negative coronavirus propaganda' by Iran's enemies; at that moment, Iran suffered eight deaths
and had the highest COVID-19 death toll outside of China (Hafezi, 2020a).
Third, the Iranian New Year – Nowruz (March 21), one of the most important holidays for Iranians with many gatherings and vacation trips for one to
two weeks. Around 1,600 casualties related to COVID-19 were reported in
Iran by March 21, 2020. Just in the two weeks of the holidays, the number
doubled (Worldometers.info). People's disregard for MHME protocols, though
hourly broadcast by State TV, forced the authority to harden the measures.
In a disciplinarian reaction, the government locked down the parks, banned
trips between cities, and traditional and religious gatherings. President Hassan
Rouhani (2013–present) also asked travellers to return to their homes (Middle
East Eye, 2020).

These measures, combined with holidays, caused a reduction of cases, and
during the first week of April both daily new cases and active cases decreased.
The lowest number was reached at the beginning of May (daily cases: 800; active
cases: 13,000). During the period, the government eased restrictions by allowing low/mid-risk business activities (Hafezi, 2020b). After these measures were
relaxed in April, the numbers of infections started to increase again in May.
Despite that, mosques/shrines were opened by mid-May. The infection distribution has become asymmetric among Iranian provinces causing re-imposition of
lockdown restrictions in affected areas. Though foreign media have questioned
provincial figures (Al-Jazeera.com, 2020), Iranian media reported the virus as
'almost under control.' At the time of finishing this chapter (mid-July 2020),
there are 31,000+ active cases in Iran, with a total number of 240,000+ infected
and 11,000+ deaths (Worldometers.info). The statistics have been challenged by
the BBC (claiming 40,000 casualties and 450,000+ infected) (August 3, 2020);

nevertheless, under these circumstances, verification of the facts is crucial but difficult.

Analysis

A time for discipline

In the absence of private and international media inside Iran, the prohibition of satellite television and the banning of some social networks, state-owned Islamic Republic of Iran Broadcasting (IRIB) seems to be the sole speaker. IRIB, under the supervision of the Supreme Leader, directly controls the information flow, shapes opinions and sets the political stance of Iran. Yet, with the explosion of new media, nobody can be the sole speaker. Except during temporary internet blackouts in Iran, like on November 16–23, 2019, rules are subverted, satellite TVs are watched, the sanctioned Zoom and Rocket-Chat, and the filtered Facebook, Telegram, Twitter and YouTube are accessed via VPN; internet disruption is probable however and the information flow is relatively slow, around 2–10 Mbit/s (Saeidi Ghaviandam, 2020). That makes IRIB/State TV not omnipotent, yet powerful and popular especially when internet infrastructures failed during home quarantine and access was almost impossible (late March–April). Pro-government commentators claimed the COVID-19 outbreak resurrected an IRIB seriously struggling to attract an audience who preferred foreign Persian TV channels like *BBC*, *VOA*, *Iran International* and *Manoto* (*Coronavirus Resurrected TV*, 2020). IRIB has four international, 12 domestic and 30 provincial channels. To paint a holistic picture of governmental policies, the data of this research is based on the scrutiny of the international and domestic plus the provincial channels of COVID-19 red zones like Qom, Tehran and Mashhad from February to early July 2020 (i.e. 22 channels).

The COVID-19 recession precipitated disciplinarian strategies for the economy and business, partly rooted in paralysing sanctions and partially in corruptions (*Iran Corruption Rank*, 2020) leading to a 'War against Corruption' campaign, *Mobarezeh ba Fesäd* (Tabnak, 2020). This campaign, popularised by Ebrahim Raisi appointed as Chief Justice (March 2019), won hourly media attention during the COVID-19 crisis. IRIB narrated how war is waged against hoarders of medicine, food, detergent, health-care products and COVID-19 supplies. Drawing affinities between 'coronavirus' and 'corruption,' their eradication, the safety of the people and the protection of treasury, *beyt-o-mäl*, were quotidian metaphors used by the highest officials of the Iranian government (Tabnak, 2020).

From the initial phase of the COVID-19 crisis to the managed crisis phase, February to May, official news and IRIB broadcast the required health-care actions daily in three stages. First, the emphasis was on symptoms and sanitation; besides TV, MHME and Red Crescent sent daily/weekly text messages to every resident in Iran (March 1 to April 17). The second phase was 'social distancing' and home quarantine (mid-March). The third was 'intelligent distancing' and the gradual reopening for business hierarchised to three levels by MHME from low- to high-risk professions by attaining a Health QR code. Depending on their risk category, they were unlocked on April 11 and 18 and May 17, 2020. IRIB covered, avowed and applauded how school and university classes were entirely held via virtual platforms and partly broadcast in *IRIB Amoozesh/Teaching* (Channel 7). Though school/university opening was optional and only white zones and graduate levels had won MHME's approval, their re-closure was announced in the second surge of COVID-19 in red zones like Tehran, Ahwaz and Mashhad on July 1, 2020.

A time for campaign

In line with the 'Against corona' campaign, with the collaboration of top Iranian universities, MHME introduced Mask mobile application on April 17 (Mask.ir); it tracks the spread in every city district, provides the user with medical information and the locations of nearby clinics. Launched on March 4 by MHME, *Salamat.gov.ir*, an electronic screening system, became the strategic government tool: it was the reference point for expert guidance, information, a threat barometer and goal-setting indicator. The disciplinary tactics of IRIB took place almost every day by commending the followers of health protocols and punishing deviant citizens either by filming how MHME inspectors sealed their shops or their remorseful and repentant comments for neglecting public health. Though MHME claimed that the required actions were justified and the objective was clear, the mandatory Health code was mildly criticised because internet infrastructures were not ready to support so many users on such a scale (*Internet Disruption*, 2020).

Since February 29, all public interactions were disciplined by two health campaign slogans, '#we_stay_at_home' and '#we_defeat_coronavirus,' decorating almost everywhere, from actual to virtual spaces. The slogans met some additions and variations. After a month, to reinforce the seriousness of the pandemic, 'still' was added to 'we_stay_at_home,' or by Ramadan, 'with God's help' either in Persian or Arabic embellishing 'we_defeat_coronavirus' – corresponding to national and Muslim tendencies. Along with the campaign, the government's ideological stance was reflected in labels like 'Ambassadors of Health' (*Safirän-e Salamat*) given to citizens who educate the public, to encourage social responsibility and 'Defenders of Health,' (*Modafeän-e Salamat*) granted to health-care personnel, to inspire the integration of the government and the people and promote regional geopolitics. Defenders of Health clearly echoes 'Defenders of the Holy Shrine,' *Modafeän-e Haram*, a term coined by the Iranian government referring to military personnel and consultants who protect Shia holy shrines, the target for destruction by Sunni rebels in Syria and Iraq battles.

The term 'Defender of Holy Shrine Martyr' emerged since December 2011 (Khodabakhsh, 2016); reiterated in 'Defenders of Health Martyr,' this title is granted to health-care casualties during the COVID-19 crisis whose martyrdom is commemorated in government-sponsored ceremonies like that of Holy Defence and Holy Shrine Defence, the official names given to the Iraq-Iran War (1980–1988), Iraqi Civil War (2014–2017), Iraqi Insurgency (2017–present) and Syrian Civil War (2011–present), respectively.

The linkage of COVID-19 to Iranian geopolitics was later reinforced with the speech the Supreme Leader (April 9) delivered for the celebration of the birth of the Twelfth Shiite Imam, Mahdi – Messiah (869 CE). Since Ramadan, the month of piety and donation was on its way, he introduced the 'Empathizing War Game' campaign, *Razmäyesh-e Hamdeli*, later retitled *Razmäyesh-e hamdeli, mosavat va komak-e momenäneh* or 'military and/or war exercise of empathy and help [carried] by the religious/pious/faithful people' (Khamenei, 2020). Though challenging to be translated to English, keywords like 'war,' 'empathy,' 'exercise,' and 'faith/religion' and the absence of 'health,' 'safety' or 'virus' can noticeably outline the government strategy: a shift of framing of fighting COVID-19 as a holy war.

COVID-19 sends messages to the nation

While the nature of the COVID-19 threat was clear, the messages sent to the people via IRIB, rather than highlighting COVID-19, were *consistently* leaning towards independence, autonomy, self-empowerment, national pride and the demise of the developed countries. The lucidity of expert guidance was covered in short reports on News and Health channels though the most-watched news was the comprehensive *14:00 News* (45–55 minutes) broadcast every day by *Channel 1* where *Corona-News* studio delivered national and international accounts (15–25 minutes). Aired from March to early June, national and international statistics were updated in *Corona-News* by the anchorperson, a medical doctor or PhD holder in medical education, and the Head of Iranian Health Ministry's Public Relations Office, Kianoush Jahanpour (February 19–June 9) and Sima Sadat Lari (June 9–present).

On a national scale, four clear message areas were delivered daily: health and quarantine; sympathy to victims; self-reliance despite sanctions and scientific improvements. Gradually, health-related news gave way to the other three. Communal help was reflected in the coverage of numerous charity and voluntary works in pictures and videos sent by people daily, the inexhaustive struggle of schoolteachers in virtual education and masked factory workers in actual life, photogenic portraits of health-care personnel, and children dedicating songs to Defenders of Health. These were some examples among many, to promote 'We Fight Coronavirus' and the 'Empathizing War Game' campaign.

The Supreme Leader's naming the New Year 'Production Leap/ Surge' campaign, *jahesh-e tolid*, linked independence, self-sufficiency, scientific improvements and overcoming the challenges of imposed sanctions under the slogan 'Turn the Threat to Opportunity' which entered the campaign lexicon under the presidency of Mahmood Ahmadinejad (2005–2013). During his presidency, the third chain of consecutive sanctions (1979; 1984; 2006–present) initiated numerous self-reliance campaigns that were reused for the COVID-19 crisis. Businesses and charitable organisations were disciplined to make masks, detergents, alcohol and COVID-19 drugs, making their shares rocket in the stock market. Besides daily medicinal and health-care improvements, news covered how natural resources were turned to technologically advanced materials that can help Iran during the COVID-19 recession. The voice of the Supreme Leader, words of the 'Production Leap' campaign and dramatic music were added to reports for artistic effect.

On the international level, the precarious and tragic situation in the world, riots, empty malls, mask theft, piled corpses of COVID-19 casualties, especially in developed countries and especially the USA and UK, were covered daily. How foreign media, mainly American and British, represent the COVID-19 pandemic in Iran won almost equal attention in Politics (News Channel) and *20:30* summarised coverage as the enemies of Iran/Islamic Revolution whitewashed their national crisis and augmented or faked the news about Iran. Titles like 'Enemy's Failed Attempt to Manufacture Crisis' (IRIB, April 7, 2020), 'Enemy's Media War,' 'Psyops,' 'Psychological Warfare' and 'Soft War' aimed at the national public trust are standard (Z. S. Hashemi, 2020a; Karkhayi, 2020; SeyedHosseini, 2020). 'Coronavirus Media Trap' criticised the biased portrayal of April and March prison riots in Iran by Western media (IRIB, April 4, 2020), 'Anti-Revolutionary TV Channels Gossip Surfing' recounts the news of a drug addict who has been reported as a COVID-19 victim left on the street (IRIB, March 12, 2020). In harmony with self-reliance as the key factor in most COVID-19 campaigns, the hardships inflicted by external forces were hardly voiced in national news, above all, how American sanctions harmed Iranians' right to health or why Google Play has removed Mask. ir app. However, numerous tweets of the officials like Mohammad Javad Zarif, Minister of Foreign Affairs (2013–present), and Jahanpour openly addressed these issues.

Discipline posed as a challenge

Since late May, though the coverage of COVID-19 was diminished to 5–15 minutes on the most popular news *14:00, 20:30* and *21:00 News* programmes (Channel 1–2), in late June, just before the second surge (2000+ daily reports), wearing masks became mandatory. Following the new disciplinary campaign, '#I-wear-mask,' whoever works for the government, if non-compliant, faced punishment by a daily wage reduction and government offices denied services to those not wearing a mask (July 5); furthermore, MHME protocols were strictly monitored in public spaces. Health topics, though short, gained momentum by being aired at the beginning of the news show. The disciplinary technique was the same, reminding the audience to follow protocols while the deviants, unmasked and gloveless, were shown apologetic and repentant more than ever.

Nevertheless, disciplining physical distance is a cultural, geopolitical and infrastructural challenge for the Iranian government. Culturally, distancing has always been a rival discourse when it comes to Iranians' prioritisation of hospitality and warmth, shaking hands and greeting kisses are an integral part of their social communication. As a solution, 'social distancing' signs in governmental offices, including public universities and semi-governmental institutions, were given a new label: *faseley-e mehrabani*, 'the kindness distance.' The 'kindness distance' is applicable in some offices. Still, when it comes to banks, that had the highest number of COVID-19 victims after the health-care personnel (Nikrouyan, 2020) and government service counters that provide COVID-19 wage subsidies, distance is unfeasible.

Similarly, following the strict discipline of one-metre distancing on public transport seemed impractical because of the weak infrastructure. To solve this problem, the government suspended the traffic reduction scheme allowing odd or even numbered licence plates in restricted zones of metropolitan cites. Though this short-term policy was extended weekly since early March until May 26, keeping Eid al-Fitr as the milestone of returning to the normal situation, some state-run news agencies[3] were critical towards its efficiency claiming that it leads to pollution, traffic congestion and even more intercity travel (IRNA, 2020; M. S. Hashemi, 2020b).

Using different disciplinary strategies and synchronised campaigns, government, IRIB and official news agencies tried to depict a unanimous body, including media, experts, scientists, commentators, politicians, religious leaders and official journalists, as the main actor. Nonetheless, the unanimity was subverted in some instances. IRIB has criticised governmental policies for social distancing in public places, temporary removal of traffic reduction and virtual schools during the gradual reopening. The 'We stay at home' campaign was promoted by 100 GB free internet (March 19–27); though the strategy seemed practical, the infrastructure was not ready for the traffic. IRIB reported how people faced frequent instances of internet crash.

Conclusion

Just before the first COVID-19 case was officially announced on February 19 amid parliamentary elections and Iran's entering the Financial Action Task Force (FATF) blacklist on February 21, Iran had experienced protests because of rises in fuel prices in November 2019 (IRIB, January 21, 2019), a drop in the currency and the assassination of Maj. Gen. Qasem Soleimani on January 3, which increased Iran–United States hostility. That is the reason why COVID-19, though a global crisis, has entered Iran rather peacefully and even farcically reflected in social network trends like '#CoronaLaughter,' 'Iranians, the survivors of Armageddon' or 'Give me more crisis!'

When crisis is piled on crisis and national media delivers news, almost every day, about the enemies of Iran juxtaposed with the beneficial outcome of clear leadership, a consistent point of reference is unattainable because they are entangled in a complicated network of internal and external factors ranging from American and European sanctions, economic corruption, weak infrastructures and social irresponsibility.

More than a health issue, COVID-19 chronicles the campaigns and disciplinary power practised upon people where politics, economy and religion are tightly woven into the fabric of public and private life. The state authority has to handle the issue with delicacy and tact due to international sanctions and national pressures. In the absence of foreign press, the state-controlled media have become the main communication channel to manage the crisis and prevent catastrophic outbreaks. Whether the future sees campaigns extend the measures taken to fight against COVID-19 or if it will be disciplined to narrate another story remains to be seen.

Notes

1 For more information about the Iranian political system, see Buchta, 2002.
2 Data provided by the Iranian MHME gathered and available at Worldometers.info.
3 IRNA, Islamic Republic News Agency, and IMNA, Iran's Metropolises News Agency.

References

Al-Jazeera.com (2020). *Iran warns of coronavirus cluster spread as 71 more die*, www.aljaze era.com/news/2020/05/iran-warns-coronavirus-cluster-spread-71-die-200514114 529520.html

BBC (2020). *Coronavirus: Iran cover-up of deaths revealed by data leak*, www.bbc.com/news /world-middle-east-53598965

Buchta, W. (2002). *Who rules Iran? The structure and power in the Islamic Republic*, Washington Institute for Near East Policy.

Coronavirus Resurrected TV (2020). How Coronavirus outbreak resurrected State TV. Khabaronline.Ir; Khabar online: Iranian analytical news agency. khabaronline.ir/ news/1357961.

IRIB (2019). *20:30* [Television News]. Tehran: IRIB Channel 2.

IRNA (2020). *Coronavirus and the controversial traffic scheme in Tehran*, www.irna.ir/news /83777481/

Hafezi, P. (2020a). Iran announces low poll turnout, blames coronavirus 'propaganda,' *Reuters.com*. www.reuters.com/article/us-iran-election-khamenei/iran-announces-low-poll-turnout-blames-coronavirus-propaganda-idUSKCN20H09Z

Hafezi, P. (2020b). Iran renews coronavirus warning as 'low risk' activities re-start, *Reuters.com*. www.reuters.com/article/us-health-coronavirus-iran/iran-renews-co ronavirus-warning-as-low-risk-activities-re-start-idUSKCN21T0AO

Hashemi, Z. S. (2020a). *The enemy's media war, aimed at public trust*, IRNA, Islamic Republic News Agency. www.irna.ir/news/83642498/

Hashemi, M. S. (2020b). *The suspension of traffic scheme caused the outbreak of Corona in central Tehran*, Iran's Metropolises News Agency (IMNA). www.imna.ir/news /424428/

Internet Disruption Blocks the Reopening for Business (2020). *Eghtesad online,* www .eghtesadonline.com/n/2CHR

Iran Corruption Rank: 2003–2019 Data (2020). *Trading economics,* https://tradingecono mics.com/iran/corruption-rank

Karkhayi, I. (2020). *Enemies wage soft war with Coronavirus,* IRNA, Islamic Republic News Agency. www.irna.ir/news/83789124/

Khamenei, S. A. (2020). *Supreme leader: speeches and news,* Khamenei.Ir, https://farsi .khamenei.ir/speech

Khodabakhsh, K. (2016). *Short accounts of the life of the first Martyr of the Holy Shrine defender,* Raja News. rajanews.com/node/260757

Lilleker, D. (2014). *Political communication and cognition,* Palgrave MacMillan, New York.

MHME, M. of H. and M. E. (2020). *Infographics: the pattern of provinces reported Coronavirus cases,* Iranian Students' News Agency (ISNA). www.isna.ir/news/98120705410/

Middle East Eye (2020). *Coronavirus: Iran warns of second wave of infections, imposes Nowruz shutdown,* www.middleeasteye.net/news/coronavirus-iran-nowruz-ban-second-wav e-death-toll

Nikrouyan, A. (2020). *The victims of Coronavirus: from health-care personnel to bank system,* Mashregh News. mshrgh.ir/1052116

Radio Farda (2020). *Iran's Health Minister says virus came from China travel,* https://en.radi ofarda.com/a/iran-s-health-minister-says-virus-came-from-china-travel/30449759 .html

Saeidi Ghaviandam, S. (2020). *The demotion of the international rank of Iran in internet speed,* Mehr News Agency. mehrnews.com/xRK6S

SeyedHosseini, M. M. (2020). *Behind the curtain of media and psychological warfare against Iran centered around Coronavirus,* Tasnim News Agancy. https://tn.ai/2214368

Tabnak (2020). *Combat against corruption: economic corruption is as dangerous as Corona virus,* Tabnak.ir. tabnak.ir/0048j8.

Worldometers.info. *Coronavirus, countries: Iran,* www.worldometers.info/coronavirus/c ountry/iran/

Wright, R. (2020). How Iran became a new epicenter of the coronavirus outbreak, *New Yorker,* www.newyorker.com/news/our-columnists/how-iran-became-a-new-epice nter-of-the-coronavirus-outbreak

19

BRAZIL

More than just a little flu

Ícaro Joathan, Andrea Medrado and Thainã Medeiros

Political context

In early 2020, President Jair Bolsonaro had completed his first year of office. His election, in October 2018, marked a rightward political shift after 14 years of government by the left-wing Workers' Party (PT). The PT had been in power since 2003 with Lula da Silva for two terms and then Dilma Rousseff elected in 2010 and reelected in 2014. In 2016, amidst corruption scandals, the Brazilian Senate impeached Rousseff for moving funds between government budgets. Rousseff denied having done anything illegal and argued that this was a common practice amongst her predecessors.[1]

At the time of his election, Bolsonaro had been in permanent campaign for at least three years (Joathan & Rebouças, 2020), presenting himself as an anti-PT candidate and advocate of Christian values. Although he had worked as a federal legislator since 1991, he was also portrayed as being anti-establishment. Gaining strength due to Brazil's political turmoil, Bolsonaro, a former army captain, managed to gather support from influential actors, such as the military, the Evangelical churches, the economic elites, and politicians aligned with a neo-liberal agenda. He beat the PT candidate Fernando Haddad in the second round of the elections with 55.1% of valid votes.

The PT's original plan was to name Lula as a presidential candidate, but the Superior Electoral Court disqualified him under Brazil's Clean Slate Law. Ironically, three days after winning the election, Bolsonaro appointed Sergio Moro, the judge who helped arrest Lula for corruption charges, to his Justice Ministry. Since then, the president remains true to his confrontational style. In this context of ideological disputes, Brazil confirmed its first case of COVID-19 in February 2020. This chapter draws from quantitative and qualitative content analyses to address issues of governance and rhetoric during the coronavirus crises.

DOI: 10.4324/9781003120254-21

Chronology

Table 19.1 presents a summary of the dissemination of COVID-19 in Brazil and the main measures taken by the federal government between February and August 2020.

Analysis

This chapter draws from quantitative and qualitative content analyses of posts published on the Facebook pages of Brazil's Federal Government (@palaciodoplanalto) (n = 237) and Favela do Alemão's Crisis Committee page (@gabinetealemao) (n = 52). For both, we have collected posts published between February 26 and June 25. We chose Facebook because Brazilian users account to 120 million people (second only to YouTube in popularity).[2] The Planalto page represents the government's official voice, allowing citizens to follow government-led actions, projects and the president's everyday life. The @gabinetealemao page was created to report the activities of the Crisis Committee, which had been established in March by three collectives from Favela do Alemão: Coletivo Papo Reto, Voz das Comunidades and Mulheres em Ação no Alemão. We also draw from inside information from Thainã de Medeiros, one of the founders of Coletivo Papo Reto.

The Crisis Committee tapped into the collectives' networks, gathering donations and supplies from citizens and companies. The committee organised teams of volunteers to sign up residents who needed to receive assistance, such as food baskets and cleaning products. Additionally, the committee devised a communication plan, using banners, loudspeakers on cars and lampposts, WhatsApp groups and social media. The Facebook page represents a meeting point for publishing reports about the committee's activities. The aim is to inform the population on how to prevent catching the virus and how to seek help in case they become infected. We analysed the posts in relation to two main categories – frequency of communication and types of themes.

Communication frequency

Pandemic-related posts represented 71.7% of the content published on the Planalto page (170 posts) as opposed to 100% of the posts published by the Crisis Committee page (52 posts). This can be explained by the fact that an official government page needs to discuss a variety of issues. As for the Crisis Committee, the page was created to support residents during the pandemic.

Themes of communication

Ten main themes were identified, which are not mutually exclusive. These are:

(1) Reports/accountability: health, legal and social measures carried out by the government or by the Crisis Committee to fight the pandemic. This

TABLE 19.1 Brazil chronology

Date		Diffusion of COVID-19	Key official actions	Key communication events
February	26	First case confirmed – 61-year-old man from São Paulo who had returned from Lombardia.		Health Minister (HM) Luiz Mandetta held a press briefing to explain the measures to prevent the spread of the disease.
	29	Second case confirmed in São Paulo state.		
March	5	8 cases. Spread to other states (Rio de Janeiro and Espírito Santo) confirmed.		
	6	13 cases.		President Bolsonaro addressed the nation on radio and television, saying 'there was no reason to panic' and that the Ministry of Health (MH) was working in partnership with state governments and municipalities.
	11	WHO declares a pandemic.	Movement restriction measures, such as closing schools and universities, implemented in Brasília by the governor of the Federal District. Other governors in states such as Rio de Janeiro and São Paulo start to impose restrictive measures (forbidding public gatherings, for example).	
	12	First death (announced by MH as March 17 but corrected three months later).		

	24	47 deaths. 2,271 cases.	In a televised speech, Bolsonaro stated, 'with my history as an athlete, if I were infected with the virus, I would have no reason to worry. I would feel nothing, or it would be at most just a little flu."
April	2	327 deaths. 8,066 cases.	The government launches programme that enabled the distribution of a BRL 600 (approximately USD 113) emergency monthly salary for informal workers. It also announced protection measures for formal jobs, authorising the reduction of hours and wages by employers in return for the maintenance of jobs.
	16	1,952 deaths. 30,891 cases.	Mandetta got fired over clashes with Bolsonaro. The HM spoke about social distancing, supported the temporary suspension of non-essential activities for cities and stated that the government responses should be based on scientific evidence. Bolsonaro held an official ceremony to announce Nelson Teich as new HM.
May	15	14,962 deaths; 220,291 cases.	Teich resigned. He and Bolsonaro disagreed on the need for social distancing. Bolsonaro promoted the use of hydroxychloroquine, Teich refused to authorise use for patients with mild symptoms. Efforts started being led by interim replacement: Army General Eduardo Pazuello. With no medical background, unlike his predecessors, he fired specialists and named fellow military officers to top posts. Teich held a press conference to announce he was resigning as HM.

(Continued)

TABLE 19.1 (Continued)

Date	Diffusion of COVID-19	Key official actions	Key communication events
June	6 36,044 deaths. 676,494 cases.	The government stopped publishing total numbers of cases and fatalities, releasing only past 24 hours' figures. It faced criticism for two days until Supreme Court ordered publishing of data. State governors began to suspend movement restriction measures.	Bolsonaro was ironic in a press interview: 'nothing left for *Jornal Nacional* to talk about,' in a reference to the evening news programme broadcast by TV Globo not being able to access COVID-19 stats.
July	7 66,868 deaths (1,312 in 24 hours). 1,674,655 cases.		Bolsonaro gave an interview to TV Brasil (state broadcaster) and two commercial TV channels to communicate that he tested positive for COVID-19.
August	8 Death toll exceeds 100,000. Number of Infected over 3,000,000. 10th consecutive week with an average of approximately 1,000 deaths per day. In mid-August, the death rate started to decrease.		Bolsonaro tweeted the media was 'spectacularising' the pandemic.

includes sending equipment and tests to hospitals and updating the number of people infected and fatalities. It does not include economic measures, such as the emergency salary, or financial rescues to states and municipalities.

Our research indicated that 75% of the posts by the Alemão page fell into this category as opposed to 64.7% of the posts published by the Planalto page. The commitment to transparency displayed by the Alemão page, a civil society initiative led entirely by volunteers, was impressive. They posted weekly short videos with the hashtag #PrestaçãoGabinete (Committee's Accountability Report), which disclosed the number and variety of items that they received as donations, and how they distributed them in different areas. In this way, the initiative represented an attempt to fill gaps left by the city, state and federal authorities. Citing Medeiros, 'the government should be doing what the Alemão Crisis Committee are doing' (interview, June 30, 2020).

(2) Prevention/guidance: posts that inform people about what they should do to avoid catching COVID-19, as well as the symptoms of the disease.

In contrast to the Planalto page, we could see that a much higher percentage of posts by the Alemão page published health guidance and prevention information: 61.5% as opposed to 27.1% of the government page. The latter appears to be a strikingly low number because these should feature as top priorities in a context of crisis. Most of the health guidance was offered in March and April when Luiz Mandetta was still the Minister of Health. For example, in a Facebook video ad, published March 13, Mandetta spoke about the importance of being careful with hygiene habits because the 'virus has a quick transmission rate, which can cause health systems to collapse.' However, speeches that challenged the guidance provided by health bodies, such as the World Health Organisation (WHO), and even the Ministry of Health itself were frequent. On March 25, for instance, Bolsonaro stated that elderly people were the only ones that needed to worry about prevention as 'the problem lies with people above 60 or people who have a health problem.'

In a study of the COVID-19 crisis in Hong Kong, Sheen et al. (2020) demonstrate that information from non-official government sources can enhance the credibility of official government messages. In Brazil's case, the messages stemming from the government were often contradictory: the Minister warned people to be careful whilst Bolsonaro said risks were little. Hence life-saving civil society initiatives were left in the dark. Referring to the frequent appeals for favela residents to stay home, Medeiros described how difficult this was, given people's precarious living circumstances. Positive prevention examples by powerful figures became even more important. Yet, our research revealed the opposite scenario. Bolsonaro's frequent public appearances in bakeries and public rallies combined with his anti-social-distancing declarations might have worsened a situation that was already critical.

(3) Economic impact and aid: measures for retaining private sector jobs, the distribution of the BRL 600 emergency salary, the injecting of financial resources into states and municipalities.

Considerable efforts were directed to communicating the government's handing out of an emergency salary to informal workers or families that have a monthly income of half the minimum salary per person (BRL 552) or BRL 3,135 per family. In press conferences, such as the one held on April 3, Pedro Guimarães, the president of Caixa Econômica, one of Brazil's major public banks, provided details on how people could receive the funds. This is consistent with the government's rhetoric that it was mostly concerned with COVID-19's economic impact. Indeed, this category corresponded to 57.6% of their Facebook posts. In comparison, the Crisis Committee published no content that fell into this category, as this was a programme entirely managed by the federal government and they had no funds to assist favela residents nor was it their responsibility.

(4) Denial of the dangers or trivialisation of the disease: posts that advocate for a return to normal life and free movement, opposing social distancing measures, minimising risks, or spreading scientifically unfounded information.

Videos and posts that featured Bolsonaro himself often minimised the risks of COVID-19. For the Planalto page, this category corresponded to 23.5% of the posts. In a televised speech on March 24, the president famously said that 'COVID-19 was at most just a little flu.'[3] Bolsonaro's encouragement of people to break quarantine measures also translated into public gestures and actions, such as joining pro-government rallies, and not wearing face masks (or wearing them incorrectly). Such denialism might have further aggravated the health crisis, particularly for Brazilians who live in the favelas where social distancing becomes almost impossible due to a combination of overcrowded spaces and poverty. Additionally, going out to work to earn a living represents an extreme necessity for many residents. Yet, despite all these challenges, Alemão's page made significant efforts to tell residents to stay home as much as possible and it published no posts within the trivialisation category.

(5) Attacks on the media: critiques of media coverage of the COVID-19 crisis, accusing it of fear-mongering and creating hysteria.

The government's trivialisation of the pandemic was often coupled with attacks on various media outlets and journalists. The category corresponded to 12.4% for the Planalto page. This complemented Bolsonaro's denial discourses by claiming the health dangers posed by the pandemic were an exaggeration or a media creation. By discrediting media reports, the president positioned himself as someone who was being unfairly targeted in an unfriendly media environment. He was particularly vocal against the Globo Network, and the newspaper *Folha de São Paulo*, amongst others. In contrast, Alemão's page had no occurrences of posts attacking the media.

(6) Conflict with different spheres of power, such as the Supreme Court, the states and municipalities: posts that criticise measures taken by these institutions, as well as the work of health ministers.

La et al. (2020) provide useful insights on the importance of cooperation between governments, civil society, the scientific community and private individuals. They shed light on how Vietnam's political readiness to combat the pandemic since its earliest days was key to the country's successful response to the crisis. In Brazil, our content analysis unveiled a fragmented scenario. The stances taken by different actors have been contradictory, even within the government itself. Timing is one revealing element here. Whilst Mandetta held a press conference on February 26, the same day that Brazil confirmed its first COVID-19 case, Bolsonaro waited until March 6 to address the nation on TV. Unlike his first two Health Ministers, Bolsonaro made speeches discrediting the information made available by the WHO. He was also the protagonist of public rows with the Supreme Court, state governors and city mayors. This confirms Rodrigues and Azevedo's findings (2020) on how the pandemic generated a crisis in Brazil's federative units. The fact that there was no clarity in terms of the different roles that must be played by the national, state and city governments worsened this scenario.

The conflicts demonstrated a serious lack of leadership in Brazil. On average, 23.5% of the Planalto page posts had content that fell into the category of 'conflict.' One emblematic example happened on April 11. During a press conference, journalists asked Health Minister Teich about the reopening of nail salons, barber shops and gyms announced by Bolsonaro. He replied, 'Was this today? This wasn't us, this is... the president's responsibility... the decision about which activities are deemed essential is made by the Ministry of Economy.' Again, this revealed the high level of internal disagreements and lack of coordination between the various ministries and the President. In contrast to this chaotic scenario, Alemão's Committee displayed horizontal and clear dynamics of leadership. Its leaders, Raull Santiago, Rene Silva and Camila Santos featured in several videos and each represented one of the committee's founding initiatives.

(7) Treatments and drugs: information on research about and/or recommendations to use drugs to treat COVID-19.

Our empirical evidence provided a variety of examples of dubious science in government communication. This was epitomised by the president's enthusiasm for hydroxychloroquine (video published on May 14, amongst others), even though several studies questioned or denied its efficiency. The category corresponded to 20.6% or 35 posts for the Planalto page, as opposed (once again) to zero posts published by the Alemão Crisis Committee page. Gollust et al. (2020) highlighting conflicting science are frequent elements of US President Trump's communication argue, 'These have contributed toward divergent responses by media sources, partisan leaders, and the public alike, leading to different attitudes and beliefs as well as varying protective actions taken by members of the public' (2020: 1).

(8) Offers of condolences: posts that express condolences to the victims and their families and that manifest appreciation for health workers.

Another noteworthy aspect was the low percentage of posts in this category for both the Planalto and the Alemão pages – 9.4% and 0%, respectively. One exceptional example took place when Bolsonaro said in a video he was sorry for the first COVID-19 death in the State of Goiás (on March 26). Here, we can also draw parallels with attitudes of indifference by leaders in other parts of the world. Analysing the British context, for instance, Tomkins (2020: 331) reflects on the implications of the prime minister Boris Johnson's absences for his leadership: in times of crisis, 'leaders who appear not to care risk triggering powerful anxieties about betrayal and abandonment.' Such a sense of abandonment appeared as a recurrent theme in the content published by @gabinetealemao. Medeiros summarises this by saying that 'the State never helps the people, and what is worse, instead of helping, they get in our way.' Indeed, the Brazilian state has a history of neglecting its favela populations, manifesting their presence only through the policing of these areas.

(9) Public safety: messages that address the relationship between COVID-19 and its impact on issues such as the increase in domestic violence and police brutality in the favelas.

This category corresponded to 6.5% and 13.5% of the posts published on the Planalto and the Alemão page, respectively. The fact that favela residents are frequent victims of police violence and human rights violations (Medrado et al., 2020) might explain why the theme appeared twice as much in the favela page. The issues are complex and were neither lessened nor exacerbated by COVID-19.

(10) Other: posts that did not fit into any of the previous categories.

This category fits 34.1% of posts from Planalto and 34.6% for Alemão posts. The high number is explained by the wide variety of topics addressed in both pages, such as when Bolsonaro and government officials prayed to God asking for the end of the pandemic, or thanked companies that made donations, or when the

Crisis Committee publicised cultural attractions online to encourage residents to stay at home.

Conclusion

Our study indicated that Brazil developed a confusing and inefficient response to the pandemic. The government invested in rhetoric minimising the health risks and maximising the negative impacts on the country's economy. This is exemplified in Bolsonaro's words and actions with frequent speeches against social distancing, and public appearances that disrespect health authority recommendations. Our content analysis of the Planalto page confirmed these points. Whilst the category of providing accountability reports featured in 64.7% of the posts, the category of 'economic impact and aid' came in at a close second, appearing in 57.6% of the posts.

Moreover, the presence of conflicting attitudes and contradictory messages was striking. This created a sense of confusion and abandonment, worsened by the government's low emphasis on communicating solidarity with the millions of Brazilians who are falling ill and the thousands who have lost their lives. This points to the need for future studies to investigate the role that Bolsonaro's permanent campaign centring on economic regeneration and his reelection plans for 2022 may have played in choosing the denial discourses he adopted. As of the time of writing, approximately 130,000 lives have been lost and the economic impact on the population has been harsh. This might hinder Bolsonaro from using an economic revamping as (literally) his trump card. Time will tell.

Notes

1 See www.bbc.co.uk/news/world-latin-america-36028117
2 See https://datareportal.com/reports/digital-2020-brazil
3 See www.bbc.co.uk/news/world-latin-america-52040205

References

Gollust, S., Nagler, R., & Fowler, E. (2020). The emergence of COVID-19 in the U.S: A public health and political communication crisis. *Journal of Health Politics, Policy and Law*, online, 1–17.

Joathan, Í., & Rebouças, H. (2020). Campanha permanente em busca da Presidência da República: As estratégias de comunicação de Jair Bolsonaro no Facebook entre 2015 e 2018. *ECCOM*, 11(22), 377–398.

La, V., Pham, T., Ho, M., Nguyen, M., Nguyen, K., Vuong, T., Nguyen, H., Tran, T., Khuc, Q., Ho, M., & Vuong, Q. (2020). Policy response, social media and science journalism for the sustainability of the public health system amid the COVID-19 outbreak: The Vietnam lessons. *Sustainability*, 12(2931), 377–398.

Medrado, A., Souza, R., & Cabral, T. (2020). Favela digital activism: The use of social media to fight oppression and injustice in Brazil. In Martens, C. et al. (Eds.). *Digital *activism, community media, and sustainable communication in Latin America*. Palgrave Macmillan, pp. 177–201.

Rodrigues, J., & Azevedo, D. (2020). Pandemia do coronavírus e (des)coordenação federativa: Evidências de um conflito politico-territorial. *Espaço e Economia*, 18, 1–12.

Sheen, G., Tung, H., & Wu, W. (2020). Citizen journalism and credibility of authoritarian government in risk communication regarding the 2020 COVID-19 outbreak: A survey experiment. New York University, Abu Dhabi, *Division of Social Science Working Paper Series*, 40, 1–22.

Tomkins, T. (2020). Where is Boris Johnson? When and why it matters that leaders show up in a crisis. *Leadership*, *16*(3), 331–342.

20

NORWAY

From strict measures to pragmatic flexibility

Bente Kalsnes and Eli Skogerbø

Political context

Norway was in 2020 governed by a conservative minority coalition consisting of the Conservative, Liberal and Christian Conservative Party, led by Conservative Prime Minister (PM) Erna Solberg. The minority coalition had fairly low support when COVID-19 hit Norway in February. 26.8% of the Norwegian population supported the government, according to a Poll of Polls (2020). In June, almost five months later, the government was supported by 31.6% of the population, an increase mainly awarded to the Conservative Party, which had increased its support from 19 to 25% of the population, while the two minor coalition partners had fallen back slightly.

Chronology

The first confirmed COVID-19 infection in Norway came on February 26 when a woman was confirmed infected after returning from a trip to China. She was isolated at home and in good shape (Sfrintzeris & Nærum, 2020). Her fellow passengers on the plane were traced for disease control. Several news articles reported how to avoid panic after the first case. The major influx of contagions came when Norwegians returned from holiday ski trips to Italy and Austria at the end of February and first week of March.

Some measures were taken after February 26, i.e. quarantine rules for health workers who had been in infected areas, home office for everyone who could work from home and cancellation of some events with more than 500 participants, and perhaps most serious for those affected, hospital and health services reduced admittance to the most serious cases only, to prepare for the mass influx of patients suffering from the pandemic. The major measure, the

DOI: 10.4324/9781003120254-22

lockdown of the country, was implemented on March 12 when the first confirmed death from COVID-19 was reported and 206 new infections were confirmed. Norwegian health authorities announced that they could no longer
trace every infected case back to its source and control the spreading of the
disease, which at this time was very high compared to neighbouring countries. Authorised by reference to the *Act On Prevention Of Transmittable Diseases*
(Lovdata, 1994), the government imposed 'the strongest and most invasive
measures in Norway in peacetime,' a term that has been repeated numerously
in subsequent public speeches (Regjeringen, 2020a). The measures succeeded
in containing COVID-19 in the upcoming months. By September 10, 2020,
Norway had 264 confirmed COVID-19 deaths, and approximately 11.000
infected cases. March and April were the time with the highest number of contagions, while the curve flattened between May and August. After the summer
holidays the number increased, in some places to high levels.[1] Most new cases
were in local clusters, tied to holiday travel, school and university openings and
social events. Since March, identifying, testing, tracking, isolation and treatment had improved and most new strict measures were implemented locally
and temporarily.

Official actions taken by the government and institutions

On March 12, the government announced the closure of schools, universities, kindergartens and many other sectors, industries and service providers.
All workplaces had to adhere to strict measures of infection protection, thereby
slowing down and reducing the number of people able to work. Children and
students were confined to digital teaching. Hairdressers, gyms, restaurants and
sport events were immediately closed. Seats on public transport were restricted
and all travelling that was not strictly necessary was discouraged. Travelling
abroad was effectively stopped as anyone arriving was quarantined for 14 days.
Medical workers were not allowed to travel abroad at all. The border control
was already tightened, and by March 16, Norway introduced unrestricted border control.

The capital Oslo and other cities were initially hardest hit. To avoid rapid
spread of the disease to rural areas, Norwegians were strongly advised against
and finally banned from using their recreational homes, the cabins, typically
located in rural, sparsely populated areas. The government imposed 'cabin ban'
was designed to avoid overloading local health services with a potential coronavirus peak of thousands of cabin visitors. This proved very controversial. Those
who violated the ban risked prosecution and potentially a fine of up to 15,000
kroner ($1,320) or ten days in prison (The Local, 2020). Similar local and con-
troversial restrictions during the spring 2020 included the so-called 'southerners'
quarantine,' a nickname for local quarantine requirements imposed on travellers
from southern Norway to some northern municipalities where the infection rate
was low. These were eventually removed by government intervention. Even

though they were strict measures, Norwegians were not under curfew as people were free to go for walks, exercise or shopping since most stores remained open.

The government started easing the measures on April 20, five weeks after they were set in place. Reopening of day care for toddlers, hairdressers and psychologists and the cabin ban disappeared. The week after, on April 27, schools got reopened for 1st– 4th grade, and new rules demanding more space between each passenger on public transport and airplanes were introduced. On May 11, the announcement to reopen all schools came, but universities and colleges remained mostly closed until the summer break in July.

The most important communication moments and media events

The spread of COVID-19 was reported in Norway in a short article written by the daily *Dagbladet* on January 3 (Ihle, 2020). The article reported a SARS scare in China after a mysterious outbreak in Wuhan. A group of researchers had temporarily concluded that it probably was a new type of coronavirus. On January 17, NTB ran an article about 'the mysterious lung virus' that apparently had caused two deaths in Wuhan. The article also stated that it had not been proved whether the virus had human-to-human transmission, but it could not be ruled out. After this date, there was daily coverage of the new virus in Norwegian media, according to the media archive Retriever. The story about the Wuhan doctor Li Wenliang who warned about the dangers of the virus got substantial attention in Norwegian news media, both when he acted as a whistle-blower against Chinese authorities and when he fell ill and eventually died on February 6.

March 12 marked the central communication moment in Norway as PM Erna Solberg along with leaders from the health authorities gave a press conference where she outlined the lockdown and invoked the people in Norway to take part in the 'dugnad,' a collective action to combat COVID-19. By 'dugnad,' they appealed to the public for solidarity and sacrifice for the greater good by emphasising the importance of everyone doing their share. This proved an effective and initially successful strategic communication instrument. The simple and effective measures were washing hands, socially distancing and coughing into the elbow – messages repeated endlessly in the next few months, but also accepting heavy restrictions on free movement (Graver, 2020), mass unemployment, overloaded health and welfare services and grave economic recession.

The main political and social issues

In order to act swiftly, on March 18 the government proposed a specific *Corona Act*, giving the government wide authorities to issue regulations. The act was a temporary extension of the *Act on Prevention of Transmittable Diseases*. On March 24, Parliament agreed the act; however, they heavily adjusted it. While the government had proposed that it should be in place for six months, Parliament decided that the statutory state of emergency could only last for one month. Nevertheless, the law gave the government wide powers to deal with the crisis and potentially set aside 62 different laws, among them possibilities for suspending regulation of working hours, overtime, workload and requirements for court cases proceeding, as well as authorities' right to requisition buildings and move public employees to other agencies.

Several economic measures were taken to secure jobs, help businesses and people, and the Parliament approved several extensive economic packages (March 13, March 20, March 27, April 3, May 12 and May 29). Preliminary figures suggested that the crisis had weakened the national budget balance for 2020 by NOK 245 billion (approx. USD 26.5 billion) (Regjeringen, 2020b).

The number of unemployed increased from 2.3% in February to 10.7% in March, basically meaning 235,000 more people registered unemployed during March, the highest increase in one month ever (Høgseth et al., 2020). The tourist industry, airline companies, the event and culture industry, sport centres and different types of service industries were severely hit while IT and the health sector did comparatively well, although the major effects will probably not be visible until 2021–2. The Norwegian Labour and Welfare Administration (NAV), the institution managing welfare benefits, suffered massive overload and inability to keep up with the record number of applications for unemployment and sickness benefits. As lockdown was eased, unemployment decreased and production of goods and services increased, but the levels were by September 2020 considerably different from what they were at the beginning of March, and tens of thousands of people had still not received compensation for temporary and permanent lay-offs.

Analysis

Norway is known for its system of solving disagreement through negotiation and cooperation (Engelstad & Hagelund, 2016). The cooperation and common trust among different institutions and actors have also been important during the COVID-19 crisis, even though strong disagreements have been visible as well; particular in terms of what appropriate measures should be applied at what time. Since March, it has also become public that clear disagreements existed between some health experts and political leaders regarding implementing measures.

The measures described above were implemented by a shifting coalition of politicians, bureaucrats and experts, and meticulously examined by the news media. The leadership for the crisis was confirmed during the first two weeks after COVID-19 arrived in Norway as being between The Norwegian Directorate of Health (HD) and The Norwegian Institute of Public Health (FHI), the two main professional public health actors. FHI provides recommendations based on academic, professional knowledge, while HD evaluates FHI advice against social and economic concerns. The heads of these agencies soon developed high media profiles. Worth mentioning is the Assistant Health Director who received much praise and media attention for his abilities to explain complicated medical information to the public, and a fan page on Facebook with more than 25,000 members was created (Facebook, 2020).

But on March 12, the government took charge. As the extent of the COVID-19 crisis became apparent, the political leaders took the lead in the daily press briefings. Each day from then on, either the Prime Minister or government ministers attended. The main actors from the government were the PM, the Minister of Health and Care Services, the Minister of Finance and the Minister of Education. The Minister of Health particularly received a lot of praise for his pedagogical and balanced way of communicating (Dagsavisen, 2020). The opposition at the parliament, Stortinget, also played a central role in adjusting and improving the proposals from the government, such as the Labour Party, the Centre Party, and newcomers in opposition after they recently left the government, the Progress Party.

In the days before March 12, commentators and opposition politicians criticised PM Erna Solberg for doing too little too late (Eikefjord, 2020; Karlsen & Gilbrant, 2020), demonstrated in press briefings where representatives from the health institutions were present but were only sporadically attended by the politicians. The government was criticised for being unclear, weak, acting too slowly and proposing the wrong measures to counter the emerging crisis. Compared to neighbour Denmark, the criticism was to the point. Denmark introduced measures earlier and locked down the country on March 11, one day before Norway (Stephensen & Hansen, 2020). More striking and unexpected, was that Sweden, in sharp contrast to its Nordic neighbours, chose a lenient approach, relying on strong recommendations, but fewer restrictions on movement, travelling and no lockdown, despite high rates of infections and deaths caused by COVID-19. The differences between the approaches taken across the Nordic countries have caused continuous media coverage through the entire period.

The news media hence prove to be a very important actor. The COVID-19 crisis is a double-edged sword as the interest in news has never been higher while revenues from advertising plummeted. The high news interest during the pandemic has steered many viewers towards the two national broadcasters. The Norwegian public broadcaster, NRK, and the commercial TV2 received the highest trust ratings. 83% said they had very or fairly high trust in the news from NRK while 70% said they had very or fairly high trust in the news from TV2. Other national news outlets have also experienced high trust such as the daily *Aftenposten*, viewed as trustworthy by 60% while local or regional newspapers were deemed very or fairly trustworthy by 51% of the population during the COVID-19 crisis (Andersen, 2020).

NRK's remit states that the public broadcaster has a specific responsibility to 'facilitate broadcasting to the population from authorities during national crises and catastrophes' (NRK, 2020), highlighted for instance in its massive and continuous news broadcasts and airing of 'posters' from the government during the time when emergency measures were imposed. However, NRK also provided critical and controversial coverage that has been praised and criticised. One current affairs programme broadcast an interview with a very alarmed researcher who predicted massive death tolls as a result of COVID-19, raising significant debate. The programme was later criticised for being unbalanced and too uncritical of the doctor's predictions. Another controversy appeared after NRK published an article by a Norwegian researcher (Svaar, 2020) that stated that COVID-19 does not have a natural origin but was likely developed by Chinese and American researchers. The article was heavily criticised for being published with too few sources and based on unpublished research material.

Another media institution that stands out is the commercial VG which have received acclamation for its corona tracker, Corona Special, which is constantly updated and visualises the numbers of people infected, tested, hospitalised, in intensive care, on respirators and deceased. The Corona Special was started on March 9, three days before the country closed down. By April, it was VG's most read and used product in the history of the newspaper (Saur, 2020).

Pragmatism, flexibility and failures and experiments

In the aftermath of the dramatic spring of 2020, some of the measures initially imposed have been heavily debated among experts, heavily covered by the news media and attracting massive social media attention, too. Closing day care and schools for the youngest children was one of the most controversial measures, others were the cabin ban and closing of the borders. The director of FHI was critical of the closing of day care and schools (Folkvord & Fjellanger, 2020). She argued the decision was not based on factual, academic knowledge. The decision was taken on March 11 by the Director of the Norwegian Directorate of Health in collaboration with the Minister of Health and Care Services. There was also some disagreement on the expressed strategy to fight the virus. The Minister of Health on March 24 stated the new strategy was to 'knock it down,' not only to 'slow it down.' It was unclear what was exactly meant by those terms, or the differences between them and what they implied. For a while, it also seemed like the politicians disagreed with the experts. Since the measures were the same, how was it possible that the government had changed strategy in fighting the virus, or was it mainly a change of communication? To clarify, in an op-ed the health authorities refuted that the politicians had acted against the experts' advice. They argued that they 'supported the government's decision on the measures and the strategy was to knock down the spread of infections as much as possible,' and openly admitted disagreement among experts on how to best do this.

A third topic that has caused uncertainty was face mask wearing. Initially, the experts argued against face masks except for health staff treating patients. The lack of equipment, experience and expertise wearing a face mask were the arguments against it. Later, face masks became mandatory on planes and strongly recommended on public transport in localities with high infection rates. These shifting recommendations and adaptations illustrate the situation that the

Norwegian health expertise has called 'a large experiment': no-one has the blue-print for how the COVID-19 crisis should be managed until an effective and safe vaccine is developed (Braaten & Fossheim, 2020).

Nevertheless, the news media, politicians and health authorities have learned some lessons from previous pandemic scares such as bird flu, swine flu and SARS, typically covered with dramatic headlines and alarming scenarios (Hornmoen, 2011). There has been space for critical perspectives of the authorities and experts, and laypersons' points of view are taken into account, due to the massive health, social and economic consequences of the situation.

The number of cases and deaths from COVID-19 fell flat during the late spring but started to climb again in August 2020. At the time of writing, new cases per day have reached significant numbers as local outbreaks flourish. Travel, social gatherings and more lax attitudes towards the measures during the summer holiday were said to cause the 'second wave' of infections. Increased testing, tracing and isolation of cases have been implemented locally, as well as targeted, temporary closures of affected schools, companies or organisations.

Conclusion

COVID-19 has posed a large challenge for Norwegian society. The virus has killed 264 people at the time of writing or 4.9 out of 100K citizens (as of September 1), which is one of the lowest numbers in Europe. Similar to most other countries, the economy has taken a hard hit, but swift and generous financial support from the government to companies and selected sectors have mitigated the damage to industries. Nevertheless, more than 200,000 individuals have lost their livelihood and unemployment and economic recession is expected to continue.

So far, it seems the health authorities and politicians have managed to communicate the risks and threats of the pandemic in a fairly clear, understandable manner despite all the uncertainty surrounding COVID-19. Hence, we describe the Norwegian approach as pragmatic, adjusting to the constantly shifting situations. New measures have been introduced, eased or removed, according to the current situation and the latest knowledge about the disease and to date this seems to have proved effective.

Note

1 See https://www.fhi.no/en/id/infectious-diseases/coronavirus/daily-reports/daily -reports-COVID19/ for full details.

References

Andersen, J. (2020). Nordmenn har høyest tillit til nyhetene fra NRK1 og TV 2 under koronakrisen. https://kampanje.com/medier/2020/03/nordmenn-har-hoyest-tillit -til-nyhetene-fra-nrk1-og-tv-2-under-koronakrisen/

Braaten, M. and Fossheim, K. (2020). I praksis er dette et stort eksperiment. www.tv2.no/a/11321879/.

Dagsavisen. (2020). Vi MA beholde roen. https://www.dagsavisen.no/debatt/leder/vi-ma-beholde-roen-1.1673342.

Eikefjord, E. (2020). Eirin Eikefjord: Vi trenger ledelse, ikke tåkeprat. www.bt.no/btmeninger/kommentar/i/70GjWV/vi-trenger-ledelse-ikke-taakeprat

Engelstad, F. and Hagelund, A. 2016. *Cooperation and conflict the Nordic way, work, welfare, and institutional change in Scandinavia*. Berlin, Germany: De Gruyter.

Facebook. (2020). Vi som heier på assisterende helsedirektør Espen Rostrup Nakstad. www.facebook.com/groups/513033566031933/

Folkvord, M. and Fjellanger, R. (2020). FHI-direktør kritisk til prosessen da Norge ble stengt ned. www.vg.no/nyheter/innenriks/i/op4677/fhi-direktoer-kritisk-til-prosessen-da-norge-ble-stengt-ned

Graver, H. P. (2020). *Pandemi og unntakstilstand – hva covid-19 sier om den norske rettsstaten*. Oslo, Norway: Dreyers forlag.

Høgseth, M., Johnsen, A., Buggeland, S. and Haugan, B. (2020). Over 400,000 helt og delvis ledige i Norge. https://e24.no/norsk-oekonomi/i/K3mLj6/over-400000-helt-og-delvis-ledige-i-norge.

Hornmoen, H. (2011). 'Pandemisk paranoia'? – En analyse av nyhetsomtalen av 'svineinfluensaen' i norske aviser. *Tidsskrift for samfunnsforskning*, 1(52), 33–66.

Ihle, M. (2020). Full alarm etter mystisk sykdomsutbrudd. Dagbladet. https://www.dagbladet.no/nyheter/full-alarm-etter-mystisk-sykdomsutbrudd/71984548.

Karlsen, K., & Gilbrant, J. (2020). Krever klare råd og kraftpakke. https://www.dagbladet.no/nyheter/krever-klare-rad-og-kraftpakke/72229947.

Lovdata. (1994). Lov om vern mot smittsomme sykdommer [smittevernloven]. https://lovdata.no/dokument/NL/lov/1994-08-05-55

NRK. (2020). NRK-plakaten. https://www.nrk.no/informasjon/nrk-plakaten-1.12253428

Poll of polls. (2020). http://www.pollofpolls.no/

Regjeringen. (2020a). Statsministerens innledning på pressekonferanse om nye tiltak mot koronasmitte. https://www.regjeringen.no/no/aktuelt/statsministerens-innledning-pa-pressekonferanse-om-nye-tiltak-mot-koronasmitte/id2693335/

Regjeringen. (2020b). Economic measures in Norway in response to COVID-19. https://www.regjeringen.no/en/topics/the-economy/economic-policy/economic-measures-in-norway-in-response-to-covid-19/id2703484/

Saur, O. (2020). Korona-spesialen tidenes mest leste VG-produkt. https://www.medier24.no/artikler/korona-spesialen-tidenes-mest-leste-vg-produkt/490287.

Sfrintzeris, Y. and Nærum, A. (2020). Coronasmittet kvinne i Tromsø: – Hun lider kanskje mest av kjedsomhet. https://www.vg.no/nyheter/innenriks/i/naK20J/coronasmittet-kvinne-i-tromsoe-hun-lider-kanskje-mest-av-kjedsomhet

Stephensen, E., & Hansen, T. (2020). Danmark lukker ned: Her er regeringens nye tiltag. https://nyheder.tv2.dk/samfund/2020-03-11-danmark-lukker-ned-her-er-regeringens-nye-tiltag.

Svaar, P. (2020). Norsk forsker skaper strid om virusets opphav: – Dette viruset har ikke en naturlig opprinnelse. https://www.nrk.no/norge/norsk-forsker-skaper-strid-om-virusets-opphav_-_-dette-viruset-har-ikke-en-naturlig-opprinnelse-1.15043634.

The Local. (2020). Norway bans cabin stays to save rural hospitals from coronavirus peak. https://www.thelocal.no/20200319/norway-bans-cabin-stays-to-save-rural-hospitals-from-coronavirus.

21

ICELAND

No lockdown and experts at the forefront

Jón Gunnar Ólafsson

Political context

Iceland is a small country with around 360,000 inhabitants (Statistics Iceland, 2020). Historically, there have been four main parties in the Icelandic political system. They consist of a conservative party (the Independence Party), an agrarian/centre party (the Progressive Party), a social democratic party (now called the Social Democratic Alliance) and a left-socialist/communist party (now called the Left-Green Movement). Until the election in 2013, the four established parties usually received in combination around 85–90% of the vote in parliamentary elections, but this had decreased to 65% in 2017. There are currently eight political parties in the Icelandic parliament, which is a record number (Önnudóttir & Harðarson, 2018).

The post-financial crisis period of political instability has involved frequent elections and challenges in forming governments. After the election of 2017, there was much talk of the need for stability, which led to the formation of a 'grand coalition' between three of the four traditional parties: the Independence Party, the Progressive Party, and the Left-Green Movement. The government is led by Katrín Jakobsdóttir, the first Icelandic Prime Minister from the left/socialist wing of Icelandic politics and the second female to lead a government in Iceland (New Left-Green led, 2017). According to Gallup, 78% supported the government shortly after it was formed in December 2017. The support has hovered around 50% for most of the term, but since the COVID-19 pandemic it has been measuring closer to 60% (Stuðningur við ríkisstjórn, 2020). This increased support can most likely be attributed to the government's pandemic response, which most Icelanders have been satisfied with, as illustrated in this chapter.

DOI: 10.4324/9781003120254-23

Chronology

The first case of COVID-19 in Iceland, reported on February 28, was a man who had arrived from Northern Italy. At the time of writing in September 2020, there have been 2,206 confirmed domestic infections and ten deaths (COVID-19 in Iceland, 2020). The contagion statistics in Iceland need to be examined in relation to the fact that much emphasis was placed on testing as many people as possible. Tests were carried out early on by health authorities specifically on those who showed COVID-19 symptoms. Soon, however, the biotech company deCODE offered to help by screening people who had no symptoms, or mild ones. This led to a vast increase in people being tested, with many cases picked up which would otherwise have been missed. These screening measures confirmed that the novel coronavirus was spreading in the community but at a slow rate. By May 17, 15.5% of the Icelandic population had been tested, whilst a comparative figure in the United States was 3.4% (Kolbert, 2020). By mid-September, 27.2% of the Icelandic population had been tested. Moreover, Iceland's death rate from COVID-19 has been one of the lowest in the world (COVID-19 in Iceland, 2020).

The highest number of contagions was in March and April, with hardly any domestic contagions in May and June. Since the end of July, there have been some new cases, with many being tied to specific events and places. At the time of writing, this 'second wave' has been much smaller than the first one. At the peak in April, there were over 1,000 people in isolation with COVID-19, whilst in late summer the highest daily number was 102 (COVID-19 in Iceland, 2020).

Official actions taken

Unlike many countries, Iceland never imposed a lockdown. Authorities did not see a need for it. This was due to the fact that the early cases of the novel coronavirus were detected soon after arrival in Iceland. The office of the Chief Epidemiologist, in coordination with the Department of Civil Protection and Emergency Management, organised contact tracing which managed to quarantine many of those who had been exposed to the pathogen (Kolbert, 2020). Icelandic authorities have used evidence-based measures, which, apart from quarantine, include isolation for infected persons and early diagnosis of infection, and much effort has been put into effective information disclosure to the public. The objectives of the official actions taken by Icelandic authorities served a clear purpose from the start. As stated on *covid.is* (a website set up by the Directorate of Health and the Department of Civil Protection and Emergency Management on March 13), the goal has been to ensure that the necessary infrastructure in the country, particularly the healthcare system, is able to withstand the strain that the illness will cause in Iceland. On March 6, the highest alert level – an emergency phase – was declared in Iceland as a result of COVID-19. This was done in accordance with the Pandemic National Response Plan (Iceland's Response, 2020).

A ban on gatherings for 100 persons or more was implemented on March 14. Upper secondary schools (high schools) and universities were closed. Operation of kindergartens and primary schools was limited but these were not closed. On March 24, the number of people allowed to come together was limited further to only 20 people and various businesses like hair salons and gyms were closed but most restaurants and shops remained open but had to follow strict guidelines. With infections going down, restrictions were lifted on May 4 when the limit of people coming together was increased to 50. Salons reopened, as did upper secondary schools and universities. On May 25 the number of people coming together was increased to 200 and gyms were reopened (with 50% of the normal capacity). The 'two-metre rule,' which had been strictly enforced since March 14, was from May 25 interpreted more as a social norm and courtesy (Iceland's Response, 2020).

Iceland is an isolated island and thus relies heavily on air-travel. On March 19, all countries were defined as having high-risk for infection. Since this time, Icelandic citizens and residents in Iceland arriving from abroad were required to undergo self-quarantine for 14 days. This changed, however, on June 15 when travellers arriving in Iceland could choose between quarantine for two weeks or to be tested for COVID-19 at the airport. Travellers were required to fill out a pre-registration form before arrival, adhere to rules regarding infection control and encouraged to download the tracing app, Rakning C-19 (Information for travellers, 2020). The number of people allowed to come together was increased to 500 on June 15 and more domestic restrictions were lifted (Iceland's Response, 2020).

Following the rise in infections in late July, further restrictions were introduced on July 30. The number of people coming together was again limited to 100 and the two-metre rule was re-introduced. In places where it was not possible for adults to adhere to the rule (such as hair salons), people were required to wear a mask (this was the first time that masks were introduced in relation to the restrictions) (Hafstað, 2020a). High schools, universities and various businesses were not closed as they had been in the stricter measures during the 'first wave.' On August 19, the rules on the border were tightened. From this day, travellers arriving in Iceland had a choice between a two-week quarantine, or undergoing two COVID-19 tests, with a four to five-day quarantine between tests. Prior to this, the double screening had only applied to Icelanders, residents and visitors staying longer than ten days (Hafstað, 2020b). Domestic restrictions were again lifted on August 28, when the number of adults allowed to come together was increased to 200 and the two-metre rule was replaced by a one-metre rule (Iceland's Response, 2020).

The most important communication moments and media events

News reports concerning COVID-19 started to appear in the Icelandic media in January following the outbreak in Wuhan and the news coverage entered a new phase on February 27 when Iceland's Director of Emergency Management, Víðir Reynisson; its Chief Epidemiologist, Þórólfur Guðnason and Iceland's Director of Health, Alma Möller, had their first joint COVID-19 press conference. Following this they held daily briefings at 2 pm, broadcast on TV, the radio and online (Hilmarsdóttir, 2020). These press conferences quickly became the most important overall communication moments concerning COVID-19 in Iceland and guided much of the news reporting. The final daily briefing took place on May 25 but the press conferences were resumed (but not on a daily basis) at the end of July following the increase in infections.

Icelandic politicians have mostly taken a back seat in communication with the public on COVID-19 and instead have made room for relevant experts. Ministers have, however, been centre stage during key moments such as during press conferences when restrictions were announced and lifted, and when economic support packages were announced. A key communication moment took place on March 13 when Prime Minister Katrín Jakobsdóttir announced the first set of restrictions, alongside Minister of Health, Svandís Svavarsdóttir, the Minister of Education, Culture and Science, Lilja Alfreðsdóttir, and Chief Epidemiologist, Þórólfur Guðnason. In addition, the President of Iceland (a mostly ceremonial role), Guðni Th. Jóhannesson, gave an address to the nation on April 12 and Prime Minister Jakobsdóttir gave an address on May 3 to discuss the lifting of restrictions.

Early on, much emphasis was placed on solidarity and getting the whole population to participate in the fight against COVID-19. This was discussed with the popular tag line: *Við erum öll almannavarnir* (Civil defence is in our hands) (Community pledge, 2020). People shared this on social media and encouraged others to wash their hands, abide by the 2-metre rule and follow other guidelines and rules. Surveys show that most people, to begin with, did what authorities expected them to do. During April and May, between 80–90% said that they followed the rules and guidelines, but these numbers fell to closer to 70% towards the end of the first wave, and they have been closer to 60% at the time of writing in September (Félagsvísindastofnun, 2020).

Analysis

Leadership, point of reference and key actors

Icelandic authorities, with Prime Minister Jakobsdóttir in charge, made a political decision early on to allow the experts to communicate directly with the public. Iceland's Director of Emergency Management, its Chief Epidemiologist and Iceland's Director of Health were interviewed on numerous occasions in January and February and on February 27 they had their first joint press conference as previously mentioned. This became *the consistent point of reference* concerning COVID-19 in Iceland. Every day, at 2 pm, they were on live TV to discuss the latest figures of those infected and in hospital, emphasising important protective measures for the public to take and to answer questions from journalists. They often invited guests that focused on specific topics, such as care for the elderly, the school system and the hospitals in Iceland. 'The trio' as they were called, quickly became household names in Iceland, the public faces of the COVID-19 response, and known simply by their first names: Alma, Víðir and Þórólfur. They often highlighted some words of encouragement, thanked people for doing a good job of abiding by scientific advice and even managed to crack a joke or two on occasion. The press conferences became the most talked about television broadcast in Iceland during this period and it was particularly emphasised how many of Iceland's elder generation would watch every single day. At one of the press conferences, the Chairwoman of the Senior Citizen's Society in Iceland likened the press conferences to how it used to be when she had sat glued to her screen to watch the soap opera *Dallas* (Valsson, 2020). The trio even teamed up with several well-known Icelandic musicians to deliver public health advice in the form of the social-distancing anthem 'Travel indoors.' The whole performance was executed remotely through video chats and emphasised the two-metre rule, respecting the gathering ban and to have 'adventures at home' over Easter rather than travel (Askham, 2020).

The website *covid.is* was updated every day one hour before the trio's press conference. There, the latest numbers of those infected, in hospital and quarantine, were announced, as well as how many people had been tested. More information was made available, focusing for example on the origin of infection and infections/quarantine by region. Various other pieces of information are available on the website, such as advice, announcements and a listing of the restrictions put in place at any given time. In addition to Icelandic, the website has information in ten languages.

Apart from the trio, a key actor involved in influencing the debate and public communication was Kári Stefánsson, the CEO of deCODE genetics. He was often vocal in the media and highlighted the importance of testing as many people as possible. His company sequenced the virus from every Icelander who came back positive. As the virus is passed from person from person, it picks up random mutations. The genome sequencing carried out by deCODE has served as an important technique for improving our knowledge of the virus, but it has also improved the quality of contact tracing. Stefánsson emphasised this in the media and discussed different strains of the virus coming from Europe and the United States and deCODE also made inferences about how the virus spread. The company, for example, found hardly any examples of children infecting adults but there were many examples of adults infecting children. Despite his often-vocal criticism on particular details of the pandemic response, Stefánsson discussed in an interview how Icelandic authorities had pretty much done everything right. As he said,

> The remarkable thing about this whole affair is that in Iceland it has been run entirely by the public health authorities. They came up with the plan,

and they just instituted it. And we were fortunate that our politicians managed to control themselves.

(Kolbert, 2020)

Iceland's Prime Minister, Katrín Jakobsdóttir and Svandís Svavarsdóttir, the Minister of Health, have been the key politicians that have influenced the debate and public communication and made decisions that focused on allowing the experts to 'do their job.' Each decision concerning bans on gatherings and associated domestic issues has been taken by Svavarsdóttir. She has received recommendations from Chief Epidemiologist Guðnason, and every single time she followed them. Svavarsdóttir has also made COVID-19-related decisions concerning Iceland's border, with input and advice from Guðnason. Issues concerning border controls have been coordinated by the Prime Minister's Office, since they involve other ministries, like the Ministry of Justice.

Message, consistency and how actions were justified

Each member of the trio had specific roles at the daily briefings, particularly during the first wave, and these official sources were very much in unison. Reynisson was in charge of the meetings and would discuss general aspects concerning the gathering bans and issues related to people's behaviour. Guðnason discussed the virus and COVID-19 and highlighted possible developments and new measures that he might suggest to the Minister of Health. Möller mainly focused on discussing how the health care system was dealing with the situation.

The trio, particularly Guðnason and Möller, stressed repeatedly that anyone could contract the virus, but the vast majority would not become seriously ill. Older people and those with underlying medical conditions would, however, be most vulnerable. To protect these groups, it was emphasised that the spread must be *slowed down* (Iceland's Response, 2020). In other words: *To flatten the curve*. This message was very clear from the start. It was highlighted how the aim was for Iceland's infrastructure, particularly the health care system, to be able to withstand the strain the virus would cause. In relation to this, the trio repeatedly stressed how individuals could do their part by washing their hands and abiding by the two-metre rule.

Since the main peak of infections in Iceland, there have been a few occasions when the message presented needed to be re-emphasised due to confusion, such as when the two-metre rule stopped being strictly enforced. Guðnason stated that he had not done a good enough job of explaining this change and so he explained it again at the daily press conference in late May (Proppé, 2020). During the second wave, there was again some confusion as to how to define the two-metre rule, but this time concerning how to define those who it did *not* apply to (members of the same household, friends, close colleagues), with Guðnason again needing to re-emphasise the key points. This became a hot topic when the Minister of Tourism, Industry and Innovation, Þórdís Kolbrún

Reykfjörð Gylfadóttir, was tagged in photos on Instagram with a large group of friends, with much less than two metres between them (Kristjánsdóttir, 2020).

The restrictions were from the start clearly justified in relation to the objective of slowing down the virus. This changed when the actions were gradually lifted. The objective then started to shift more towards re-starting the economy and this became a very prevalent theme following the June 15 change in rules concerning the testing of passengers arriving in Iceland. At this time, there was some discussion that authorities had put economic concerns ahead of the health and well-being of the population. Following harsher restrictions in late summer there has been much criticism in the media from the tourism sector and some have started to question what the main aim of the measures really is. Opposition politicians such as former Prime Minister Sigmundur Davíð Gunnlaugsson have asked if Icelandic authorities have moved from the aim of 'flattening the curve' to a 'completely virus free society' (Sóttvarnaraðgerðir svo lengi, 2020).

In an international Gallup survey conducted in April, Iceland ranked highest out of 17 countries (including Germany and South-Korea) when respondents were asked if they were satisfied with how authorities in their country were dealing with the situation. 96% of Icelanders said that they were satisfied with how the Icelandic government was dealing with the COVID-19 pandemic, whilst for example a comparative figure for the United States was 50% (COVID-19 rannsókn, 2020). More recent surveys seem to indicate that Icelanders are very satisfied with how authorities have been handling the pandemic. Despite increased criticism in the media from the tourism sector, only around 10% of Icelanders were in favour of looser restrictions at the border according to a survey conducted in August (Ólafsdóttir et al., 2020). In two surveys conducted in June and August, the trio and their press conferences were trusted by an overwhelming 95% of the population to convey reliable information on COVID-19. The government communication also received high trust numbers of close to 70%. Over 80% of Icelanders trusted Icelandic media outlets to deliver reliable information, and respondents mentioned that if they saw false or misleading information on COVID-19, it was usually on social media or from foreign news outlets (Skýrsla vinnuhóps, 2020).

Conclusion

The Icelandic government's response to the COVID-19 pandemic has focused on enabling relevant experts to disseminate important information to the public on a daily basis and ministers have followed scientific advice. Politicians were present at press briefings to announce new restrictions, but they have let the scientists speak directly to the public concerning the disease and the virus. The trio's daily press conferences have been very well received by the public, with over 95% of Icelanders trusting these briefings to deliver reliable information on COVID-19.

Overall, Icelandic authorities acted quickly before the virus arrived in Iceland. The trio's press conferences started before the first infection was reported, and with heavy testing and tracing in place, Icelandic authorities did not need to impose a lockdown. The input from the company deCODE genetics played a big role in enabling the mass testing that took place in Iceland. Primary schools and kindergartens remained open, as did many restaurants and shops. Iceland has one of the lowest COVID-19 death rates in the world and the health care system was able to withstand the pressure during the pandemic's peak in March and April.

Iceland is a small and remote island, and this undoubtedly helped in its quick and effective response to the pandemic. With short chains of command, authorities were quickly able to coordinate effective strategies, which so far have been, by most comparative measures, a success.

References

Askham, P. (2020). COVID-19 Response Trio Stars in Social-Distancing Song. *The Reykjavík Grapevine*, 8 April. https://grapevine.is/news/2020/04/08/covid-19-resp onse-trio-stars-in-social-distancing-song/.

Community Pledge (2020). *Covid.is*. www.covid.is/community.

COVID-19 in Iceland (2020). *Covid.is*. www.covid.is/data.

COVID-19 Rannsókn (2020). *Gallup*. www.gallup.is/frettir/covid-19-rannsokn-saman burdur-milli-landa/.

Félagsvísindastofnun (2020). *COVID rakning*. https://fel.hi.is/is/covid-rakning.

Hafstað, V. (2020a). When to Use Face Masks in Iceland. *Iceland Monitor*, 31 July. https ://icelandmonitor.mbl.is/news/news/2020/07/31/when_to_use_face_masks_in_ice land/.

Hafstað, V. (2020b). Travelers to Iceland to Be Tested Twice, Starting August 19. *Iceland Monitor*, 14 August. https://icelandmonitor.mbl.is/news/politics_and_society/2020 /08/14/travelers_to_iceland_to_be_tested_twice_starting_au/.

Hilmarsdóttir, S. K. (2020). Sendingin frá Kína sem reyndist allt annað en hættulaus. *Vísir*, 22 May. www.visir.is/g/20201704098d.

Iceland's Response (2020). *Covid.is*. www.covid.is/sub-categories/icelands-response.

Information for Travellers Arriving in Iceland from 15 June (2020). *Government of Iceland*, 5 June. www.government.is/diplomatic-missions/embassy-article/2020/06/05/ Information-for-travellers-arriving-in-Iceland-from-15-June-2020/.

Kolbert, E. (2020). How Iceland Beat the Coronavirus: The Country Didn't Just Flatten the Curve; it Virtually Eliminated it. *New Yorker*, 8 June. www.newyorker.com/ma gazine/2020/06/08/how-iceland-beat-the-coronavirus.

Kristjánsdóttir, I. L. (2020). Ráðherra á vinkonudjammi í gær. *Fréttablaðið*, 16 August. www.frettabladid.is/frettir/radherra-vinkonudjammi-i-gaer/.

New Left-Green Led Grand Coalition Enjoys 78% Approval Rating (2017). *Iceland Magazine*, 6 December. https://icelandmag.is/article/report-new-left-green-led-gran d-coalition-enjoys-78-approval-rating.

Ólafsdóttir, S., Torfason, M. T., Bernburg, J. G., & Jónsdóttir, G. A. (2020). Hvað finnst almenningi um sóttvarnaraðgerðir? *Vísindavefurinn*, 2 September. http://visindavefur .is/svar.php?id=80004.

Önnudóttur, E. H., & Harðarson, Ó. Þ. (2018). Political Cleavages, Party Voter Linkages and the Impact of Voters' Socio-Economic Status on Vote-Choice in Iceland, 1983–2016/17. *Icelandic Review of Politics & Administration*, *14*(1), 101–130.

Proppé, Ó. (2020). Ný skilgreining á tveggja metra reglu: Leyfilegt að sitja og standa þétt saman. *Fréttablaðið*, 22 May. www.frettabladid.is/frettir/ny-skilgreining-tveggja-met ra-reglu-leyfilegt-ad-sitja-og-standa-thett-saman/.

Sóttvarnaraðgerðir svo lengi sem faraldurinn geisar (2020). *Mbl*, 13 September. www.m bl.is/frettir/innlent/2020/09/13/sottvarnaradgerdir_svo_lengi_sem_faraldurinn_ge isar/.

Statistics Iceland (2020). The Population Increased by 1,400 in the Fourth Quarter of 2019. www.statice.is/publications/news-archive/inhabitants/population-in-the-4th-quarter-2019/.

Stuðningur við ríkisstjórn (2020). *Gallup*. www.gallup.is/nidurstodur/thjodarpuls/st udningur-vid-rikisstjorn/.

Skýrsla vinnuhóps þjóðaröryggisráðs um upplýsingaóreiðu og COVID-19 (2020). Stjórnarráð Íslands: Þjóðaröryggisráð. www.stjornarradid.is/library/01--Frettatengt---myndir -og-skrar/FOR/Fylgiskjol-i-frett/Upplydingaoreida_covid19_05-10-20.pdf.

Valsson, A. Y. (2020). Þríeykið fastur liður á óvissutímum – en ekki í dag. *RÚV,* 14 April. www.ruv.is/frett/2020/04/14/thrieykid-fastur-lidur-a-ovissutimum-en-ekki-i-dag.

22

IRELAND

Solid swansong from caretaker government

Dawn Wheatley

Political context

Any discussion of Ireland's political communication COVID-19 response should start with the general election on February 8, 2020, which saw the three biggest parties (Fine Gael, Fianna Fáil and Sinn Féin) each secure 20–25% support. As no government was immediately formed, the leader and ministers overseeing the early stage of the crisis were part of a caretaker administration, continuing in their Departments until late June.

As ongoing coalition negotiations took a backseat, the political focus remained on the outgoing government led by the centre-right Fine Gael, in power since 2011. Taoiseach Leo Varadkar (equivalent to prime minister) was leader since 2017, with no certainty that he would return to office. As Taoiseach, 41-year-old Varadkar was somewhat divisive. For some, he illustrated Ireland's progression from an inward-looking, social conservativism; Varadkar is the son of an Indian migrant and appears publicly with his male partner. For others, however, Varadkar represents a Dublin-centric neoliberal elite: privately educated, doctor, supposedly with little understanding or empathy for those struggling with low incomes and poor housing.

It took until June 15 for an agreed programme for government between the two centre-right parties, Fine Gael and Fianna Fáil, and the Green Party. Fianna Fáil leader Micheál Martin took over as Taoiseach on June 27, just two days before some of the most severe COVID-19 restrictions were lifted, with Varadkar taking on the deputy prime minister role (Tánaiste). This change in leadership was, of course, a pivotal moment: overall, the public had responded positively to the outgoing government's handling of the pandemic. Fine Gael, which polled 21% of first-preference votes in February's election, reached 37% support in an *Irish Times* opinion poll in mid-June. It showed 75% personal

DOI: 10.4324/9781003120254-24

approval for Varadkar, a national level only exceeded in the 1990s following the Northern Ireland peace process. This period of change in late June would, therefore, be a critical juncture in Ireland's response, feeling like the natural end of the initial COVID-19 chapter given the new faces in Cabinet and the easing of many restrictions.

Chronology

Initial Irish media reports unsurprisingly focused on China, and the first case in the Republic of Ireland was March 11. A few days previously, March 8, the *Business Post* newspaper's front-page headline caused a stir: 'Irish health authorities predict 1.9m will fall ill with coronavirus.' There was some backlash suggesting this was fearmongering, but the editor responded saying, 'The headline is an accurate reflection of predictions…I agree it is scary but it is being repeated by other credible sources this morning so it is not irresponsible' (Oakley, 2020). See Table 22.1.

Regarding official public addresses, March 12 marked the most serious one up to that point. Taoiseach Leo Varadkar, in Washington DC for the annual St Patrick's Day trip, announced that childcare, schools and universities would close. On St Patrick's Day itself (March 17), the Taoiseach gave another televised address from the Government Buildings podium in Dublin. He was widely praised for this 11-minute address, with one PR analysis describing it as a 'career-defining speech': '[It was delivered in] a confident and disciplined manner that has achieved its aim of reassuring Irish citizens while also creating a stronger sense of unity that will be needed in the coming months' (Rosney, 2020). Varadkar gave a similar-style address on March 27, announcing the most stringent 2km restrictions, drawing on Ireland's political history by acknowledging how 'freedom was hard-won in our country, and it jars with us to restrict and limit individual liberties' (MerrionStreet.ie, 2020). Throughout April, cases would rise steeply, moving from 3,235 total cases (71 total deaths) on April 1, up to 20,253 total cases (1,190 deaths) on April 30.

On May 1, the government announced the five-phase 'Roadmap for reopening society and business,' spanning three-week intervals between May and August (later adjusted with many restrictions eased in late June). Varadkar provided this information in another national address rather than a press conference which frustrated those arguing that the plans' significance warranted journalistic scrutiny. Instead, Varadkar appeared on the RTÉ television chat show, *The Late Late Show*, that night.

Political and social issues

Ireland went through similar concerns as other countries regarding personal protective equipment (PPE) and testing efficiency, especially in the initial period when fear and uncertainty were rampant. Outbreaks in nursing/care homes were

TABLE 22.1 Ireland chronology

Date		Diffusion of COVID-19	Key official actions	Key communication events
January	5			First Irish media reports. Headline on TheJournal.ie: 'Mysterious Pneumonia Outbreak in China Is Not the Return of SARS Virus, Officials Say.'.
	27		National Public Health Emergency Team (NPHET) for COVID-19 established in Department of Health.	
February	20		Health Service Executive adds COVID-19 to list of notifiable diseases.	
	28	First confirmed case on island (in Northern Ireland. Travelled via Dublin Airport).		
	29	First case confirmed in Republic, associated with trip to Italy.		Daily Department of Health/NPHET daily media briefings begin.
March	8		St Patrick's Day (March 17) festivities cancelled.	
	11	First COVID-19 death in Republic (35 total cases).		
	12		Closure of schools, universities and childcare. Mass gatherings cancelled.	Speech from Leo Varadkar in Washington DC: 'This is unchartered territory. We said we would take the right actions at the right time. We have to move now to have the greatest impact.'

	Event	Statistics	Address / Interview
13	Department of Foreign Affairs advises 'a high degree of caution' before travelling to other EU states.		
15	Pubs ordered to close.	Total cases exceed 100.	
17			St Patrick's Day address from Varadkar: 'In years to come let them say of us, when things were at their worst, we were at our best.'
24	Closure of non-essential retailers/services (eg, gyms, hairdressers, cinemas). Cafes and restaurants limited to take away. Sports events cancelled.	1,125 total cases. 6 deaths.	
24	Temporary COVID-19 employment schemes announced.		
27	People ordered to stay at home for two weeks except for essential travel. Exercise within 2km.	Total: 1,819 cases. 19 deaths.	TV address from Varadkar: 'These are radical actions aimed at saving as many lives as possible…I am asking us for a time, to forego our personal liberties and freedoms for a greater cause.'
April			
4		Death toll reaches 100.+	
6		Total cases exceed 5,000.	
8	Garda (police) law passes to allow officers to redirect people home if caught in breach of guidelines.		
10	2km lockdown period extended.		
18		7,393 cases. 263 deaths.	
20		Cases total 15,000+ (610 deaths).	Chief Medical Officer claims the 'curve has flattened' during TV interview.

(Continued)

TABLE 22.1 (Continued)

Date		Diffusion of COVID-19	Key official actions	Key communication events
May	30	Cases 20,000+ (1,190 deaths).		
	1		Publication of five-phase 'Roadmap for reopening society and business' restrictions slowly lifted mid-May–mid-August.	Varadkar avoids journalists' questions on plan, instead appears on TV chat show.
	5		Exercise extended to 5km from home.	
	8		June's Leaving Certificate state exams cancelled.	
	15	Total deaths exceed 1,500.		
	18		Phase 1: can meet groups of 4 outdoors. Garden/hardware shops reopen.	
June	2	Total cases 25,000 (1,650 deaths).		
	8		Phase 2: travel within 20km and/or within own county allowed. Meet up to 6 people indoors/outdoors allowed. Most retail reopens.	
	23			Varadkar's final TV appearance as Taoiseach: discusses what he would have done different, citing better PPE stockpiling and earlier testing in nursing/care homes.
	27		New government/Cabinet takes power: Micheál Martin new Taoiseach, Varadkar now deputy leader (Tánaiste). New Minister for Health appointed.	
	29	25,417 cases. 1,731 deaths.	Phase 3: travel anywhere in the country allowed. Certain pubs (serving food), gyms, hairdressers etc. reopen.	

also a crucial dimension, with scrutiny shifting to clusters in meat-processing factories and direct provision asylum centres later in the summer.

In late March, the government announced the Wage Subsidy Scheme for employers to top-up salaries, and the weekly €350 Pandemic Payment Support for those who lost jobs. In its June update, the national statistics office noted standard unemployment of 5.6%, but a COVID-inclusive measure of 26.1%, reaching 51% for those aged 15–24 (Central Statistics Office, 2020). Varadkar caused a backlash at one point after suggesting some people were profiting from the €350 scheme, reigniting his anti-welfare reputation.

Various public information campaigns were prominent and effective regarding hand hygiene and social distancing. Another campaign targeting healthcare workers entitled 'Be on call for Ireland' aimed to fast-track recruitment, while the 'Answer Ireland's call' campaign targeted Irish healthcare workers overseas. Other campaigns included the 'In this together: stay connected, stay apart' and 'stay local' messaging. Small initiatives were also evident from state agencies, e.g. the national postal service issued every household with two postcards to post for free with a 'sending love' message, while RTÉ broadcast education-based programming as part of its 'Home School Hub' for children. One notable civil-society initiative was the Feed the Heroes campaign which took donations for takeaway/restaurant food to healthcare workers. It ended on June 9, having raised €1.37m and delivering 180,000 meals to front-line staff over 11 weeks.

Analysis

The main faces

Despite the election result, there was no real question over the legitimacy of the Taoiseach and ministers overseeing COVID-19. Although hashtags such as #notmytaoiseach were used by frustrated individuals who felt the outgoing administration had no mandate, it was never a dominant narrative as their presence until new government formation is constitutionally sound. Elsewhere, all regulations were initially applicable on a nationwide level with no regional government/federal factors at play (beyond minor council-level decisions, for example regarding parks) meaning the focus remained on national figures.

Varadkar was at the fore, regularly accompanied at press conferences alongside Cabinet colleagues such as Minister for Health Simon Harris and others. Throughout the pandemic's peak, daily press conferences (starting on February 29) featured the Chief Medical Officer (CMO) Tony Holohan and/or other senior health officials and journalists. They were typically held around the same time (early evening) each day, providing a sense of consistency on latest case/death figures. On June 5, the Department of Health announced that these briefings would be reduced to twice a week, with daily figures provided through press releases. During these daily media briefings, CMO Holohan rose from a relatively unknown figure to a key voice with mass admiration for his calm, reassuring demeanour. He earned further respect for his dedication despite personal challenges after announcing in early July that he was temporarily stepping aside to be with his wife who had entered palliative care. The Taoiseach paid tribute: 'Every home in Ireland has come to know Dr Tony Holohan…As a country, we owe him and his family a great debt of gratitude.' Holohan also chaired NPHET (National Public Health Emergency Team) which provided advice to the government. The Taoiseach and ministers repeatedly said they based decisions on public health advice, but this led some critics to suggest that unelected NPHET officials – not the government – were running the country (Ryan, 2020).

Regardless of the dynamics behind the scenes, for many onlookers, Varadkar's leadership was praiseworthy, particularly his early communication, highlighting the challenges ahead. During a radio panel discussion assessing the Taoiseach's response, political journalist Lise Hand noted Varadkar and (Minister for Health) Simon Harris 'decided that communication and laying all the cards of the table was key to bring everybody along with them' (RTE .ie, 2020). Writer Peter Sheridan, on the same panel, suggested Varadkar was 'head and shoulders above' Boris Johnson and Donald Trump combined and as a doctor Varadkar 'knows how to speak to people around medical issues and there's an empathy there, but there's also a strictness there…he did it really brilliantly.' Sheridan's comments raise two important points. First, Ireland was regularly compared with the US and UK, two countries from which Irish audiences consume much media. Secondly, Sheridan highlighted Varadkar's medical qualifications, perhaps a factor in public trust. Varadkar also gained international attention after re-registering as a doctor and working one shift a week on a patient helpline.

As mentioned, following the May 1 speech announcing the five-phase roadmap, Varadkar avoided journalists' questioning, instead appearing on chat show *The Late, Late Show*. For one question, the Taoiseach had to check details and pull notes from his pocket. Some interpreted this as poor preparation, not instilling confidence in his leadership and the planned phases, but many onlookers were more sympathetic. A Twitter poll by broadcaster Eoghan McDermott asked, 'Did Leo checking his notes bother you?' 96% of the 6,660 respondents were 'not bothered,' with many saying they prefer having accurate information rather than bluffing (McDermott, 2020). Of course, Varadkar did not escape criticism. Some pointed out how he simply read speeches probably written by others, while his inclusion of pop-culture quotes (such as *Lord of the Rings* and *Terminator*) was questioned. In particular, using a line from the *Mean Girls* teen film ('The limit does not exist') as part of a celebrity bet irked some, and Varadkar even ended up defending this in his final *Prime Time* interview as Taoiseach.

Many opposition politicians did not get much media space during the crisis; given it was the aftermath of an election, there was perhaps less at stake. Moreover, they were effectively squeezed out by scientific/medical experts who provided insight and critique on government decisions. One example was immunologist Prof. Luke O'Neill who regularly appeared in media advocating for mandatory face masks in public places, at odds with government guidelines.

Consistency and accuracy

All schools closed in March with ambiguity over reopening as many parents, balancing work and care, were left frustrated at the 'dithering' (O'Connell, 2020). The Leaving Certificate exams, which take place in early June and determine university access, faced uncertainty since March. Despite repeated official suggestions that they would take place, the exams were eventually cancelled on May 7.

Some media outlets tackled misinformation circulating on social media (Bohan, 2020), while the Taoiseach advised people to 'seek information only from trusted sources' (Varadkar, 2020). Thankfully, there were few major examples of officials providing inaccurate information, and any missteps were relatively short-lived. One Friday evening (March 27), the Taoiseach announced the closure of non-essential workplaces from midnight, but the list of workplaces was not published until the following day causing uncertainty for employers/ staff. Elsewhere, Minister for Health Simon Harris, generally praised, slipped up on radio referencing 18 previous coronaviruses (instead of '-19' coming from 2019). The Chief Medical Officer corrected it during a press conference, and Harris posted a Twitter video owning up to his mistake and apologising, saying he can be an 'awful old idiot at times,' citing 'cabin fever' and workload (Carswell, 2020).

Yet the communication issue which may have had the most significant impact relates to face masks, with Harris admitting in early June that guidance had been unclear. He told the Dáil (parliament): 'I accept that the evidence, and maybe even the messaging on this, has changed over time. Perhaps it has been confusing for people and has not got through in the clear way it needs to' (Harris, 2020). Furthermore, it seems the resistance towards enforcement was at odds with public opinion: one mid-June poll showed 68% supported the mandatory wearing of face masks in enclosed public spaces (Ireland Thinks, 2020). Although further facemask regulations would come later in the summer, the early ambiguity and associated debates were potentially damaging.

Appropriate action?

In late February, no formal government decisions had been taken regarding closures or cancelling events, inaction criticised by those fearful of the looming threat. Attention fixed on an Ireland–Italy Six Nations rugby match scheduled for Dublin on March 7; concerns focused on the influx of visitors from COVID-hotspot Italy, alongside visions of 50,000 fans inside a stadium. Ultimately, on February 25, the Department of Health recommended the game's postponement, with the IRFU rugby federation initially appearing resistant before eventually cancelling.

As March began, media discussed whether St Patrick's Day festival events (around the March 17 national holiday) should proceed. Eventually, on March 8, the government announced all festivities were cancelled. Many felt this was too late coming – some towns had already cancelled theirs – and a similar pattern was evident the following week regarding pubs and restaurants. Restaurant Association of Ireland chairman Adrian Cummins pleaded with Varadkar and two other ministers on March 14: 'I am appealing to you – trigger the closure of licenced premises – Our staff are appealing for it. #SocialDistancing not being observed by customers. It's responsible and it's leadership,' while #closethepubs was trending that day. Given pub culture's popularity in Ireland, especially around St Patrick's Day, it appeared the government lagged behind the public mood.

Overall, there was little resistance to the restrictions. However, in May, two journalists-turned-activists took a High Court case challenging the constitutionality of some legislation. The judge scathingly dismissed Gemma O'Doherty and John Waters' case, drawing on the misinformation zeitgeist, noting the applicants' lack of scientific expertise: 'Unsubstantiated opinions, speeches, empty rhetoric and a bogus historical parallel are not a substitute for facts' (O'Faolain, 2020). O'Doherty and Waters are well known so the case received media attention but little public backing, perhaps because both have reputations for questionable alt-right nationalistic movements which have little support in Ireland.

Conversely, some scientists feared things were returning to normal too soon and Ireland should take the opportunity to 'crush the curve,' acknowledging that thus far, the public supported the restrictions and 'they clearly understood the need.' However, as they wrote in early June, now there was 'a fork in the road,' forming the basis of their petition garnering more than 1,300 signatures, led by the science and medical field (O'Sullivan, 2020).

Conclusion

During a June 25 press conference, Varadkar identified two areas in which the official COVID-19 response could have improved: firstly, better PPE stockpiling and, secondly, more early testing in nursing/care homes. Despite this, polling figures ultimately showed broad support for government actions. Varadkar is known for valuing strategic communication – some critics suggest he is spin-obsessed – but was effective here. At almost all times, the public broadly understood the guidance regarding hygiene, work, travel, visiting family and gathering in public. As well as the consistency of daily briefings, May's 'five phases' provided a clear schedule. Throughout, NPHET's support to the government gave the impression of cohesion and evidence-based decision-making; politicians informed by – not at odds with – health experts. Of course, the legacy of COVID-19 decision-making may only fully surface in years to come when, for example, the repercussions of suspending medical procedures such as breast cancer screenings are understood, and a more contextualised assessment is made regarding the effective shutdown of the country.

This chapter focuses on the early response. Ireland was at a crossroads in late June 2020: the trust and confidence associated with Varadkar and senior ministers were reset as new politicians took over these key roles. While the successful launch of the contact-tracing app was one of July's positives, cracks continued to appear during the summer ensuring it was challenging for the newer political figures to establish such positive relations with the public. General fatigue towards some regulations, confusion over travel guidelines, a gradual second wave of cases (although deaths remained low), the return of serious restrictive measures at some local county levels and backward moves on social gathering rules triggered frustration. One high-profile GP on Twitter, Dr Maitiú Ó Tuathail, summed it up with the question:

> What's different now to March? In short, the messaging! In March it was clear what we were trying to do, there was a plan – we were aiming to flatten the curve…At the moment we are stumbling from one set of restrictions to another.
>
> *(Ó Tuathail, 2020)*

Public anger peaked in late August after some senior political figures attended a parliamentary golf society dinner breaching public health guidelines, leading to resignations by a minister and a European Commissioner. The revelations infuriated many who had made huge personal sacrifices over the previous six months; restoring public trust would be a major challenge facing the new government ahead of the virus's autumn-winter phase.

References

Bohan, C. (2020). Why those messages you're getting on WhatsApp about coronavirus cases in Ireland are (probably) not true. www.thejournal.ie/misinformation-covid-19 -coronavirus-ireland-whatsapp-facebook-5025117-Feb2020/.

Carswell, S. (2020) Simon Harris sorry for 'awful boo-boo' about 18 viruses before COVID-19. www.irishtimes.com/news/health/simon-harris-sorry-for-awful-boo -boo-about-18-viruses-before-covid-19-1.4235478.

Central Statistics Office (2020). CSO statistical release. www.cso.ie/en/releasesandpubli cations/er/mue/monthlyunemploymentmay2020/.

Harris, S. (2020). Dáil Éireann debate – Thursday, 11 Jun 2020. Vol. 993 No. 10. www .oireachtas.ie/en/debates/debate/dail/2020-06-11/3/.

Ireland Thinks (2020). Support for making facemasks mandatory in enclosed public spaces at 68% to 21%… *Tweet.* June 25. https://twitter.com/ireland_thinks/status /1276020294633705472.

McDermott, E. (2020). Did Leo checking his notes bother you?… *Tweet.* May 1. https:/ /twitter.com/eoghanmcdermo/status/1256335991771553792.

MerrionStreet.ie (2020). Speech of Taoiseach Leo Varadkar 27 March 2020. https://me rrionstreet.ie/en/News-Room/News/Speech_of_Taoiseach_Leo_Varadkar_27_M arch_2020.html.

Oakley, R. (2020). The article explains all of the questions you are asking... *Tweet*. March 8. https://twitter.com/roakleyIRL/status/1236621757328642048.

O'Connell, J. (2020). Endless dithering on children and education is unconscionable. www.irishtimes.com/opinion/jennifer-o-connell-endless-dithering-on-children -and-education-is-unconscionable-1.4254439.

O'Faolain, A. (2020). High Court rejects legal challenge by Gemma O'Doherty and John Waters to COVID-19 laws. www.thejournal.ie/gemma-judicial-review-50974 00-May2020/.

O'Sullivan, K. (2020). COVID-19: Letter signed by Irish researchers seeks policy rethink. www.irishtimes.com/news/health/covid-19-letter-signed-by-irish-researc hers-seeks-policy-rethink-1.4273936.

Ó Tuathail, M. (2020). What's different now to March? In short, the messaging!... Tweet. August 19, 2020. https://twitter.com/DrZeroCraic/status/1296075544996515840

Rosney, M. (2020). The St Patrick's Day Address – An Taoiseach's career defining coronavirus speech. www.reputation-inc.com/our-thinking/the-st-patricks-day -address-an-taoiseachs-career-defining-coronavirus-speech.

RTE.ie (2020). Newspaper Panel – Brendan O'Connor. www.rte.ie/radio/radioplayer/ html5/#/radio1/21791763.

Ryan, P. (2020). Inside the all-powerful coronavirus taskforce – Ireland's decision-makers in a crisis. *Sunday Independent*. www.independent.ie/world-news/coronaviru s/inside-the-all-powerful-coronavirus-taskforce-irelands-decision-makers-in-a-cr isis-39103497.html.

Varadkar, L. (2020). Useful.tips to deal with the sudden and constant stream of news which can cause anxiety and worry. *Tweet*. March 15. https://twitter.com/LeoVa radkar/status/1239258428129902593.

23

THE CZECH REPUBLIC

Self-proclaimed role models

Otto Eibl and Miloš Gregor

Political context

At the beginning of 2020, the political scene in the Czech Republic was polarised but stable. Party preferences had barely changed since the general elections in 2017, which had resulted in a minority coalition government led by billionaire Andrej Babiš and his entrepreneurial party ANO (Hloušek & Kopeček, 2019) together with the Social Democrats (ČSSD). The government was officially supported by the Communists and unofficially by the far-right populist SPD. This coalition of unlikely partners was the result of Babiš's scandals (i.e. criminal prosecution, conflict of interests and suspicion of EU-subsidy fraud), which led other parties to refuse to cooperate with him. Despite this, ANO constantly leads in the polls by a substantive margin, with support around 30%.

The ideological position of ANO is not clear; it holds a pragmatic approach to politics, which means it does not take any strong ideological stance, with the exception of its flagship policy – fighting corruption. Concurrently, it perceives permanent communication with voters to be of crucial importance – Andrej Babiš never misses an opportunity to present himself as a non-politician, manager and saviour of the country.

Chronology

See Table 23.1.

Communication moments and media events

The period from February 25 to the end of May was characterised by a huge number of press conferences organised by the government and ministries.

DOI: 10.4324/9781003120254-25

TABLE 23.1 Czech Republic chronology

	Date	Diffusion of COVID-19	Key official actions	Key communication events
February	25			PM Andrej Babiš (ANO) recommends citizens not travel to the most affected parts of Italy at a press conference.
	28			PM Andrej Babiš (ANO) says during a press conference that there is no reason to panic, no need to buy food supplies and face masks.
March	1	First case confirmed.		
	7		Obligatory quarantine for people returning from Italy.	Minister of Health Vojtěch (ANO) forced by PM Babiš (ANO) during a press conference to name from whom he had received misinformation.
	10		Prohibition on meetings of 100+ people.	
	11		Schools and universities close.	
	12		Declaration of a state of emergency.	
	13		Prohibition on meetings of 30+ people.	
	14		Closure of restaurants and shops (with a few exceptions, e.g. grocery stores).	
	15	100 new cases/day.		Change in the ČSSD communication strategy. Jan Hamáček becomes a leader dressed in jeans and a red sweater. PM Andrej Babiš (ANO) says 'we are at war with the virus' to the media.
	16		Closure of state borders, restriction on movement outside of home and work, establishment of the Central Crisis Staff.	
	19		Mandatory wearing of face masks outside of home.	President Miloš Zeman addresses the nation.
	22	First confirmed death.		
	23			PM Andrej Babiš (ANO) addresses the nation for the first time and partially restores his image.

	27	Peak of new cases 373/day. — Jan Hamáček (ČSSD) and Adam Vojtěch (ANO) argue on Twitter.
	28	PM Andrej Babiš (ANO) addresses the nation for the second time.
April	8	4,600 active cases, 100 deaths.
	9	
	11	Peak of the active cases (4,750).
	20	The first easing of restrictions: craft shops and farmer markets open.
	23	Testing capacity exceeds 2,000 tests/day. — The court annuls some government measures – they were not declared correctly according to the crisis law.
	27	Testing capacity exceeds 5,000/day.
The turn of April and May – the number of recoveries begins to permanently exceed the number of active cases.		
May	5	Conducted tests peak at 9,383/day.
	11	Partial reopening of schools, cinemas, theatres etc. (for up to 100 people).
	18	End of the state of emergency.
	19	300 deaths from COVID-19.
	25	Opening of restaurants and allowing of events up to 300 people.
June	4	Opening of borders with Slovakia.
	5	Opening of borders with Austria, Hungary and Germany.
July	1	Wearing of face masks outside of home no longer mandatory.

Without exception, three or four press conferences were held daily, weekends included, ranging from early morning to midnight. Some were accompanied by remarkable moments, which will be the main focus of our analysis.

President Miloš Zeman addressed the nation on March 19 (iDnes.cz, 2020a). In his speech, Zeman showed support for the government, called on the Czech nation to be brave, and thanked China for supplying (meaning selling) the country medical equipment, which was widely criticised. In fact, the whole government was criticised for buying overpriced medical equipment and expressing undignified gratitude. An illustrative example was the delivery of supplements from China on March 21 where Babiš, Hamáček and other ministers welcomed China's plane and bowed at the airport (iDnes.cz, 2020b). Andrej Babiš also addressed citizens through two speeches broadcast by television stations on March 23 and April 9. While the first one resembled a supra-party and presidential speech, that is, without presenting clear outlines of the government's strategy (Seznam TV, 2020a), the second was more in line with the position of the prime minister (PM) and provided citizens with a government plan (Seznam TV, 2020b).

Political and social issues

The first moment the novel coronavirus topic appeared on the Czech political scene can be traced to the end of January 2020 when the opposition asked the government about its readiness for a possible outbreak in the Czech Republic. Minister of Health Adam Vojtěch (ANO) replied that a delivery of 25,000 face masks was about to take place and that one Czech manufacturer had a million in stock; thus, they assured, there was no danger of a shortage. Despite Vojtěch's assurances, there was barely any protective equipment in the state stocks. Since private retail sold out of masks and respirators within a few days, the government had missed an opportunity to solve the situation in advance and be ready for the virus striking. Despite repeated reminders by the opposition of the government's laxity, the public was mostly satisfied with the government's measures (ČT24 April 4, 2020).

On March 12, the government declared a state of emergency (Ministry of the Interior, 2020) across the whole country, which resulted in, among other things, a ban on the retail sale of goods and services (with some exceptions), orders limited to takeaway from restaurants and pubs and restrictions on free movement. The original government resolution expired on March 24 and was immediately prolonged. However, this time the measures were not declared by the government and regulated by the *Crisis Management Act* (Act No. 240/2000 Coll.) but by the Ministry of Health under Act No. 258/2000 Coll., on the protection of public health. The reasons why the government moved the regime, despite having the same measures, is not clear. Lawyers and opposition politicians saw this as an attempt to avoid paying compensation for the damage to businesses affected by the measures in the original implementation. The Prague Municipal

Court cancelled some of these measures on April 23 for being illegal as they were not implemented under the crisis act (Fraňková, 2020). Following this decision, the government adopted the measures once again, this time under the *Crisis Management Act*.

The establishment of a Central Crisis Staff (CCS) was another subject of dispute within the coalition. Even though the *Crisis Management Act* presupposes its creation, and Jan Hamáček had called for its establishment at the start of March, the government did not activate it until March 16. A change in the law preceded the establishment of the CCS itself so that the Deputy Ministry of Health, Roman Prymula, close to ANO, could be appointed by the leadership of the CCS instead of the Minister of the Interior. The situation was settled when Hamáček replaced Prymula at the end of March. The CCS ceased operations on June 11.

Social network and the web

A number of essential activities were united under the COVID19CZ (covid19cz .cz) initiative, which served as an umbrella platform for tech and IT savvy persons, firms and other organisations. They started operating in mid-March and their intention was to help the government accelerate the development of smart IT solutions which would be helpful in fighting the virus. Their goals were threefold: to develop a smart quarantine (part of which were projects like eMask, GPS tracking in Czech map applications and the creation of memory-maps), to provide medical staff with reliable protection gear (3D printed shields, work on CoroVent lung ventilators, and supporting the logistics of medical supplies via DobroVoz), and to inform the public about the disease and minimalise its impact (i.e. the 1212 hotline, the hashtag #stopcovidcz and the translation of various materials from abroad).

The Ministry of Health together with COVID19CZ created a dedicated webpage where they published the latest data and updates. However, the publication of raw data was criticised because it was reported on an aggregate level and thus too general. They therefore failed to provide sufficient localised detail even though the government had this data at its disposal.

Besides that, many brands and celebrities started their own COVID-19 related projects. One of the most influential and internationally relevant was the 'Mask4ALL' campaign aiming to convince people that wearing a simple (even homemade) face mask could help with slowing down the spread of the virus. To do so, the founders published a video (Ludwig, March 27, 2020) in which they explained the meaning of wearing a mask. The video was widely shared on social media; Prime Minister Babiš even tweeted it to Donald Trump (Babiš, March 29, 2020). Many others contributed as well, but, in comparison with this particular campaign, their reach was significantly smaller.

The internet, however, was also full of half-truths, disinformation and lies. Some of them were similar to those published abroad (see Chapter 1 on the

WHO), but there was also Czech-specific fake news. The most visible was the case of Jaroslav Dušek, a well-known actor who, in a YouTube video together with healer and shaman Milan Calábek, advised people that COVID-19 can be treated through a combination of herbs, red wine and Antabus, a drug used to treat alcohol addiction. The video was withdrawn from YouTube and other video platforms upon request from the Centre Against Terrorism and Hybrid Threats (CTHT) at the Ministry of the Interior. Other fake news included cases where martial law was supposedly being planned in areas of restricted movement due to the increased incidence of the virus (Magdoňová, 2020). Chain emails targeted the elderly with messages accusing the European Union (EU) of being incompetent, inconsistent and unwilling to help. Other emails accused the body of abusing the pandemic to smuggle more refugees into Europe, which had been a prominent issue within the Czech political scene since 2014. Although the response to COVID-19 was not related to EU policy, the EU is the most common target of fake news in the Czech Republic, and thus arouses emotions.

Analysis

From the very beginning of the crisis, the Czech government communicated intensively. The constant flow of information and the presence of prominent state representatives at press conferences were aimed at creating an image of a government with everything under control. It was evident that Andrej Babiš enjoyed his media presence. The moment which symbolises the pandemic period as well as the way the government works came during a press conference on March 7 when Minister of Health Adam Vojtěch apologised to a doctor who he had previously mistakenly claimed had contracted COVID-19, pointing out he was misinformed. In a supplementary question, PM Babiš indiscriminately pressed him in front of the television cameras with the words 'Don't be polite, tell the truth. Who gave you the information? Say the name!' Vojtěch hesitated at first to reveal the identity of the source; however, Babiš's authority coerced him to do just that.

A week later, Babiš appeared visibly tired and exhausted – he struggled with Czech, mixing Slovak and Czech together, and his statements became harder to understand. His ministers had to explain what the PM intended to say. The highlight of this period was a joint press conference of PM Babiš and several ministers on March 15. While other members of the government appeared in front of the media in suits, Minister of the Interior Jan Hamáček (ČSSD) came dressed in jeans and a red sweater. Next to a very tired Babiš, Hamáček was suddenly perceived as a man of action, not as a classic 'white collar' bureaucrat. He started to dress informally for press conferences regularly and the sweater became a trending topic among people and a symbol of the crisis.

At the end of March, Babiš addressed the nation with his first speech during the pandemic, which quickly helped restore his partially damaged image.

However, from this point on, he no longer took part in all the press conferences and left the opportunity to 'shine' to his colleagues.

Communicational chaos

Regardless of Babiš's presence, the permanent communication exposed the unpreparedness of the Czech state in facing the crisis. The problem was not the lack of information but its quality and the predictability of further necessary steps. The government did not follow any pandemic plan and was therefore swayed by the flow of events. Members of the government appeared more reactive than proactive; they were not able to explain clearly when and how the measures would be introduced or lifted. Some of the steps remain widely misunderstood; for example, why, during Easter, the government decided to open hobby markets but not churches. This constant flow of inconsistent information resulted in misunderstandings and behavioural errors. Sometimes, contradictory statements were even published, having to be later corrected. Furthermore, it was not exceptional that the ministries of ANO and ČSSD argued among themselves on social networks, which did not contribute to the clarity of already adopted measures. Other weak points in the government's communication included attempts to ignore reality, as in the case of the lack of protective equipment, or to present governmental steps in a far more positive light than evidence suggested.

The relationship between the government and the opposition is also worth noting. The opposition parties agreed to create necessary space for the government. They also proposed a number of policies and measures, which the government regularly negated immediately. Given the polarised nature of Czech politics, this is unsurprising. However, a series of odd situations occurred whereby the government presented the same ideas as their own a few weeks later. Later, when the epidemic situation had improved and the economy became a more salient issue, the opposition started criticising the government for lacking a clear plan to return to normal and restore the economy in general.

Unavailable protective equipment: DIY

As said, the government tried to cover up the lack of the protective equipment, and PM Babiš, at a press conference on March 14, appeared emotional and annoyed, claiming, 'It is not true that our medical staff do not have respirators. Tell me where there is a lack of supply, and I personally will deliver it there today' (Bartoníček, 2020). Over the course of the day, he had to admit that there were no respirators available. Health Minister Vojtěch added that the supplies were 'several hundred thousand or even one million respirators short.' We observed a very similar pattern in the discussion about sufficient testing for COVID-19 – the reality differed from the government announcements substantially, and testing capacities improved only slowly.

On March 19, a paradox emerged. Despite face masks being unavailable, covering one's nose and mouth became mandatory. Nevertheless, the people managed to equip themselves with DIY face masks within a few days. A fitting symbol of this period was people queuing in lines in front of haberdashers, waiting for the opportunity to buy fabrics from which they could sew masks. The face mask became the symbol of extraordinary times and of the Czech nation's unity. Babiš applauded citizens for being so capable, considerate of others and caring for elders and other at-risk groups. He turned a clear disadvantage into an advantage for his government and did not hesitate to talk about (t)his success internationally.

We are at war: rhetoric, promises and the reality

One further characteristic of the Czech government's handling of the pandemic was the visible discrepancy between what the government was saying and the reality. Some examples have already been mentioned, but there were many more. From late March, the government started to use metaphors of war to describe the situation. Phrases such as 'people on the front line' or even 'we are at war with the virus' could be heard from the ministries (Echo24, 2020). The narrative was soon adopted even by the media. Another example of exaggeration on the part of PM Babiš was his often repeated claim the Czech Republic was handling the virus better than anyone else in the world and even that other states should learn from the Czech example. The fact is the Czech Republic did belong to the group of successful countries. However, there were countries handling the pandemic better according to many international comparisons (Tiefengraber, 2020; Bremmer, 2020).

The discrepancy is even more visible when it comes to the economic help following the epidemiological measures. In April, the government announced the state had already spent CZK 1.2 trillion (approximately EUR 45 billion) to support the economy, which represents more than 20% of the national GDP. The support was to include social aid to employees, money for local governments, and direct assistance to entrepreneurs as well as guaranteed loans. Despite the bold proclamations, actual use of the funds has fallen far short (0.9% of GDP in financial support and 0.2% of GDP in liquidity guarantees by June 22) and has been accompanied by bureaucratic difficulties (hlidacstatu.cz, 2020).

Conclusion

Measures introduced by the Czech government resulted in flattening the curve and only slightly over 11,000 people were infected (with only 350 deaths) by the end of June. From this perspective, the Czech government performed well. Now they must take a further step and do everything possible to stimulate recovery and prepare for a possible second wave. Unfortunately, local outbreaks during the summer proved that the so-called smart quarantine was not working properly.

The number of new cases per day rose to 500+ with a peak of 1,164 cases on September 8; therefore, measures valid for the whole country, such as mandatory face masks on public transport, have been adopted again.

At the communication level, the Czech prime minister and his colleagues created something which can be called permanent chaos. Very often, it was not clear what the next step would be or even what a minister's statement actually meant. The government did not offer a clear plan on how to return the country to normal and, even in cases when further steps were introduced, they were changed several times. The government representatives were frequently disunited, presented (even) opposing positions and did not offer logical and simple explanations for their steps. Sometimes, they did not reflect the reality and tried to make things look far better than the situation actually was. Many people even felt that the crisis was handled through a series of lucky accidents, supported by the hard work of paramedics, organisations and individuals from the COVID19CZ initiative.

However, from the government's perspective, the strategy worked. Despite all the communication flaws, ANO's support in the polls increased, and the introduction of the restrictions was not accompanied by noticeable public debate. Citizens were driven by fear and wished for a resolute solution to the unprecedented situation. This is exactly what Babiš's government offered when they shut down the state (even opposition parties agreed on most steps taken by the government). Moreover, it helped Babiš suppress some of his scandals and strengthened his perception as a capable manager whose intentions are to secure a better future for all of us.

References

Babiš, A. (2020). 29 March. https://twitter.com/AndrejBabis/status/1244147274298654 720.

Bartoníček, R. (2020). Rozvezu respirátory, tvrdil Babiš. Poté přiznal, že chybí. V Číně je shání Hamáček. *Aktuálně.cz*, 15 March. https://zpravy.aktualne.cz/domaci/jak-ha macek-bude-shanet-respiratory-a-rousky-ktere-podle-bab/r~0126d77a667f11eaa6 f6ac1f6b220ee8/.

Bremmer, I. (2020). The best global responses to COVID-19 pandemic. *Time*, 12 June. https://time.com/5851633/best-global-responses-covid-19.

Crisis Management Act 2000. 240/2000. www.zakonyprolidi.cz/cs/2000-240.

ČT24 (2020). Průzkum: Nařízení ohledně epidemie jsou podle většiny adekvátní. Lidé nejvíc věří Prymulovi. *Česká televize – ČT24.* 4 April. https://ct24.ceskatelevize.cz/ domaci/3071922-pruzkum-narizeni-ohledne-epidemie-jsou-podle-vetsiny-adekvat ni-lide-nejvic-veri.

Echo24. (2020). Jsme jako ve válce. *Možná dnes zavedeme karanténu, řekl Babiš*, 15 March. www.echo24.cz/a/SVVcV/jsme-jako-ve-valce-mozna-dnes-zavedeme-karantenu -rekl-babis.

Fraňková, R. (2020). Prague court cancels anti-coronavirus restrictions on free movement, retail sales. *Czech Radio*, 23 April. https://english.radio.cz/prague-court -cancels-anti-coronavirus-restrictions-free-movement-retail-sales-8102105.

Hlídač státu. (2020). *Jaká je slibovaná a jaká je skutečná pomoc státu v dobách koronavirové epidemie?* https://www.hlidacstatu.cz/report/27.

Hloušek, V., & Kopeček, L. (2019). How to run an efficient political machine: the billionaire Andrej Babiš and his political-business project. *Politics in Central Europe, 15*(1), 35–54.

iDnes.cz. (2020a). Čína nám jediná pomohla, řekl Zeman. Ocenil dobrovolníky, kritizoval opozici. *iDnes.cz,* 19 March. www.idnes.cz/zpravy/domaci/projev-prezid ent-milos-zeman-koronavirus-tv-prima.A200318_150920_domaci_blj.

iDnes.cz. (2020b). Letadlo naděje dosedlo. Ruslan dopravil miliony roušek a respirátorů. *iDnes.cz,* 21 March. www.idnes.cz/zpravy/domaci/ruslan-letiste-pardubice-rousky-r espiratory-priletel-z-ciny.A200321_170815_domaci_chtl.

Ludwig, P. (2020). *How to significantly slow Coronavirus? #Masks4All.* https://youtu.be/ HhNo_IOPOtU.

Magdoňová, J. (2020). Koronavirové dezinformace neměly v Česku vážné dopady. Týkaly se uzavřených obcí nebo Evropské unie. *iRozhlas.cz,* 28 May. www.irozhl as.cz/zpravy-domov/koronavirus-dezinformace-stanne-pravo-karantena_20052812 31_zit.

Ministry of Interior (2020). *State of emergency.* www.mvcr.cz/mvcren/article/state-of -emergency.aspx.

On the Protection of Public Health 2000. 258/2000. www.zakonyprolidi.cz/cs/2000-258.

Seznam TV (2020a). *Projev premiéra Andreje Babiše ohledě epidemiologue nového typu koronaviru.* www.televizeseznam.cz/video/domaci-9257/projev-premiera-andreje-b abise-ohledne-epidemie-noveho-typu-koronaviru-64047731.

Seznam TV (2020b). *Projev premiéra Andreje Babiše.* www.televizeseznam.cz/video/do maci-9257/projev-premiera-andreje-babise-64052626.

Tiefengraber, S. (2020). What's your country's COVID-19 safety ranking? *Kongres,* 24 April. https://kongres-magazine.eu/2020/04/whats-your-countrys-covid-19-safety -ranking.

24

HUNGARY

Illiberal crisis management[1]

Norbert Merkovity, Márton Bene and Xénia Farkas

Political context

The ruling Fidesz–KDNP parties won a two-thirds supermajority in the National Assembly three elections in a row since 2010. However, in the local elections of 2019 Fidesz suffered sensitive losses unprecedented since the birth of the regime, and when united, the opposition proved it could win in several larger cities including the capital. While there is extensive public and academic debate about the character of the Orbán-regime, its illiberal nature is widely accepted including by Prime Minister (PM), Viktor Orbán himself in his famous speech in 2014 (Buzogány, 2017: 1307–1308). To support the ideal of the illiberal state, the ruling coalition often uses the label 'liberal' against the critics of the government, by which it proves that they are defending the nation from mainstream international actors that would sell out the country to the International Monetary Fund (IMF) or other transnational institutions. These conflicts are often framed in crisis narratives such as the lingering economic collapse of 2008 or the refugee/migration wave of 2015 (see Körösényi et al., 2020). The crises are utilised to justify campaigns against the so-called liberal mainstream such as 'Brussels,' NGOs, international media, the Obama-administration or George Soros. The most durable campaigns were against immigration and included billboards, radio, TV and internet ads raising awareness of the risks of uncontrolled immigration. The government often initiates 'national consultation' in topics that are owned by the government which become government-sponsored opinion polls with the entire population as its sample. The results of consultations are used to strengthen the narrative of a strong and credible government defending Hungarian people's interests.

DOI: 10.4324/9781003120254-26

Chronology

At the early phase, the Operational Group (OG) responsible for the control of COVID-19 was set up by government decree the end of January. The course of events is summarised in Table 24.1.

From January, the first cases in China were described in Hungarian newspapers as a 'mysterious respiratory disease.' The opposition news dealt a lot with the spreading of the virus, while pro-government media were more sceptical about it, often claiming that it was less dangerous than it was presented in the international and opposition news. Also, pro-government media outlets often accused opposition media of devoting too much attention to it and causing unjustified panic. The Prime Minister also claimed at the end of February that 'At present the coronavirus is attracting all the attention, but the historic challenge we're living with continues to be migration' (Kormany.hu, 2020a; see also Kormany .hu, 2020b). The government argued there was enough protective equipment in health care facilities for effective defence, a claim frequently challenged by the opposition. A recurring concern on the pro-government side during this first phase was the presence of fake news around the topic.

During the second phase, after the first cases were confirmed, a dominant topic on the pro-government side was the link between illegal migration and the coronavirus epidemic, which was fuelled by the fact that the first cases were students from Iran. This link was highly challenged by the opposition camp. At the same time, the opposition media and Hungarian Medical Chamber (MOK) warned 'the already squeezed Hungarian healthcare faces the coronavirus without reserves' (Sarkadi, 2020). However, it was highly disputed and attacked by the government and the pro-government media who highlighted the country and health care system was well prepared. Effective protection against the virus and the need for various restrictions became an important topic in this period.

In the third phase, after the first restrictions were announced on March 11, the pro-government side emphasised the importance of national unity and strongly attacked the opposition for threatening this. Also, the timing and determination of government action were praised. Meanwhile, the opposition media argued the quality of government communication was insufficient, and often challenged government measures and their implementation. At the end of March, the so-called 'Enabling' or *COVID-19 Act* sparked strong criticism and protests by internal and non-domestic opponents of the regime. They warned the law contravened essential human rights and fundamental freedoms. In contrast, the pro-government side emphasised the necessity for effective defence and claimed the European elite, international liberal mainstream, NGOs and Hungarian opposition, which they aligned with George Soros, were making a coordinated political attack intending to bring down the Hungarian government.

From April, a further central discourse was the conflict between the government and Gergely Karácsony, the opposition mayor of Budapest. Referring to the high number of infections in a nursing home in Budapest, the pro-government

TABLE 24.1 Hungary chronology

	Date	Diffusion of COVID-19	Key official actions	Key communication events
January	30		**Start Phase 1**. The Operational Group (OG) is formed.	
March	4	COVID-19 reaches Hungary: two infected Iranian citizens studying in Hungary.	**Start Phase 2**. COVID-19 reaches Hungary.	
	10			Orbán, in a conference call with the European Union heads of state and government, draws attention to the economic impacts and the connections between the coronavirus and migration.
	11	The number of infections is 13.	**Start Phase 3**. After the Operational Group proposed the emergency order to the government, the government proclaims a state of emergency (including stay-at-home order) in the entire country.	
	13			Viktor Orbán announced in a live Facebook video address that the schools, kindergartens and nurseries will be closed, and remote teaching will start.
	15	The first patient dies.		
	16		Schools, kindergartens, baby day care close.	
	21	The number of new infections: 103 people. 7 cured and 4 died from the virus.		Viktor Orbán's Facebook page gained more than 200 thousand new followers (the final number is above 1 million by the end of the first wave).

(Continued)

TABLE 24.1 (Continued)

Date		Diffusion of COVID-19	Key official actions	Key communication events
	23		The opposition votes against the urgency of the time-unlimited coronavirus law that is often referred to as the 'Enabling' Act by the critics.	
	30		With 138 votes for, and 53 against, the Hungarian Parliament passes the 'Enabling' or COVID-19 Act and President János Áder signs the bill in record time.	
	31		The government announces that they would release the infection map which shows that most of the infections happened in the capital and the county around the city.	
April	4		On the 4th and the 6th, the government announces its economic and epidemic protection program.	
	9		The Prime Minister announces that the curfew would be extended indefinitely.	
	13	The number of infected people is 1,458, death number is at 109.		
	29	1,891 active cases in Hungary.	Prime Minister announces in his Facebook video address that the restart of the country can begin without Budapest and its surrounding areas. As the outbreak is the most intense in the mentioned territories, the stay-at-home order remains in effect in the capital and Pest county.	

May	3	The expected peak. Fatalities rise to 340. 629 have recovered. 2,029 active cases; 2,998 registered infected.
	15	'I felt important now that I manage this defence personally' – Viktor Orbán said in a radio interview.
	16	Restrictions would be eased in Budapest from the 18th, Viktor Orbán announces on Facebook.
	18	The prevalence of COVID-19 infections is low in Hungary, according to a joint, representative study of medical universities.
	27	The repeal of the 'enabling' or coronavirus law is submitted to the parliament and accepted on June 16.
June	18	107 days after the first infections, the state of emergency ends. The number of confirmed cases: 4,079. 568 deaths, 2,564 had recovered. The number of active infections is 947. 199 cases require hospital, 15 on ventilators.

side heavily attacked the mayor arguing he was personally responsible for this central hub of the pandemic. However, Karácsony claimed the municipality acted prudently, they purchased tests and protective equipment, as the government did not ensure these, and government did not inform him properly about the situation.

Another controversial topic was the decision of the Minister of Human Resources to evacuate at least 60% of publicly funded hospital beds to make space for COVID-19 patients. In response, the government referred to its philosophy of 'prepare for the worst but hope for the best' as this way they could avoid situations seen in other Western countries. In contrast, the opposition attacked the government for ignoring chronic patients falling out of the shrinking health care system.

Another highly discussed topic was the European and global political consequences and lessons of the pandemic. The pro-government side often claimed the failure of the Western liberal world and contrasted it with the success of the Central and Eatern European (CEE) region. They also argued that the coronavirus showed the inefficiency of the European Union (EU) in a crisis. The crisis could only be handled by strong nation-states and real political leaders, and the most effective form of international collaboration during the crisis is the bilateral cooperation between countries. They also claimed that these lessons should have long-term consequences on the global and European political order. On the other hand, the opposition side often stressed that many European countries acted faster or more efficiently than Hungary.

Social network sites, especially Facebook, were intensively used by political actors, media outlets and ordinary citizens during the crisis. This is well illustrated by the fact that one of the most important information resources of the crisis, Viktor Orbán's Facebook page, gained more than 200 thousand new followers during the first weeks of the crisis, and his Instagram account was also heavily used. On the one hand, Facebook has become one of the most important information resources for citizens as the heightened engagement over this topic made countless related information pieces widely visible. At the same time, numerous fake news items also spread widely. Many of them were unveiled and corrected by mainstream media outlets, and in several cases, the police arrested the publishers of fake news by the means of the newly enacted *COVID-19 Act*. A few of these incidents provoked lively controversy in the public about the state of freedom of speech and its alleged violation. On the other hand, social media platforms were efficient tools for ordinary citizens to organise their work and life while maintaining social distance. Solidarity and civic political self-organisation actions were prevalent on the platform. Several groups coordinated voluntary and supportive actions but protests against the controversial *COVID-19 Act* including petitions and an online protest event also took place on the platform.

Analysis

One of the most important features of Hungarian crisis management was the clear prominence of Viktor Orbán's leadership during the pandemic. This is not surprising since Körösényi et al. (2020) demonstrate that crisis discourse, whether exogenous or endogenous, is an inherent feature of the Orbán-regime. This is what triggers the emergence of the charismatic leadership that the regime is based on (p. 38). Nonetheless, at the first latent phase of the crisis before the virus broke into the country, the Prime Minister seemed to stay away from the COVID-19 topic. However, since the virus reached Hungary, Orbán soon became the prime decision-maker, information resource and face of the Hungarian crisis management.

Orbán's main communication platform was his own Facebook page where he kept his followers informed about day-to-day crisis management. The most important information was delivered in video format in his own words, from the first death through the restrictions and regulations to the economic measures, often from his office. Further, as is usual in general, the Prime Minister gave more detailed interviews on each Friday on the national radio, where he offered more elaborate explanations for measures and evaluations of the current situation and its political context. His third main communication platform was the parliament where he directly answered opposition critics five times until the end of May. Overall, the PM's communication on these platforms largely shaped the public discourse around COVID-19 as the most important information of the crisis and arguments for its management appeared in his posts which in turn were echoed frequently on both sides of the political spectrum. Even the government's crisis management advertisement campaign and the main slogans used during the pandemic were built around Orbán's speeches.

Beyond this discursive dominance, the prominence of leadership was manifested in the one-man and highly hierarchical decision-making structure. This was explicitly claimed by Orbán in one of his radio interviews: 'I felt it important that I now manage this defence personally' (Mediaklikk, 2020b). From the beginning of the crisis, he kept talking about measures in the first person singular as his own decisions. However, this one-person decision-making, responsibility-taking, omnipotent role does not mean an omnicompetent image of leadership. Orbán often emphasised he is not competent in managing pandemics and viruses, therefore his main task as a leader is to collect all scientific evidence and expert opinions on the topic. However, these expert opinions are not able to directly lead political measures, these should be decided and made by the leader drawing upon his common sense, properly informed by evidence and scientific predictions. He explicitly justified the one-man leadership of the crisis management by this argument when he continued the above-cited sentence about his leadership: 'And this is not because I'm competent in health care policy – I cannot be accused of it-, but I have common sense' (Mediaklikk, 2020b).

For these reasons, the constant, active and information-collecting presence is an important part of his leadership image which was primarily and intensively reported on his Facebook and Instagram page. Several short video spots showed him unexpectedly visiting hospitals[2] and other state institutions where he was shown asking for information from the directors, staff or even patients. He said in one radio interview that even if these visits may be unnecessary from a rational point of view, 'my instinct suggests that I have to go' (Mediaklikk, 2020a) to collect information. Also, many posts portrayed official meetings with experts and staff members. The image of hard-working leadership was depicted by the timing of these events, often recorded in the description of social media posts. Many posts reported meetings in the very early morning and the late at night, and even on Easter Sunday morning the PM visited a hospital in the countryside.

This charisma-based and hard-working leadership image was further emphasised by contrasting his political activity with other political actors. While these contrasts appeared mostly in the communication of other governmental politicians and pro-government media, in some cases Orbán highlighted some contrasting points himself. The main contrast was drawn with the opposition party mayor of the capital, Gergely Karácsony, who was shown as an indecisive, responsibility-avoiding, inactive leader who was mostly communicating rather than acting during the crisis. An explicit contrast was evident when Orbán said in one of his radio interviews that Karácsony is a 'theoretical-minded' leader who may be able to write 'great studies' about the events, but was unable to make effective and firm decisions. Orbán argued that the management of a crisis requires 'practical-minded' leaders who can act and take responsibility (Mediaklikk, 2020c).

Another characteristic contrast was often made with the political class of the European Union who were claimed to be ineffective in crisis management but active in 'political attacks' against the 'country.' This contrast was made explicitly by Orbán when he kept claiming in interviews and open letters to European leaders that he did not have time to deal with political critics and controversies during the crisis, because effective crisis management requires all the energies he has. Recurring further contrasts were drawn with the crisis management of the previous left-wing governments that were shown as wrong and ineffective as opposed to Orbán's successful management of the crisis, but this contrast was mostly related to the economic measures.

A last but important feature of the crisis leadership of Orbán is the personal style of his communication. On his social media communication, ordinary people, personal stories and remarks and celebrities often appeared and, in his interviews, he often talked about the everyday difficulties and pleasures of ordinary people in a rather personal way. Overall, he used a highly mundane language to explain measures, political dilemmas and complicated arguments.

Beyond Orbán, one of the other prominent actors during the crisis was the Minister of Foreign Affairs, Péter Szijjártó, whose main issues included bringing back Hungarian citizens stuck abroad, coordinating the foreign, mainly Chinese, acquisition of protective equipment and the donations to other countries, and especially liaising with Hungarian communities beyond the borders. The performances in these areas were presented as some of the most important political achievements during the crisis, and they were intensively communicated across several platforms. These messages fit well with the main official slogans of the crisis management such as 'no Hungarian is alone' and 'every Hungarian is responsible for every Hungarian.' Péter Szijjártó was also active in the international defence of the Hungarian government's position on the question of the *COVID-19 Act*. In this area, other members of the government such as the Minister of Justice, Judit Varga and the State Secretary of International Communication and Relations, Zoltán Kovács were also prominent and appeared on several international media outlets to react to international critics. In turn, these reactions have become important reference points in the domestic discourse to show how the government was struggling with international political 'attacks.' Ministers responsible for the economy were also prominent actors during the crisis, concerning their specific areas. However, it is noticeable that members of the government officially responsible for the health care policy were hardly visible in the public discourse.

An important actor in official communication was the Operational Group (OG); one of their most important tasks was day-to-day information provision through daily press conferences and on an online website. Although the members who publicly represented the OG were leaders of law enforcement bodies and health care professionals rather than politicians, the judgement of their work was divisive in the public discourse. While the pro-government public was supportive of their work and personalities, the opposition discourse was more critical of the quality of the information provided.

Another main actor was Gergely Karácsony, the opposition party mayor of the capital. Besides his contrasting role to the Prime Minister, he was highly critical of the crisis management of the government, but sometimes he publicly expressed his support for some of its measures. He also heavily used his Facebook page to react to his critics and defend his position, attack the government and present his city-level crisis management often as a contrast to the government's approach.

Experts and scientists were prominent actors during the crisis. On the one hand, both pro- and anti-government media outlets were keen to give space for experts such as virologists, doctors and economists. However, media outlets selected experts carefully based on their political leanings. In the pro-government media outlets, only experts who were supportive of government measures appeared, while in the opposition media outlets experts who were critical of government were given a platform. On the other hand, as discussed above, the government also drew extensively upon experts, even if the PM made it clear their expertise cannot replace political decisions. Nonetheless, Orbán often referred to the opinions and advice of experts when explaining his decisions, and while the latter provoked much criticism from the opposition, the underlying expert arguments were rarely challenged.

Although there were no major contradictions of information provided by officials, some decisions caused confusion. For instance, originally the government was against the closure of schools, kindergartens and baby nurseries. On the morning of the day when the PM announced the closures, he argued on the national radio that closures are not necessary as it would endanger the school year, teachers would go on unpaid leave and parents would stay home to take care of their children. However, at 9 pm, Orbán announced in a live Facebook video address that the schools, kindergartens and nurseries would close, and remote teaching would start.

Further confusion was caused by territorial infection data. At the beginning of the epidemic, this information was not made public. Mayors, heads of regional or municipal institutions and ordinary citizens published some data based on the knowledge they had alone. At the end of March, the infection map was released. But otherwise, the messages from officials regarding the threat and the handling of the crisis and the objectives of the measures were clear.

Since mid-May, the government has kept declaring the Hungarian management of the crisis was incredibly successful. While many oppositional actors reject this claim, according to some of the polls, crisis management is positively evaluated by the majority of the voters (HVG, 2020). At the end of May, Viktor Orbán announced the government would launch a 'national consultation' about the management of the crisis. It is highly likely this will validate this leadership further.

Notes

1 The research was supported by the Incubator program of the Center for Social Sciences, Eötvös Loránd Research Network (project number: 03013645). Further, Márton Bene is a recipient of a Bolyai János Research Fellowship awarded by the Hungarian Academy of Sciences (BO/334_20), and Xénia Farkas is a recipient of a ÚNKP Fellowship (ÚNKP-20-3-II-CORVINUS-10).

2 E.g.: www.facebook.com/298090296092/videos/641754303067234 or https://www.facebook.com/watch/?v=625470641338034.

References

Buzogány, A. (2017). Illiberal democracy in Hungary: Authoritarian diffusion or domestic causation? *Democratization*, *24*(7), 1307–1325.

HVG (2020). Medián: A járvány enyhül, a Fidesz erősödik, de a 30 év alattiak közt elvérezne. *HVG.hu*, 10 June. https://hvg.hu/360/20200610_A_jarvany_enyhule sevel_erosodott_a_Fidesz_de_a_30_ev_alattiak_kozt_elverezne.

Kormany.hu (2020a). Prime Minister Viktor Orbán on the Kossuth Radio programme 'Good morning Hungary.' *Kormany.hu*, 28 February. www.kormany.hu/en/the-pri me-minister/the-prime-minister-s-speeches/prime-minister-viktor-orban-on-the -kossuth-radio-programme-good-morning-hungary-20200228.

Kormany.hu (2020b). Prime Minister Viktor Orbán informed his EU counterparts about situation in Hungary. *Kormany.hu*, 10 March. www.kormany.hu/en/the-prime-mi nister/news/prime-minister-viktor-orban-informed-his-eu-counterparts-about-situation-in-hungary

Körösényi, A., Illés, G. & Gyulai, A. (2020). *The Orbán regime: Plebiscitary leader democracy in the making*. Routledge.

Mediaklikk (2020a). Orbán Viktor – miniszterelnöki interjú (Jó reggelt, Magyarország! – április 10.). *Mediaklikk.hu*, 10 April. https://mediaklikk.hu/miniszterelnoki-interju

k/cikk/2020/04/09/orban-viktor-miniszterelnoki-interju-jo-reggelt-magyarorszag-aprilis-10/.

Mediaklikk (2020b). Orbán Viktor – miniszterelnöki interjú (Jó reggelt, Magyarország! – május 8.). *Mediaklikk.hu*, 15 May. https://mediaklikk.hu/miniszterelnoki-interju k/cikk/2020/05/08/orban-viktor-miniszterelnoki-interju-jo-reggelt-magyarorszag-majus-8/.

Mediaklikk (2020c). Orbán Viktor – miniszterelnöki interjú (Jó reggelt, Magyarország! – május 15.). *Mediaklikk.hu*, 15 May. https://mediaklikk.hu/miniszterelnoki-interju k/cikk/2020/05/14/orban-viktor-miniszterelnoki-interju-jo-reggelt-magyarorszag-majus-15/.

Sarkadi, Z. S. (2020). Tartalékok nélkül néz szembe az eleve kifacsart magyar egészségügy a koronavírussal. 13 March. https://444.hu/2020/03/13/tartalekok-nelkul-nez-sz embe-az-eleve-kifacsart-magyar-egeszsegugy-a-koronavirussal.

25

POLAND

Protecting the nation while struggling to maintain power

Michał Jacuński

Political context

The political system in Poland is based on the duality of the executive branch, characteristic of a semi-presidential regime, and on a bicameral legislature. Due to high electoral support, from 2015 to 2019 political power lay in the hands of the right-wing coalition. Electoral success and the persistent popularity of the Law and Justice political party (PiS) introduced widely beneficial welfare benefit programmes accompanied by a strong populist rhetoric. The consistence in expansion of individual social policies, including an extremely popular child subsidy and raising state pensions, translated into long-lasting governmental credibility.

However, the political landscape started to undergo certain changes several months prior to the outbreak of the epidemic. On the one hand, the political situation at the beginning of 2020 still appeared to be stable; on the other hand, however, symptoms of political change could be sensed. The stability on the part of government and parliamentary majority was affected by the fact that there had been parliamentary elections held in the autumn of 2019, won by the ruling right-wing coalition. However, the upper house of parliament, the Senate, was taken over by the opposition, which managed to appoint the Speaker of the Senate. After several years of independent rule by the PiS party, there appeared an institutional and political counterpoint, likely to complicate the governance.

The changing balance of power meant the PiS were determined to ensure they retained the presidency, an important role occupied by Andrzej Duda from PiS from 2015 to 2020. For the PiS, orchestrating the incumbent's swift re-election was a key issue, which, as it turned out, took on a new meaning with the outbreak of COVID-19.

DOI: 10.4324/9781003120254-27

Chronology

Although in January 2020 there were already the first cases of the coronavirus infection in Europe, neither the media, politicians nor the general public attached importance to the impending threat. In the last week of January, the Chief of the Sanitary Inspectorate gave a few interviews in the national mainstream media (Zaborski, 2020), in which he expressed hopes that Poland could avoid the coronavirus and that there was no reason to panic. During January and February, however, the first meetings of crisis-management teams were held and an inventory of supplies available in the health care and sanitary services and in laboratories started to be compiled. The first case of COVID-19 was officially confirmed on March 4. Ten days later, the Polish authorities introduced a state of epidemic emergency, and soon afterwards, on March 21, a state of epidemic was announced. This gave the government authority to implement restrictions on movement and freedoms. Press conferences and briefings by the prime minister (PM) Mateusz Morawiecki (PiS), the minister of health Łukasz Szumowski (MP, elected on the PiS list) and other government officials started to be held on a daily basis to communicate the rationale for those socially vital decisions. The government also announced protective measures for the economy.

In the face of the festering political dispute regarding the presidential elections, and the growing discontentment around the limitations on civil liberties, the government decided that covering one's nose and mouth in public spaces would become mandatory as of April 16 while other restrictions would gradually be lifted.

Table 25.1 summarises the development of the epidemic in Poland.

Analysis

With the appearance of COVID-19 in Poland, the government relatively quickly assumed the communicative initiative. During the first few weeks, the government made and communicated unhesitating decisions led, on the one hand, by the World Health Organisation (WHO) announcing a global pandemic, and on the other hand, by the fact that the first Pole was diagnosed with the virus. The key figures in the first days and weeks of the crisis were the prime minister Mateusz Morawiecki and the minister of health Łukasz Szumowski. Important decisions regarding the closing of borders, schools and institutions of higher education were delivered by the relevant ministers. Politicians representing the governing camp argued that the tools chosen to battle the coronavirus were selected appropriately and if Poles observed the rules of isolation and restrictions on social contact, they would ensure safety for themselves and others. The underlying aim according to the government was avoiding the Italian scenario, meaning a high ratio of infections and a high death toll, resulting from what the Polish Government perceived as the lax approach taken in Italy. The communicative initiative was accompanied by a controversial decision to ban doctors serving as

TABLE 25.1 Poland chronology

Date		Diffusion of COVID-19	Key official actions	Key communication events
January	30			The first conference on the epidemic threat in the Ministry of Health (MH). Chief Sanitary Inspector expresses hope that Poland could avoid the coronavirus.
February	2	2 planes with Poles evacuated from China.	Conducting laboratory tests begins.	
	19	12 hospitalised, 13 quarantined and 1,000 monitored.		
	23			Live coverage of pandemic in top Polish news media.
	25			Government-held information website concerning pandemic initiated.
	27		Visits to hospitals forbidden.	
	29	307 tests performed.		MH refuses to state how many test kits were available in Polish laboratories.
March	2		Special-act, which allows the use of all the necessary measures in the fight against COVID-19 and its effects.	
	4	The first infection confirmed.	First meeting of the Government Crisis Management Team.	MH starts daily updates on infections.
			MH ensures that country's capability reaches 2K tests per day.	MH claims that 9 laboratories were ready to carry out testing. Journalist proves that only 4 were ready.

7		The government imposes cancelling of mass events.	The discussion about the closure of churches is sweeping through the country.
10	Local transmission of COVID-19 detected.	Preparation of lockdown-type control measures started.	President's 1st televised address to the nation.
12	The first casualty of the coronavirus in Poland.	First lockdown measures taken. The government closes all schools, universities, kindergartens and nurseries.	
13		State of an epidemic emergency.	PM's televised address to the nation.
14	103 infected.		Government press conferences to take place online, without media presence.
15		Polish borders closed for 10 days. Extended to mid-June.	Promotion of the #StayatHome.
18	The first infected person cured and released home.		
20	Infections are registered in all regions.	State of epidemic announced.	President's 2nd televised address to the nation.
24	Death toll 10. 20,127 tests performed.	Second lockdown measures are taken. Far-reaching restrictions on motility introduced.	The media and political opposition accuse government of insufficient number of tests performed.
25		Schools switch to distance learning.	
26			Numerous candidates and influencers start voicing about the need to postpone the election date.

(Continued)

TABLE 25.1 (Continued)

Date	Diffusion of COVID-19	Key official actions	Key communication events
27	1,340 Infected.		Doctors acting as national consultants banned to speak in the media about the pandemic.
31		First anti-crisis legislation package adopted. The list of restrictions that will tighten the rigour of leaving the household announced.	
		A government package of protective solutions Anti-Crisis Shield v. 1.0 is signed.	
April 3		Access to state forests prohibited.	Coronavirus and internal security become the leitmotivs of the presidential campaign.
5	3,834 infected, death toll close to 100.		
6		New law on correspondence voting in presidential elections.	
16		Obligatory to cover mouth and nose in public places.	
17			MH claims that the only safe form of elections is postal elections.
18		Anti-Crisis Shield 2.0.	
19	545 new infections and 13 deaths.		

20	Restrictions reduced. More people can enter the stores. Forests and parks reopen.	ProteGO Safe application launched.
24	Daily death toll 40. Total death toll exceeds 500.	
25		Public media start broadcasts of non-paid presidential ads. Public and institutional dispute over the postal elections. Very critical opinions related to legal instability issued by the OSCE Office for Democratic Institutions and Human Rights (ODIHR) and the Polish Supreme Court.
29	12,640 infections, 624 died since the first infection.	Financial Shield of PLN 100 billion (27 billion USD) allocated to entrepreneurs.
30		Presidential elections by correspondence to be held May 10. Postmen to distribute millions of election packages.
May 4		The second stage of defrosting the economy.
6		Leaders of the coalition parties announce a political consensus that there will be no elections on May 10.
10		The scheduled presidential vote does not take place.
16		Anti-Crisis Shield 3.0.
18		Third stage of easing the restrictions.

(Continued)

TABLE 25.1 (Continued)

Date		Diffusion of COVID-19	Key official actions	Key communication events
	20	19,739 infections. Death toll 962.		
	27		PM Morawiecki presents another plan to lift part of the restrictions.	
June	3		The new date for the 2020 presidential election set to be on June 28.	The election campaign starts all over again.
	4	25,048 infections. Death toll 1,117.		
	6	Regional outbreaks of infections appear.		
	25			
	28			First round of presidential elections.
	30	34,393 infections. Death toll 1,463. Quarantined 83,499.	Anti-Crisis Shield 4.0.	The second round of presidential elections is to be held on July 12. Presidential campaign carries on.

Source: own elaboration, based on data from the Polish Ministry of Health website and Polish Government Portal, www.gov.pl/web/koronawirus

infectious disease consultants from commenting on the situation. Medical workers were deprived of influence on the organisation or communication of the anti-crisis effort. In the words of the chairman of the Superior Council of Doctors (Matyja, 2020: 4) 'a state of caricature asymmetry' was reached as 'several people [at the central level] gather and concoct what to communicate at a press conference.' Next, the decisions made in the cabinets 'are presented in the spotlight while NHS institutions are left to their own devices.'

As of March 14, all press conferences related to the government's handling of the epidemic began to be streamed live on Facebook and Twitter with the media a virtual presence only. COVID-19 generated strong interest in the Polish social media, with approximately 400k mentions daily (Mierzyńska, 2020).

In crisis management, when public safety is a concern, crisis response strategies have to take into account people's information needs. The initial reactions of the government were organised accordingly around two functions: instructing and adjusting information (Sturges, 1994). The role of instructing information was to educate people what they should do to protect themselves from a crisis. Adjusting information aimed to help people to cope with the crisis psychologically.

On March 16, Morawiecki was interviewed by a popular Polish YouTuber nicknamed Blowek (Blowek, 2020), addressing the issue of fake news regarding COVID-19, and the recording soon reached two million views. The government launched a crisis webpage and prepared infographics, aimed at fighting misinformation, similar to the tools used by Obama in 2008 during the 'fight the smear' campaign (Folkenflik, 2008). The Ministry of Digitalisation from April 20 promoted a free exposure notification application for mobile devices named ProteGO Safe. It was downloaded over 150K times via Google Play and AppStore. The Prime Minister's Office spent €100,000 over three months on the promotion of 71 posts on social media. Most of them pertained to the prevention of COVID-19 infections, the information campaign #StopFakeNews and the promotion of content posted on the government site.

The government maintained an information advantage also because the first two-day parliament session was not held until March 26. For almost three weeks the government managed to position itself as the key independent actor in the fight against COVID-19. Public and commercial media assumed the roles of interpreter and informer, framing news, discussing events and disseminating guidelines (Ulmer et al., 2019: 18–23).

News framing consisted of the daily covering of the progression of the epidemic, often in the form of a 'Daily Report.' Special editions of programmes introduced dedicated content, based on the expertise of virologists and epidemic experts. The media also reported on events, reactively covering government decisions and single events (e.g. the passing of the Anti-Crisis Shield) or pseudo-events (e.g. the arrival of the cargo aircraft carrying medical supplies from China, greeted at the airport by senior government officials). Disseminating information and guidelines had two foci: national and international. The national news drew upon statistics relating to infections, deaths and the people under quarantine, delivered by the Ministry of Health (MH). Overnight, the chief of this ministry became a point of reference for the general public and opinion-forming media. In April 2020, Szumowski enjoyed greater public trust than the president and the prime minister, and in May he still ranked among the three most trusted politicians in Poland. Diffusion of news from abroad encompassed mainly dramatic reporting from countries with the higher diagnosed cases and casualties (Italy and Spain) and about the situation in the United States. It is worth mentioning here that public media in Poland has recently been characterised by political instrumentalisation by the ruling party. Present in this media is entrenched journalism, meaning journalism that clearly takes sides, with the media playing a political role (López-Escobar et al., 2008: 185), which results in extremely biased reporting, favourable for the government and negative for the opposition. The epidemic in Poland therefore became an opportunity to emphasise the differences between those in power and the opposition. Also, the authorities in Poland and the media supporting them juxtaposed what they perceived as effective and decisive actions on their part, confirmed by the low number of infections, with the inaction and incompetence of the European Union.

Political opponents and media critical of the government served as a watchdog, monitoring the government's actions quite impassively during the first few weeks, relinquishing the communicative initiative. During this time, the main accusation levelled against the government was not disclosing whether Poland possessed enough respirators and test kits to meet needs. The authorities consistently refused to address this issue, claiming that tests are administered as needed among those possibly infected. Prior to the first case diagnosed with COVID-19 on March 4, 584 tests had been done. In the first few weeks of the biggest growth in infections, about 2% of tests proved positive (Pawłowska, 2020). Up until April 2, all over Poland about 50k tests had been done, resulting in 2k confirmed infections according to the Ministry of Health (TVN24). What raised doubts was the small scale of testing, limited only to those suspected of being infected. Another criticism was the inconsistency in introducing bans and contradictory media statements, e.g. on March 18 the PM Morawiecki stated that 'Poland started preparations to fight coronavirus several months ago' only to say on March 19 that 'we are faced with circumstances that nobody could foresee a month ago, that nobody knew about two months ago.' Apart from some rare cases, government communication until May 10, the planned election date, evolved around repeating statements claiming success in the fight against the epidemic, accompanied by forecasts of the growing risk of economic crisis and the collapse of public finances, both of which were claimed to be prevented by the government's measures.

After several weeks of 'national isolation,' the government aimed to give a semblance of normalcy and being in control of the situation, which would legitimise holding elections on May 10, likely resulting in re-electing Andrzej Duda, who was enjoying widespread support. However, the peak in the number of infections was not over yet: while the daily ratio of infections flattened, the number of those diagnosed with coronavirus did not decline. The elections were not postponed, the ballot papers were printed and the candidates showed up at the televised debates. On May 6, there was a surprising twist. Leaders of the coalition parties announced a political consensus that there would be no elections on May 10. This happened four days ahead of the State Election Committee decision that it would be impossible to vote safely. Nobody went to vote. The election date was rescheduled to June 28.

The first serious rift appeared at the end of April, when the MH voiced support for postal elections, speaking as a politician, backing his political camp, rather than as a doctor. Next, on May 18 journalists revealed Szumowski and his family's business connections with public funds and his ministry's dubious purchasing decisions concerning protective and medical equipment. In order to keep its reputation, the government had no other choice than to curb Szumowski's media exposure and move the communication focus from its hitherto pandemic fight frontman to economic matters. Amid the re-starting of the election campaign in June, red-herring topics started to appear, aimed at changing the focus and polarising voters' opinions around social values, including legalising same-sex marriages or fighting LGBT 'ideology.'

Here it can be assumed the government employed the logic of decision theory and diffusion theory (Fearn-Banks, 2016: 11–20), being aware that the crisis situation in the days preceding presidential elections might result in an image crisis and a lasting drop in public support. As explained by Coombes (2012: 62), 'reputation and crisis communication have a very strong bond' so ineffective crisis communication 'can create a further need for risk communication, issues management and reputation management.'

During the first phase of the fight against the epidemic, which entailed numerous restrictions, social anxiety and frustration, and the slowing down of the economy, the government resorted to two image restoration strategies (Benoit, 1997: 179). The first one involved reducing public concern through cancelling of or gradual easing of restrictions. The other consisted of introducing compensation mechanisms and corrective actions, in the form of financial aid and the Anti-Crisis Shield.

After three months of government communication, the crisis was at the phase of continuous containment and mitigation of negative effects through government intervention and public financial aid, supported by a slogan coined by the PM: '100 billion PLN [approx. USD 27 billion] for 100 days of the epidemic.'

Was the government successful in its efforts to manage the crisis? This question has an ambiguous answer. Opinion polls (Smith, May 2020) show that the government's performance ratings were strongly polarised: after two months of fighting the crisis, 53% view the government's actions negatively, with 39% supporting them. Social Changes, an opinion research centre cooperating with pro-government media (WPolityce, 2020), established, however, that the public assessment of the government's actions remains stable, since 44% of those participating in the poll viewed those actions positively and 42% negatively.

By the end of June, 34,393 infections were recorded in Poland, with the death toll of 1,463. Compared to other European countries the infections and deaths indicators were low, but one needs to bear in mind that the number of tests per capita in Poland was lower than that of 22 other members of the European Union.

Poles were significantly affected by the restrictions imposed in the first stages of the epidemic. The threat was taken seriously however and both on an individual and collective level, the restrictions were observed. When after several weeks ,the Poles saw that the epidemic did not follow the Italian or Spanish scenario but the government showed no intention of relaxing the lockdown regulations while it was aiming for presidential elections at the beginning of May, more and more questions started to be publicly asked. Did the government not go too far in limiting civic liberties? Was it necessary to drastically restrict the activities of many sectors of the economy? Was the government's crisis management not aimed at achieving political goals?

It is hard to accuse the government of bad intentions. However, it is certain that the looming political crisis, caused by ineffective fight against the pandemic, paired with the possibility of economic collapse and of the loss of the presidential office were all significant factors which influenced what decisions were made. Undoubtedly, the ruling majority strived for elections at all costs. However, heated debates broadcast by the media regarding the legitimacy of presidential elections and safe voting continued, which led to the postponement of the elections by almost two months. In the meantime, restrictions were relaxed, and the government introduced subsequent versions of the Anti-Crisis Shield, which have been accompanied by extensive public support for entrepreneurs and social security measures. So far, despite criticism, the government is coming out of the crisis successfully. In July, Andrzej Duda was elected president for a second term. Five weeks later, the minister of health resigned.

References

Benoit, W. L. (1997). Image repair discourse and crisis communication. *Public Relations Review*, 23(2), 177–186, https://doi.org/10.1016/S0363-8111(97)90023-0

Blowek (2020). Czy miasta zostaną zamknięte? *Interview with PM Mateusz Morawiecki*, March 15, http://tiny.cc/bitssz

Coombes, T. (2012). Crisis communication and its allied fields. In W. T. Coombs & S. J. Holladay (Eds.), *The Handbook of Crisis Communication* (pp. 54–64). Blackwell Publishing.

Fearn-Banks, K. (2016). *Crisis Communications: A Casebook Approach*. Routledge.

Folkenflik, D. (2008). Obama campaign opens anti-smear web site. *NPR*, June 12, http://tiny.cc/aitssz

López-Escobar, E., Sádaba, T. & Zugasti, R. (2008). Election coverage in Spain: From Franco's death to the Atocha Massacre. In J. Strömbäck & L. L. Kaid (Eds.), *The Handbook of Election News Coverage Around the World* (pp. 175–191). Routledge.

Matyja, A. (2020). Co by tu jeszcze odmrozić, panowie? *Gazeta Lekarska*, June, p. 4.

Mierzyńska (2020). Epidemia dezinformacji w Polsce. *OKO.press*, March 14, https://oko.press/koronawirus-wywolal-dezinformacyjna-powodz/

Pawłowska, D. (2020). Testy na koronawirusa. *Biqdata.pl*, April 2, http://tiny.cc/4jvhrz

Polish Ministry of Health Website. www.gov.pl/web/zdrowie/

Polish Government Portal. www.gov.pl/web/koronawirus

Smith, W. (2020). International COVID-19 tracker update. *YouGov*, May 18, http://tiny.cc/zwvhrz

Sturges, D. L. (1994). Communicating through crisis: A strategy for organizational survival. *Management Communication Quarterly*, 7, 297–316.

Ulmer, R. R., Sellnow, T. L. & Seeger M. W. (2019). *Effective Crisis Communication: Moving From Crisis to Opportunity*. SAGE Publications.

WPolityce (2020). *Jak Polacy oceniają działania rządu ws. epidemii koronawirusa?* May 18, http://tiny.cc/bsvhrz

Zaborski, M. (2020). W Polsce nie ma tego wirusa. *Interview on RMF FM Radio*, January 30, http://tiny.cc/32ejrz

26

GHANA

Political expediency or competent leadership?

Sally Osei-Appiah

Political context

When the World Health Organisation (WHO) declared COVID-19 a global pandemic on March 11, Ghana was yet to confirm any cases. The next day, the Ministers of Health and Information announced the first two cases, both of which were imported cases from Norway and Turkey. By then, Ghanaians had already witnessed the pandemic's slow but sure progress across the world and the increasing death toll that accompanied its journey. About 80 countries had confirmed cases. China had recorded over 80,000 cases with approximately 3,000 deaths, while other countries like Italy, where many Ghanaians live, were fast approaching 15,000 cases and over 1,000 deaths. In Africa, 137 cases had already been recorded across 12 countries.

Before March 12, there had been some apprehension about how the country would fare against the pandemic. It is true that many consider Ghana a shining example in Africa (Bawa & Sanyare, 2013) given its relatively stable political history and growing economy. However, like other African countries, Ghana's healthcare infrastructure has many challenges including shortage of healthcare workers, facilities and medical supplies, weak health information systems and governance, and inadequate financial investment in healthcare (Adua et al., 2017; Nyarko et al., 2015). The fact that wealthier, Western countries like Italy and Spain seemed overwhelmed by the pandemic gave cause for grave concern. Besides that, the Ghanaian culture is deeply communal with much interpersonal interaction occurring at festivals, weddings, funerals, church services and other cultural events. Thus, the onset of a virus that transcends borders and demands social distancing was going to pose a challenge not just to the country's porous borders, relatively weak healthcare system and growing but still very young economy, but also its socio-cultural lifestyle. This is the challenge that

DOI: 10.4324/9781003120254-28

Nana Akufo-Addo faced as president and head of government. Since assuming office in December 2016, he has enjoyed much public support due to his policies. Notably, he had introduced Free Senior High School education which allowed many poor parents to educate their children beyond Junior High, as well as starting a local industrialisation drive dubbed 'One District One Factory,' a plan to build one factory in every district in Ghana.

As an incumbent working towards re-election in December 2020, the emergence of the COVID-19 pandemic complicated Akufo-Addo's re-election ambitions. Ansell et al. (2014) note that leaders are defined according to how they perform in times of crises. How Akufo-Addo managed the pandemic in the country, or was perceived to manage it, would not only significantly impact public confidence in his leadership but also, consequently, impact his electoral goals. Leading a country through a crisis of such proportion as a global pandemic presents its own hurdles. When that is coupled with campaigning for re-election, the pressure to perform and gain legitimacy as a worthy candidate in the eyes of the electorate increases considerably. Ghana's case therefore presents a study on how political leaders can navigate the murky waters of campaigning during a crisis in ways that ensure public support. This chapter thus explores Nana Akufo-Addo's response to COVID-19 in the first few months of its occurrence in Ghana, focusing on his communication approach and its likely impact on his candidature.

Chronology

Before Ghana's first confirmed case, media coverage of the pandemic was minimal, comprising mainly general updates from China and other affected countries. Regionally, only Kenya, Algeria, Nigeria and Senegal had cases. The lack of importance was reflected in the sometimes-humorous reporting such as the attention given to the 'Wuhan shake,' an alternative way of shaking hands which involved elbow or foot taps. The government stance, however, was necessarily serious, aimed primarily at reassuring citizens of the president's capability to adequately handle the pandemic. Consequently, government communication at this time focused on preparation and education. For example, Ghana was among the first countries to start screening inbound travellers at airports from January 24 when China's death toll was only 9 and before the WHO declared COVID-19 a pandemic. Besides screening, travellers were also required to complete a health card to enable subsequent contact tracing if necessary. After the first case was confirmed, the government moved swiftly to contain its spread by initiating several interventions which mainly focused on social mobility regulations.

Arguably, Akufo-Addo's swift and decisive response might have been facilitated by the country's prior experience with the 2015 Ebola scare in which three close West African countries had been affected, making Ghana highly vulnerable. Many of the stakeholder recommendations at the time mirrored Akufo-Addo's COVID-19 directives: investment in healthcare infrastructure, border closure, coherent messaging from government, provision of securities for frontline workers and engagement with local religious and community leaders to develop contextually informed solutions (Nyarko et al., 2015; Oleribe et al., 2015). While all COVID-19 measures were generally well received, the main opposition party, the National Democratic Party (NDC) did raise questions about whether Akufo-Addo was exploiting the crisis for his re-election ambitions. Already, government had secured loans from the World Bank and International Monetary Fund (IMF), and the NDC sought accountability for how funds were disbursed. However, these issues did not gain much traction in the media. There were some criticisms of the media for their fawning coverage of the government's COVID-19 policies (Mensah, 2020), as it seemed that journalists were too eager to sanction government actions rather than critically assess their feasibility or sustainability for the period of the pandemic which was yet unknown. See Table 26.1.

Pre-emptive communication and its benefits

According to Ansell et al. (2014: 419), 'crisis leadership differs from leadership in routine times. Its stakes are much higher, the public is much more attentive, its mood more volatile, and institutional constraints on elite decision making are considerably lower.' As president, Akufo-Addo became the key focus of attention as Ghanaians looked to him for direction. However, COVID-19 presented a disruption to normalcy. Not only did he have to lead the country through a crisis, but he also had to campaign for his re-election. Faced with this challenge, Akufo-Addo adopted a communication strategy that was politically expedient as well as being contextually informed, relevant and impactful. As Aelst and Walgrave (2017: 4) argue, politicians are 'strategic actors with specific goals and ambitions that try to pursue those goals as good as they can.' Even during a global pandemic, Akufo-Addo managed to exploit the situation in ways that benefited his political ambitions.

The communication approach adopted by Akufo-Addo was highly coordinated. He sought to control the national narrative on COVID-19 from the onset. The day *before* the first cases were announced on March 12, Akufo-Addo gave his first national update across all broadcast media and his Facebook account, in which he emphasised three key things: none of the 57 suspected cases had tested positive so Ghana was still COVID-19 free so far; several measures were in place to ensure public safety and security; and the nation needed to unite to 'defeat the spread of the virus' (Akufo-Addo, 2020a). In using this pre-emptive tactic to foreground what government was *already* doing even before any cases were confirmed, Akufo-Addo cleverly took control of the narrative by filling the information void the crisis will likely create (Coombs, 1999). By the time the confirmed cases were announced the next day, the public discussion that ensued could be situated within what government was doing. This was a clever manoeuvre that significantly reduced the likely negative impact of the confirmed

TABLE 26.1 Ghana chronology

Date		Diffusion of COVID-19	Key official actions	Key communication events
January	12			WHO confirms COVID-19 cases in Wuhan China as a respiratory disease.
	22			Ministry of Health (MoH) announces airport screening of inbound travellers from China.
	24		Airport screening of inbound travellers from China begins.	
	25		Airport screening of inbound travellers extended to all countries.	Deputy Ambassador to China advises suspension of all travel to China.
	27		MoH designates 2 main hospitals as COVID-19 centres.	
	28		Ministry of Foreign Affairs sets up dedicated phone lines for families with wards in China.	
	31		COVID-19 sensitisation programme begins at the national port in Tema.	
February	5			Ghanaian students in China appeal to government in 7-page statement to be evacuated as other countries begin evacuations of their citizens.
	12		Minority party leaders in parliament call on government to evacuate Ghanaian students in Wuhan.	Health Minister tours international airport in Accra with journalists to evidence government's preparedness for the pandemic.
	16		Upper East region put on high alert due to its many travel entry points.	Health Minster announces that all 15 suspected COVID-19 cases test negative.
	19			Foreign Affairs Minister announces it will not be evacuating Ghanaian students from China.

(*Continued*)

TABLE 26.1 (Continued)

Date		Diffusion of COVID-19	Key official actions	Key communication events
	28		Consular services in Italy suspended following high COVID-19 infection and mortality.	
	29			Health Minister asks Ghanaians not to panic as Nigeria records first case; reaffirms government's preparedness.
March	11	First case confirmed.		President gives 1st national COVID-19 update.
	12	2 more infections confirmed.		
	13			
	15		President institutes 4-week ban on all social gatherings; schools and universities closed except for final year Junior and Senior secondary students. Passport services suspended.	President gives 2nd national COVID-19 update.
	19	Total confirmed infections 9.		
	21	Infections rise to 21; 1 death recorded.		President gives 3rd national COVID-19 update.
	23		2-week closure of border and beaches begins; 137 markets to be disinfected in Accra.	
	25	Infected cases rise to 52; 2 deaths recorded.	President organises a national day of prayer and fasting; Electoral Commission suspends nationwide voter registration amidst fears of facilitating COVID-19 spread.	
	26	First COVID-19 recovery.		

	27	Total infected cases rise to 137; 2 deaths and 1 recovery.	President announces partial lockdown in COVID-19 epicentres Accra, Tema and Kumasi.	President gives 4th national COVID-19 update.
	28	Infections rise to 141 with 5 deaths.		MoH announces special life cover for frontline health workers.
	29		Government sets up quarantine centres in Tamale following rapid rise in area infections; COVID-19 Trust Fund inaugurated.	
	30		Partial lockdown in Accra, Tema and Kumasi begins; presidential appointees donate 50% of salary to COVID-19 Trust Fund.	Information Ministry begins 'stay-at home' campaign.
April	3		Education Ministry begins virtual learning for secondary students on dedicated state TV channel; Parliament passes COVID-19 National Trust Fund bill.	
	5		Border closure extended for 2 weeks; government to absorb citizen's water bills for 3 months.	President gives 5th national COVID-19 update.
	8	Death toll rises to 6.	Gender Minister announces provision of free meals for vulnerable groups.	
	9	Confirmed infections rise to 378.	Government announces absorption of citizen's electricity bills for lifeline consumers for 3 months; movement restrictions extended for a further 1 week; border closure to remain indefinitely.	President gives 6th national COVID-19 update.
	12		Ban on social gatherings extended for 2 weeks.	

(Continued)

TABLE 26.1 (Continued)

	Date	Diffusion of COVID-19	Key official actions	Key communication events
	16	Infections rise to 641 with 83 recoveries and 8 deaths.	Government implements tax reliefs for health workers.	
	19		Partial lockdown in Accra, Tema and Kumasi lifted; nose mask wearing in public made mandatory.	President gives 7th national COVID-19 update.
	26		Ban on social gatherings extended for further 2 weeks.	President gives 8th national COVID-19 update.
	30	Total infections 2,074 with 17 deaths and 212 recoveries.		
May	1		Ban on social gatherings extended further to end of May.	President gives 9th national COVID-19 update.
	11		Hotels, bars and restaurants allowed to open under strict social distancing procedures.	
	31	Total infections reach 7,881 with 36 deaths and 2,841 recoveries.		President gives 10th national COVID-19 update.
June	14		Schools reopen partially.	President gives 11th national COVID-19 update.
	21		Incentive package for health workers extended for 3 months.	President gives 12th national COVID-19 update.
	28	Total infections 7,351; 12,994 recovered and 112 deaths.		President gives 13th national COVID-19 update

cases on news reports. An examination of the March 13 newspapers headlines revealed only five of 15 newspapers led with COVID-19. Even then, almost all the headlines were tempered in tone, devoid of the emotive language one would have expected to accompany the arrival of a virus that had caused much havoc in countries with better healthcare systems. These headlines ranged from 'Stop Spreading COVID-19 Fake News – GTA' (*Ghanaian Times*), 'COVID-19: Ghana Combat-Ready – Akufo-Addo Assures' (*The Informer*), 'Ghana Confirms First Cases of COVID-19' to 'Judgement Day; Deadly Virus Finally Arrives in Ghana…As Government Faces Accusation of Hiding Facts on Disease' (*The Herald)* (MyJoyOnline.com, 2020). Thus, from the onset, President Akufo-Addo was able to deploy a pre-emptive communication strategy to portray himself as both decisive and competent.

Because Akufo-Addo framed COVID-19 as a fight in his first national update, it allowed him to justify the swift, proactive and decisive approach that he seemed to be taking to ensure public safety. This approach aligns with Strömbäck and Nord's (2006) argument that prompt and forceful response to a crisis helps leaders shape the way the crisis is framed. Brewer et al. (2003) also suggest that despite any criticisms, the media and citizens tend to rally around their leaders in times of crisis. By framing the pandemic as something that needed a united national effort in order to defeat it, Akufo-Addo sought to suppress criticisms, to position critics as national enemies pursuing their own interests and not the country's. This way, he could more likely elicit the support of people rather than their criticism while also strategically projecting himself as a leader who cared for his people.

Disseminating information during a crisis

Akufo-Addo's national updates became the big headliners. These regular updates – a total of 13 between March 11 to June 28 – were as dramatic as they were unusual. They were all broadcast late in the evening, always began with 'Fellow Ghanaians.' a greeting that soon became synonymous with Akufo-Addo, and in a format rarely used by presidents to address the nation directly. Presented at key points of the ongoing crisis, the updates covered major measures the president had taken such as the partial lockdown and ban on international travel. This approach seemed less tedious but more dramatic than the daily updates that other countries opted for. Through these updates, Akufo-Addo positioned himself as the manager of the pandemic and focused public attention on him.

The presidential updates were complemented by more regular updates from the Information Minister often accompanied by the Health Minister. The communication strategy established was as follows: after each presidential update, the Information Minister was then responsible for extrapolating and clarifying key issues raised by the president as well as answering questions from journalists. To complement the updates, infographics of key updates were circulated on the social media accounts of the president and Information Minister. In fact, besides the president, the Information Minister was regarded as the face of COVID-19 as he became the key government source. Through his ministerial press briefings, 'Ask the minister' sessions on both traditional and social media as well as several other media interviews, the Information Minister further amplified Akufo-Addo's directives. In keeping with Coombs's (1999) model of crisis response, communication was quick and consistent, seeking to provide clear information about what measures the government was taking. However, the government did not just provide information about measures but also addressed public concerns raised on social media or through phone-in segments during live programmes, particularly on radio. For instance, before the partial lockdown in the three main cities was announced, several prominent people suggested the resulting media attention led to mass panic buying. Both the president and Information Minister responded, directly denying such a decision had been taken while also reassuring the public of prior consultation and warning before any lockdown is announced.

Akufo-Addo also projected himself as a trustworthy leader by ensuring that his 'talk' was backed by actions. Strömbäck and Nord (2006) argue confidence in political leaders is affected not just by how they manage a crisis but the perception of crisis management. If the public thinks the crisis is being managed well, political confidence is increased. However, if they think the contrary, then confidence drops. Therefore, to appeal to the public's cognitive consciousness, Akufo-Addo visually demonstrated some of the measures he mentioned in his updates. To prove that his decisions were supported by science as well as expert advice from relevant stakeholders, accounts of him consulting with various groups including leadership of parliament, medical and media professionals, religious leaders and heads of markets and local industries were circulated on his and the Information Minister's Facebook and Twitter accounts to complement news reports. Images of the president observing social distancing in his meetings where all wore face masks served as visual evidence that he was observing the rules himself to encourage citizens to do the same. Research shows that media images shape evaluations of politicians while influencing voter decisions (Coleman, 2010). In fact, information processing research suggests that the human brain prefers to process visual information over the verbal (Esser, 2008). By combining verbal and visual elements in his communication, Akufo-Addo maximised the effects of his political communication while also presenting himself as an authentic leader.

National and international acclaim

The success of Akufo-Addo's handling of the pandemic during the first months can perhaps be measured by the national and international acclaim he received. Nationally, he received public support across traditional and social media (Donkor, 2020; Nyavor, 2020; Pulejo & Querubin, 2020). During a briefing with the president on April 21 to discuss the government's COVID-19 strategy, the Chairperson of the Council of State, Nana Otuo Sriboe II, was quoted as saying 'We are lucky, as a country, to have you as President at such a time as this' (*Daily Graphic*, 2020). This level of commendation, coming from the leader of the council of state, the highest advisory body to the president, was a good endorsement for the president which he used to his advantage to signal his popularity during campaign messages. Beyond the country, Akufo-Addo received praise from dignitaries and media personnel. Notably, one of the quotes from his March 27 national address, 'we know how to bring the economy back to life. What we don't know is how to bring people back to life' (Akufo-Addo, 2020b) which was posted on his social media accounts received international affirmation. WHO Director General, Tedros Adhanom Ghebreyesus, described the quote as 'powerful,' while the Chairperson of Global Public Health, Devi Sridhar, similarly tweeted her commendations for Akufo-Addo's leadership. In the UK, host of ITV's *Good Morning Britain*, Piers Morgan, both tweeted and discussed the quote during one of the shows. Perhaps the most significant acclaim was a viral video by a British Airways cabin crew member who praised Ghana's, a supposed third world country, preparedness as much more effective than Britain's, a so-called developed country. Having gone through the international airport in Accra and Heathrow, he noted the screening taking place in the former which was conspicuously absent in the latter. Whether as a consequence of his leadership or not, The United Nations selected Ghana together with Egypt and South Africa as regional humanitarian hubs for the pandemic. Together, these further legitimised Akufo-Addo's leadership, providing (unintended) support for his re-election ambitions.

Conclusion

The COVID-19 pandemic disrupted normalcy. For political leaders due for re-election the same year, its emergence presented a double challenge that required strategic manoeuvring if they were to emerge victorious. Being in such a position, Akufo-Addo's response to the pandemic presents a useful case study on how politicians can strategically navigate considerably challenging situations to their advantage. His contextually relevant communication approach, coupled with his swift, pre-emptive and decisive measures helped him establish his leadership in handling the pandemic, ensure public safety and endear himself not only to Ghanaians but also to the rest of the world. Given the country's economic, socio-cultural and health vulnerabilities compared to more established, wealthier Western countries, Akufo-Addo's ability to quickly contain the virus seemed commendable. As to whether he can sustain and maximise the national goodwill he has garnered so far to get re-elected in December 2020 remains to be seen.

References

Adua, E., Frimpong, K., Li, X., & Wang, W. (2017). Emerging issues in public health: a perspective on Ghana's healthcare expenditure, policies and outcomes. *EPMA Journal*, 8(3), 197–206. https://doi.org/10.1007/s13167-017-0109-3

Akufo-Addo, N. A. D. (2020a). Address to the nation: update No. 1. www.ghanaweb .com/GhanaHomePage/NewsArchive/Infographics-Akufo-Addo-s-address-to-the -nation-on-coronavirus-892870

Akufo-Addo, N. A. D. (2020b). Address to the nation: update No. 4. www.myjoyo nline.com/news/national/full-text-of-akufo-addos-fourth-address-on-coronavirus -pandemic/

Ansell, C., Boin, A., & Hart, P. T. (2014). Political leadership in times of crisis. In *The Oxford Handbook of Political Leadership*. doi:10.1093/oxfordhb/9780199653881.013.035

Bawa, S., & Sanyare, F. (2013). Women's participation and representation in politics: perspectives from Ghana. *International Journal of Public Administration*, 36(4), 282–291.

Brewer, P., Aday, S., & Gross, K. (2003). Rallies all around: the dynamics of system support. In Norris, P., Kern, M., & Just, M. (Eds.), *Framing Terrorism. The News Media, the Government, and the Public*. Routledge.

Coleman, R. (2010). Framing the pictures in our heads. In D'Angelo, P., & Kuypers, J. A. (Eds.), *Doing News Framing Analysis: Empirical and Theoretical Perspectives*, 233–261. Routledge.

Coombs, W. T. (1999). *Ongoing Crisis Communication: Planning, Managing, and Responding.* SAGE.

Daily Graphic. (2020). 'Ghana is lucky to have you as President at this time' – Council of State. 22 April. www.graphic.com.gh/news/general-news/ghana-is-lucky-to-have-you-as-president-at-this-time-council-of-state-chairperson.html

Donkor, A. (2020). Ghana President shows exemplary leadership in COVID-19 fight. https://africaupclose.wilsoncenter.org/ghana-president-shows-exemplary-leadership -in-covid-19-fight/

Esser, F. (2008). Dimensions of political news cultures: sound bite and image bite news in France, Germany, Great Britain, and the United States. *The International Journal of Press/Politics*, 13(4),401–428.

Mensah, K. (2020). In the fight against COVID-19, has Akufo Addo landed the crucial free-kick? https://thebusiness24online.net/2020/04/16/in-the-fight-against-covid-19-has-akufo-addo-landed-the-crucial-free-kick/

MyJoyOnline.com. (2020). Today's front pages: Friday, March 13, 2020. 13 March. www .myjoyonline.com/news/todays-front-pages-friday-march-13-2020/

Nyarko, Y., Goldfrank, L., Ogedegbe, G., Soghoian, S., Aikins, A. D. G., & NYU-UG-KBTH, G. E. W. (2015). Preparing for Ebola virus disease in West African countries not yet affected: perspectives from Ghanaian health professionals. *Globalization and Health*, 11(1), 7.

Nyavor, G. (2020). Leadership experts praise Akufo-Addo's handling of coronavirus crisis in Ghana. www.myjoyonline.com/news/politics/leadership-experts-praise-akufo-addos-handling-of-coronavirus-crisis-in-ghana/

Oleribe, O. O., Salako, B. L., Ka, M. M., Akpalu, A., McConnochie, M., Foster, M., & Taylor-Robinson, S. D. (2015). Ebola virus disease epidemic in West Africa: lessons learned and issues arising from West African countries. *Clinical Medicine*, 15(1), 54.

Pulejo, M., & Querubín, P. (2020). *Electoral Concerns Reduce Restrictive Measures during the COVID-19 Pandemic, (No. w27498)*. National Bureau of Economic Research.

Strömbäck, J., & Nord, L. W. (2006). Mismanagement, mistrust and missed opportunities: a study of the 2004 tsunami and Swedish political communication. *Media, Culture & Society*, 28(5),789–800.

van Aelst, P., & Walgrave, S. (Eds.) (2017). *How Political Actors Use the Media – A Functional Analysis of the Media's Role in Politics*. Palgrave Macmillan.

27

SOUTH AFRICA

A united front? A divided government

Robert Mattes and Ian Glenn

Political context

In January 2020, one would not have thought that South Africa was a country well placed to respond to a pandemic. While it had accumulated invaluable experience in its public health response to the HIV/AIDS pandemic, the country was still marked by high levels of enduring poverty 25 years after the fall of *apartheid*, with continuing racial and new class cleavages. These economic inequalities were reflected in sharp health inequalities and very different abilities to implement non-medical interventions such as social distancing and frequent handwashing (Mattes et al., 2020). Public health facilities, in spite of significant strengths in some areas, had too few nurses, doctors and beds, and deteriorating facilities in several provinces. And while the population was very young, many people had underlying health issues, with high rates of obesity and hypertension and, in particular, large numbers with tuberculosis and HIV/AIDS.

South Africa was also in an economically parlous situation. What President Cyril Ramaphosa himself called the 'nine wasted years' of the previous government of Jacob Zuma had left a state marked by increasing levels of corruption, mounting debt and a credit rating downgraded to junk status by major international ratings agencies.

While Ramaphosa enjoyed a surge in support and optimism ('Ramaphoria') after Zuma's resignation, he laboured under significant constraints in trying to right the ship of state. First, while South Africa's chief executive is called President, the title is misleading. The country's 1996 Constitution designed an executive much closer to a Westminster style prime minister than an American, or French, president. Thus, while he was expected to lead the government response to COVID-19, and speak to and for the nation, the fact that he was directly elected by parliament (not the voters), and could be removed by a simple

DOI: 10.4324/9781003120254-29

parliamentary vote of no confidence, forced him at least in theory to govern with the consent of his Cabinet and party parliamentary caucus. Moreover, because South Africa's legislators are elected proportionally from large party lists, and can be removed from parliament at any time after their election, the central committee of the governing African National Congress (ANC) exercises an exceptionally large degree of control over government. Its national executive committee has 'recalled' both of Ramaphosa's immediate predecessors, Thabo Mbeki and Jacob Zuma, without a formal parliamentary vote.

While the ANC won 58% of the vote in the 2019 election, this was its smallest vote share since the country's first inclusive election in 1994. Moreover, Ramaphosa won the party's presidential nomination by a razor thin margin over Nkosazana Dlamini-Zuma, former wife of the previous President (Jacob Zuma), whose supporters control almost as many seats on the party's central committee as Ramaphosa. In January 2020, rumours circulated that the pro-Zuma faction was going to attempt to 'recall' Ramaphosa at the upcoming (June) party conference (Ndletyana, 2020). Thus, the divided state of the party not only led Ramaphosa to construct his Cabinet carefully to represent the Zuma wing, but also gave Dlamini-Zuma the Cabinet portfolio of 'cooperative governance,' the ANC's preferred term for federalism, which enjoyed considerable powers.

Chronology

While there is little evidence that the South African government devoted much attention or effort to preparing for the arrival of COVID-19 in early 2020, its response, once the disease did arrive in the country in early March 2020, was swift, clear and decisive. Within three weeks of the first confirmed case, President Cyril Ramaphosa had announced a comprehensive and severe package of policies (including international and domestic travel bans, school and university closures, stay-at-home-orders and bans on the sale of tobacco and alcohol) that were supported by the leaders of all major political parties (Merton, 2020), and by a large majority of public opinion.

The number of cases and deaths remained low for weeks, and largely confined to the regions most connected to the global economy. By the end of July, however, the disease had spread across the country, and South Africa had the fifth highest number of cases in the world (over 500,000) (Meldrum, 2020), with shortages of critical care staff and beds, oxygen and personal protective equipment (PPE) in hospitals and clinics in several cities (Sparks, 2020; Harding, 2020). Yet the rate of new infections peaked and began to decline in August (Whiteside, 2020). While a total of 650,000 infections had been recorded by mid-September, some analysts concluded that the government response had shifted the peak of the epidemic to later in the winter and limited the carnage to a relatively low number of deaths (officially recorded at 15,600) (Brodie, 2020). Others countered that the substantially higher number of excess deaths over this period (44,500) placed South Africa amongst the hardest hit in the world, in per capita terms (Myers,

2020), particularly since the country experienced a net reduction in deaths in the early months of the lockdown due to sharp drops in road accidents and murders.

Many of the details of the government response, and the way they were publicly communicated, created confusion and resistance. Moreover, the extended restrictions on commerce generated devastating economic hardship. Much of this could not be helped. But once non-essential services began to open up, arbitrary decisions about specific products, and continued bans on tobacco and alcohol dealt unnecessary blows both to jobs and tax revenues normally generated. These decisions drew derision from the news media and decreased public support.

The policy response

Little thought was devoted to preparing for COVID-19 in early 2020 and few resources were set aside. Neither President Ramaphosa nor Finance Minister Tito Mboweni mentioned it in the annual February State of the Nation address or February budget speech (Sanderson-Meyer, 2020). On March 3, however, the first case, an infected tourist returning from Italy, was confirmed (Cowan, 2020). The government responded on March 15. With just 61 confirmed cases, President Ramaphosa gave his first national address on the subject declaring a National Disaster and announcing a ban on international travel, ordering the closure of schools and universities, limiting social gatherings to 50 people or less, and creating a National Command Council.

Restrictions were ratcheted upward on March 23, with the imposition of a 'hard lockdown' that banned domestic travel between provinces, and imposed a 'stay-at-home-order' for all but essential services, an 11 pm–4 am curfew was imposed and the sale of alcohol and tobacco products banned. The government extended the restrictions for another three weeks on April 9. On April 23, a five-level, risk-adjusted strategy was announced that would determine when the country could begin to ease the lockdown, with the first relaxations implemented on May 1 (moving downwards from Level 5 to 4), and further relaxations throughout the subsequent four months.

Communicating the response

As president, Cyril Ramaphosa was the public face of South Africa's response, giving 13 nationally broadcast speeches announcing the original restrictions, and providing periodic updates, as well as communicating through a weekly newsletter. But other important briefings were provided by the Health, Police, and Cooperative Governance Ministers. The government also used the head of the Medical Advisory Council, the impressive Harvard-trained Dr Salim Karim, to explain and justify decisions.

In each speech, Ramaphosa adopted a dignified demeanour, and sober but reassuring tone. In later speeches, he apologised for errors such as contradictions in policy statements, police and army brutality, and attacks on medical experts who had criticised government decisions, and extended olive branches to try to repair damage done by his colleagues.

Ramaphosa is generally regarded as an affable and engaging person, and it is not clear if these usually hour-long, stilted formal speeches were the best medium for him. Despite only 12% of adults citing English as their mother tongue, and just 13% speaking it as the main language at home (Afrobarometer, 2020), each address was delivered almost wholly in an ornate English combining elements of the pulpit and the business address (Glenn, 2020). Written by a small committee, with the significant personal involvement of Ramaphosa (Davis, 2020), the speeches were long on bureaucratic decisions and management jargon and short on inspiration.

Policy controversies

Besides its form and method, the government's communication strategy was complicated by the actual content of policy. With few exceptions, the initial package of policy responses was widely accepted and supported. However, lines of public and media criticism emerged early and grew over time. One source of dissatisfaction was the severity of the lockdown, and its collateral consequences. As early as late April, for instance, the decision to extend the lockdown was criticised by Chief Medical Adviser Karim who told *Rapport* newspaper he thought the lockdown had done what was possible to prepare medical services for the pandemic and suggested it was no longer useful (Retief, 2020). A group of prominent university academics subsequently published a piece arguing it was no longer possible to contain the spread through a lockdown, and thus almost all economic activity should be resumed (leaving limits on mass gatherings, and lockdowns of known transmission hotspots in place) (Valodia et al., 2020). Leading medical experts also pointed to the negative effects of the lockdown on other aspects of public health (Medical Brief, 2020).

Critics also disparaged government over apparently arbitrary regulations, such as the ban on outdoor exercise and dog-walking, or the early May decision to ease restrictions on some retail activities but not others. Subsequent lockdown relaxations allowed churches, and later casinos, auction houses, hairdressers and beauticians to reopen even as visits amongst family members were still illegal. Other instances gave the impression the government was willing to compromise evidence-based policy when it met resistance from constituencies important to the ruling party. For instance, minibus taxi drivers, who had been limited to 70% capacity (with windows open), went on strike in late June, after which the government decided to allow full loads. While plans originally called for primary and secondary schools to reopen fully in late July, government decided to keep them shut for a further four weeks after public complaints from African National Congress (ANC)-aligned teacher unions. Not surprisingly, many South Africans, including key journalists, saw these decisions as a sign of the government caving in to pressure groups outside or inside the government (e.g. Mthombothi, 2020; Du Toit, 2020). In perhaps the most explosive broadside, Glenda Gray, head of the South African Medical Research Council and member of the Cabinet's Medical Advisory Committee, gave an interview in which she argued that many regulations were not the product of medical advice, and criticised the overall strategy as a blunt tool trying to address a series of very different problems: 'It's almost as if someone is sucking regulations out of their thumb and implementing rubbish, quite frankly' (Basson, 2020).

No other issue, however, was a lightning rod for criticism like the bans on tobacco and alcohol. While there was certainly some questioning of these bans in the original lockdown, public criticism exploded at the end of April when, six days after Ramaphosa had announced that the sale of cigarettes would resume when the country moved to Stage 4, Minister Dlamini-Zuma said the ban would remain. Cartoonists, social media commentators and mainstream news media all seized on this as a sign of confusion and an attempt by Dlamini-Zuma to use the crisis for her own personal anti-smoking agenda (stemming from her previous service as Minister of Health in the late 1990s). More than 400,000 people signed a petition against the tobacco ban, and the tobacco industry began efforts to take the Minister to court (Sguazzin, 2020).

Analysis

Who's in charge?

While Ramaphosa's speeches were clearly cast in terms of his role as head of state and embodiment of the nation, a great deal of doubt was created by the actions and words of his Ministers. His appointment of Dlamini-Zuma to the Cooperative Governance portfolio in 2019 was important for two reasons. First, the country's existing emergency legislation, the National Disaster Act, specifically empowered the head of this ministry to issue emergency regulations. Second, the government created a powerful Cabinet committee, called the National Coronavirus Command Council (NCC), which consisted of 19 Ministers and their head civil servants, plus the heads of the policy, military and intelligence services. Importantly, the committee was co-chaired by *both* Ramaphosa and Dlamini-Zuma. While Ramaphosa originally announced that the NCC would 'coordinate' the national response to COVID-19, within two days, the Presidency's official Twitter page said the NCC would 'lead' the response (Haffajee, 2020; Pitjieng, 2020).

While Ramaphosa dutifully attributed major policy decisions to the NCC, he was often undercut by his Ministers. Besides embarrassing violations of stay-at-home orders by the Ministers of Social Development and Communications, there were at least two flagrant violations of policy decisions that had already been announced. We have already discussed Ndlamini-Zuma's reversal of the decision to end the ban on tobacco sales, as well as her efforts to keep it in place long after it could be justified. And while the first regulations issued by Ramaphosa in March had not ruled out outdoor exercise or dog-walking, Police Minister Bheki Cele unilaterally announced that it would be banned following criticism from Julius Malema, leader of the populist opposition party Economic Freedom Fighters, who argued that allowing (White) citizens to walk their dogs removed any justification for the severe lockdown.

More ominously, while Ramaphosa had decided to use not only the police but also the South African National Defence Force to enforce the lockdown measures, Cele enthusiastically defended police against accusations of heavy-handed tactics, reportedly vowing 'Wait until you see more force.' Officers using rubber bullets and leather whips (favourite tools of *apartheid*-era policing) to enforce the lockdown in Johannesburg told reporters they were following orders from 'the top' (De Villiers, 2020).

Ramaphosa did himself no favours on this issue. On March 26, he appeared before soldiers in combat uniform, the first South African President to do so, and said he was wearing the uniform to signal his 'total support' for the army and its role. Police and army forces subsequently arrested, or imposed fines on at least 300,000 people for various violations of lockdown regulations (SABC, 2020). And at least 12 people died at the hands of security forces, the most prominent and shocking case being that of Collins Khosa who was attacked on Easter Friday for drinking in his own backyard, and died in his house after being beaten by soldiers (Haffajee, 2020). Incidents of police violence led to hostile media coverage and criticism from senior ANC officials. While Ramaphosa acknowledged the validity of these criticisms, he chalked up violence to 'over enthusiasm,' and failed to condemn the brutality.

Corruption

Those trying to communicate and persuade citizens and stakeholders of the rationale for government policy had to deal with a major crisis in late July when Ramaphosa announced he had authorised the police's Special Investigating Unit (SIU) to probe emerging allegations of corruption in various aspects of the government emergency relief measures. These included fraud in unemployment insurance claims, overpricing of goods and services, collusion between government officials and service providers, violations of emergency procurement regulations, abuse of food parcel distribution and the creation of fake non-profit organisations to access relief funding. Referring to corruption during a national emergency as a 'particularly heinous type of crime,' Ramaphosa compared it to 'a pack of hyenas circling wounded pray.'

It then emerged that the SIU was examining a range of suspicious tenders from provincial health departments and municipalities to dozens of companies and individuals for things like emergency purchases of personal protective equipment, and that Ramaphosa's own spokesperson Khusela Diko was caught up in a scandal involving allegations of irregularities in two lucrative contracts between her husband and the most senior health official in the Gauteng province (Business Tech, 2020; Rampedi, 2020). Ramaphosa's inability to take decisive action was highlighted by the retort of ANC Secretary-General Ace Magashule, who argued all ANC leaders had family members who benefited from tenders and suggested it should not be seen as corruption but normal practice.

'Declining' support

Reflecting the accumulating criticism and frustration, public support for Ramaphosa and his government appears to have declined sharply. We say 'appears' because in-person surveys of representative samples of respondents were not possible during the lockdown, and large-scale random digit dialling phone surveys are inefficient and expensive in South Africa and were also hobbled by closure of call centres. However, two different surveys utilising a combination of computer-assisted telephone and online interviews concluded that approval and trust in Ramaphosa had increased at the start of the crisis, but dropped substantially, by over 20 percentage points a few months later. It should be noted, however, that because his March/April surge in approval was so great, this decline still left Ramaphosa with levels of support around 60% in late July (Ask Africa, 2020; Robert, 2020). However, neither measure included the full impacts of the corruption revelations.

How well did South Africa do medically?

South Africa was in many ways an exemplar of World Health Organisation (WHO) advice: a lockdown to 'flatten' the curve in order to buy time to prepare clinics and hospitals for an influx of patients. According to the Google COVID Community Mobility Index, the lockdown achieved a remarkable reduction in mobility in terms of transport and commerce (an average of about 60% in April and May, and 40% by the end of June), drastically cutting the total number of social interactions and opportunities for infection. It also successfully pushed the peak of infection back at least a month, at least in terms of the time between the first death and the peak (Brodie, 2020).

But while the number of officially confirmed deaths (15,600 as of mid-September) appeared to represent a relative success, especially when compared to initial fears, some analysts have pointed out that the total number of excess deaths (44,500) places South Africa amongst the most hard-hit countries in the world, in per capita terms (Myers, 2020).

Economic devastation

While there is debate about the health consequences of the South African response, the evidence related to its non-illness related human costs is clear. Economists have estimated approximately 3 million people lost their jobs during the lockdown, and an additional 1.5 million remained employed but lost their incomes (Smit, 2020). The ban on alcohol sales threatened an additional 700,000 livelihoods (Rose, 2020) linked to the fate of wine farms, distilleries, breweries and restaurants who rely on the trade. In all, 40% of households reported they had lost their main source of income, and 20% reported that someone had gone hungry (Wills et al., 2020). While food parcels ultimately reached 5 million people, the closure of schools removed daily nutrition from 9.6 million children (Wills et al., 2020), nearly doubling child hunger, and made life difficult for essential health workers with children, or other employees able to return to work (Spaull, 2020). The economic slowdown also resulted in a loss of R82 billion ($4.8 billion) in taxes, more than what South Africa borrowed from the International Monetary Fund (IMF) or African Development Bank in COVID-19-linked loans, with a significant loss of taxes from tobacco and alcohol (Naidoo, 2020). These are consequences with which the country will have to deal for years to come.

References

Afrobarometer. (2020). South Africa. www.afrobarometer.org

AskAfrika. 2020. Week 19 Results, Level 3 Advanced. *The AskAfrika Covid-19 Tracker* August 5–11.

Basson, A. (2020). The truth behind that interview with Glenda Gray.

Brodie, N. (2020). 2020, hindsight. *Medium*, 9 September. *News24*, 24 May.

Business Tech. (2020). Billions of rands looted by south Africa's 'Covidpreneurs': report. *BusinessTech*, 26 July.

Cowan, K. (2020). Insights: The first 100 days of COVID-19 in 10 graphs. *New s24*, 12 June.

Davis, G. (2020). A peek into how Ramphosa's SONA speech is written. *Eyewitness News*, 13 February.

De Villiers, S. (2020). How Ramaphosa is being undermined by his own ministerial clowns. *Financial Mail*, 17 April.

Du Toit, P. (2020). Ramaphosa evades another opportunity to lead as he caves in to unions. *New s24*, 23 July.

Glenn, I. (2020). Should President Ramaphosa fire his speechwriters? *New s24*, 7 June.

Haffajee, F. (2020). National coronavirus command council: who guards the guardians? *Daily Maverick*, 7 May.

Harding, A. (2020). Coronavirus in South Africa: inside Port Elizabeth's 'hospitals of horrors.' *BBC News*, 15 July.

Mattes, R., C. Logan, E. Gyimah-Boadi, & G. Ellison. (2020). COVID-19 in Africa: vulnerabilities and assets for an effective response. *Afrobarometer Policy Paper, no. 67.* Accra: Afrobarometer. www.afrobarometer.org.

Medical Brief. (2020). Medical experts rebel over SA's 'nonsensical' lockdown strategy. *Medical Brief: Africa's Medical Media Digest*, 20 May.

Meldrum, A. (2020). South Africa hits 500,000 infections but president hopeful. *AP News*, 3 August.

Merten, M. (2020). Covid-19 State of Disaster vs. State of Emergency: What's the Difference? *Daily Maverick*, 19 March.

Mthombothi, B. (2020). We are led by a man who has dropped the ball, and stands on the touchline. *Sunday Times*, 19 July.

Myers, J. (2020). COVID-19: After a severe epidemic, South Africa appears to be approaching some herd immunity. *Daily Maverick*, 7 October.

Naidoo, P. (2020). South African lockdown tax loss exceeds value of two virus loans. *Bloomberg Quint*, 2 August.

Ndletyana, M. (2020). Public approval is Ramaphosa's only defence against his critics. *The Conversation*, 24 January.

Pitjeng, R. (2020). Covid-19: What Exactly is the National Command Council? *Eyewitness News*, 4 May.

Rampedi, P. (2020). Husband of presidency spokesperson's R215m PPE tender bonanza. *Sunday Independent*, 19 July.

Retief, H. (2020). Woede bou op oor inperking. *Rapport*. Johannesburg, 19 April.

Roberts, B. (2020). What's Trust Got to Do With It? University of Johannesburg-Human Sciences Research Council Covid-19 Democracy Survey, Round 2 Public Launch. HSRC Seminar Series, 19 August.

Rose, R. (2020). Dlamini Zuma relied on 'unsound scientific data and hearsay.' *BusinessLive*, 3 August.

SABC. (2020). Almost 300,000 arrested for contravening lockdown regulations, crime stats. *SABC News*, 14 August.

Saunderson-Meyer, W. (2020). Ramaphoria enjoys a revival. *PoliticsWeb*, 27 March.

Sguazzin, A. (2020). Ramaphosa risks public backlash as cracks starting to show in government. *BizNews*, 5 May.

Smit, S. (2020). Three million jobs lost and hunger surging amid COVID-19 crisis – survey. *Mail & Guardian*, 15 July.

Sparks, J. Coronavirus: South Africa in the midst of a COVID-19 'storm'-and it's likely worse than data suggests. *SkyNews*, 28 July.

Spaull, N. (2020). Six reasons why schools must be open if we are to fight COVID-19. *Daily Maverick*, 22 July. www.dailymaverick.co.za/article/2020-07-22-six-reasons-why-schools-must-be-open-if-we-are-to-fight-covid-19/

Valodia, I., van den Heever, A., Allais, L. & Veller, M. (2020). South Africa's COVID-19 strategy needs updating: here's why and how. *The Conversation*, 13 May.

Whiteside, A. (2020). Covid watch: setbacks. 16 September. https://alan-whiteside.com/2020/09/16/covid-19-watch-setbacks/

Wills, G., Patel, L. & van den Berg, S. (2020). South Africa faces mass hunger if efforts to offset impact of COVID-19 are eased. *The Conversation*, 26 July.

28

KOSOVO

Political crisis, one more challenge alongside COVID-19

Dren Gërguri

Political context

Despite the global spread of COVID-19, Kosovo was in stasis with no government until early February. Internal disputes over Kosovo's tariffs on Serbian produce had produced early elections on October 6, 2019, the same issue prematurely ended the mandate of the government formed as a result. The 2019 elections were won by the Self-Determination Movement (LVV) and on February 3, 2020, the new government was formed, headed by Albin Kurti, the chairman of the LVV. The difficulties encountered during the coalition negotiations were also reflected in the functioning of the government, which lasted only until March 25, when a vote of no confidence was initiated in the Assembly by the Democratic League of Kosovo (LDK), their partner in the governing coalition. The ideological differences, the LVV is the centre-left party and the LDK is the centre-right, proved too great (Gërguri, 2019). However, the main disagreement was over the issue of the tariffs, as the LVV was determined to replace the tariff with reciprocity, while the LDK, which had introduced the same idea during the election campaign, changed its stance following a US request to remove tariffs without establishing reciprocity so that Kosovo and Serbia return to the negotiating table. The overthrow of the Kurti government makes it the shortest-lived government in the history of the state of Kosovo.

After the parties addressed the Constitutional Court, the potential existed for the formation of a new government. On June 3, a new government was formed with Hoti, the new prime minister (PM). In this difficult political situation, Kosovo also faced COVID-19.

Chronology

Kosovo had an advantage over many other countries in the fight against COVID-19 because it was among the last European countries to be affected. This allowed

DOI: 10.4324/9781003120254-30

lesson learning from other countries and allowed the government to take preemptive measures. On March 11, the Kosovo Government held an emergency meeting to determine the appropriate measures required two days before the first case was confirmed. A brief chronology of these can be found in Table 28.1.

Government measures

On March 13, the first two cases were confirmed, one in Vitia and the other in Klina. The government quarantined both cities blocking entrances and exits. This caused panic and citizens started to panic buy food products, especially flour reserves. This exacerbated an increase of infections, which doubled week to week to reach 283 in less than 30 days. By April the number 700 was exceeded, and on April 15, new measures came into force to prevent further spread including restricting the citizens from leaving home for any more than 90 minutes a day for performing essential tasks. However, by the end of April the situation improved and there were no more than ten infections confirmed per day. This created the opportunity for the relaxation of restrictions and on May 4–18, the government allowed citizens to leave home twice a day, for 90 minutes each, at set times determined by the penultimate number of their national identification number. The beginning of May marked further relaxation of restrictions. The low number of new cases ushered in the second phase when citizens could leave home twice a day for 120 minutes. Also, during this phase, as of May 18, there was a gradual reopening of the economy, initially scheduled for June but introduced early because of improvement of the situation. From May 28, leaving home was permitted from 5 am until 9 pm. The opening of religious buildings was also allowed from May 31, the premises that served as a quarantine for persons entering Kosovo from other countries were closed. Meanwhile, in the third phase, which began on June 1, other measures began to be applied that allowed the full reopening of the economy, land borders, shopping malls etc.

Criticism of the government decisions

During this period, government decisions were strongly contested by President Thaçi and opposition parties, questioning the constitutionality of decisions to restrict movement, and from the moment the fall of the Kurti government, another important political development in Kosovo received the attention of the public, until the election of the new government. Before the first two weeks of infections in Kosovo, through a no-confidence motion, on March 25, the Kosovo Assembly dismissed the LVV-LDK Government. The fall of the government nurtured fear and insecurity in the citizens, who even protested from their homes by hitting pots and pans together. The protests sent a message to political parties to work together in the fight against COVID-19 and to put aside political agendas.

TABLE 28.1 Kosovo chronology

Date		Diffusion of COVID-19	Key official actions	Key communication events
February	3		The new government was formed.	
	8	Suspicions of first case, a British tourist results negative.		National Institute of Public Health of Kosovo (IKSHPK) in an extraordinary conference, announces no infections.
	21		Infectious Disease Monitoring Committee has approved the Coronavirus Preparedness and Response Plan.	
	27			Press release of IKSHPK: There is no COVID-19 in Kosovo.
	29	33 tested, and all were negative.		
March	11		Preventive measures taken by the government. All schools and universities closed. Temporary suspension of air and land travel from high- and medium-risk countries. Restaurants, nightclubs, gyms and swimming pools close at 11 pm.	
	12		The Special Commission for the Prevention of the Spread of the COVID-19 is established.	
	13	First 2 confirmed infections (1 Kosovar and 1 Italian tourist).	Government quarantines 2 municipalities, Vitia and Klina.	
	14		Another municipality quarantined, Malisheva.	
	15		Government declares state of public health emergency.	

17		President of the Republic of Kosovo, Hashim Thaçi proposes a state of emergency. PM Kurti: 'Declaring a state of emergency is unreasonable, illogical, unnecessary, useless.'
18		
22	First confirmed Kosovar death.	
24	The movement of citizens and private vehicles is prohibited, 10 am to 4 pm and 8 pm to 6 am. Gatherings are prohibited.	
25	The overthrow of the government.	
27	Government extends restrictions on citizens and private vehicles movement, from 5 pm to 6 am.	
30		The Fiscal Emergency Package is approved
31		Government decision restricting movement ruled unconstitutional
April 5	Government extends restrictions on movement until 12 April.	
8	The government authorises the Minister of Health to issue decisions to prevent the pandemic.	
12		Incumbent Prime Minister Kurti: "Let us not give space to the coronavirus for it to take our lives afterwards"
14	A coordination group is established to address economic issues and problems facing the private sector.	Incumbent PM Kurti presents the 15 measures in the Emergency Fiscal Package.

(Continued)

TABLE 28.1 (Continued)

Date	Diffusion of COVID-19	Key official actions	Key communication events
	15	Movement of citizens restricted to 90 minutes a day, according to a weekly schedule based on the penultimate figure of citizens' personal number.	
	16 Death toll reaches 11.		
	20		Roundtable with representatives of institutions and political entities for the management of the pandemic.
	30		Acting Minister of Health, Vitia presents three phases of easing restrictions.
May	4	**Start phase 1**: government removes entry-exit ban for municipalities of Klina, Malisheva and Vitia. Movement of citizens restricted to 90 minutes, twice a day, with a weekly schedule. Partial trade opening.	
	5 Slowdown in spread, 1 new case.		
	18	**Start phase 2**: government ends most restrictions. Movement allowed twice a day for 2 hours. Some businesses reopen.	
	24 First days no infections reported.		

	25	Total cases 1,038. Deaths 30.
	28		The decision of the Constitutional Court paves the way for the formation of a new government.
June	1	**Start phase 3**: government suspends remaining restrictions. Only few minor limits remaining. **End of Lockdown**.
	3	The new government is formed.
	16	Daily infections 141, a record.	Media report alarming figures, 141 infected.
	18		The Manual for protection against the spread published.
	22	The Executive Commission for Combating, Monitoring and Responding to COVID-19 is established.
	29	Total cases: 2,799. Infected: 1,293. Death toll: 49.

Disinformation and harsh language on social media

The quarantine period boosted internet use; 93% of households in Kosovo (Eurostat, 2019) have access to the internet. Social media were used extensively, both by institutions and by citizens to learn about COVID-19, so exposing them to disinformation, such as 'Cures for COVID-19 or Ways to Eliminate It,' 'Coronavirus Is a Fraud. Masons Want to Control the World,' 'American Doctor Shakes the World, Shows the Truth of Coronavirus' (Gërguri et al., 2020). Divisions over the efficacy of government measures and reality of the threat fuelled the use of harsh language on social networks, with sides trading insults and incitement to hatred. The polarisation was also fuelled by bots or sites of unknown origin and source, increasing tensions among heavy social media users.

But the online environment was also put to positive use. On March 11, the government closed schools until March 27, and on March 23, distance learning began. Online teaching was also practised at universities. COVID-19 made online learning a feature of the entire summer semester.

Analysis

During crises, information becomes even more valuable, citizens' interest increases, but many may not be able to adequately assess correct information (Halper, 1971). In Kosovo, society was divided into two, some fearing the virus and constantly seeking information to understand more about the virus, while others discounted the dangers of the virus and considered it a seasonal flu. The adoption of these polarised positions depends not just on exposure to information but also the demographic and social position or cultural orientation (Boin et al., 2005). A serious challenge for the government was convincing all citizens they should respect quarantine restrictions. In the initial period, despite plans being in place, the government's actions were not coordinated with the local authorities. This produced dissatisfaction among citizens because conflicting information was received from local and central authorities. Due to increased vigilance (Halper, 1971), they were more aware of discrepancies.

In order to have a unified response, the government held press conferences to relay each decision as well as posting information on social media. These are effective measures as they represent an opportunity to show leadership and commitment to resolving the issue (Brataas, 2018). In order to create a positive image, former Prime Minister Kurti and former Minister of Health, Arben Vitia often led the press conferences, explaining the situation and the measures taken. These communications bolstered the image of Minister Vitia. These two were the main figures who influenced public debate; President Thaçi, Director of the National Institute of Public Health of Kosovo, Naser Ramadani and microbiologist Lul Raka were also influential.

The clash of Kurti and Thaçi

President Thaçi dominated discussions, demanded the declaration of a state of emergency and then later rejected decisions to restrict public movement taken by the Kurti government. Coordinating communication is very important for effective governance (Boin et al., 2005). In times of crisis, it is dangerous when conflicting messages are conveyed and thus, open disagreements between Prime Minister Kurti and President Thaçi created uncertainty, especially on the declaration of a state of emergency. The way these messages were received differed according to which leader the audience supported (Lilleker, 2014); Kurti supporters accepted his message and ignored Thaçi's message, and vice versa. In the first days after the outbreak of the COVID-19, President Thaçi demanded a state of emergency be declared, Kurti opposed it and on March 15, the government declared a state of emergency in public health only. Another very sensitive moment was at the end of March when the Kurti government introduced measures to restrict movement. In a press conference on March 24, President Thaçi called the decision unconstitutional and called on citizens and institutions not to respect the decision (Shehu, 2020). The Constitutional Court ruled the government's decision was unconstitutional and that 'restriction of fundamental rights and freedoms can only be done' by law 'of the Assembly of the Republic of Kosovo' (Constitutional Court, March 2020). However, due to the circumstances, the Constitutional Court ruled that the March 31 decision would take effect on April 13.

Kurti's other clash with Thaçi was over control of northern Kosovo. President Thaçi criticised the Kurti government for allowing municipalities in northern Kosovo to be illegally allowing Serbian authorities to operate within the territory of Kosovo. Government officials denied this, claiming that the Ministry of Health was involved in an emergency public health situation in the northern municipalities of North Mitrovica and Zvecan.

So, at the time of the rise of the pandemic, politics was polarised about how the situation should be managed. Some decisions of the Kurti government were opposed by their coalition partner, the LDK, as well as opposition parties and President Thaçi. The pandemic thus became overshadowed by clashes between Kurti and Thaçi as well as their political partners and opponents. Hence while Kurti and Vitia followed the edict that 'care should be a vital word in all crisis communication' (Brataas, 2018: 78), this was undermined by the hostile environment.

Political crisis during a pandemic

In crises, such as pandemics, risk communication (Ruhrmann, 2015) must take into account insecurity and responsibility-attribution (Udris, 2019). In Kosovo, during the first weeks of the pandemic, insecurity was high because society was facing an unknown enemy, there were complete unknowns about the virus and all eyes were on the government, which was expected to keep the situation under control. However, the political crisis complicated matters and aggravated the situation. Health concerns, just 52 days after the formation of the new government, added to the concern about what new political developments, new elections or new government will produce. The overthrow of the government and the creation of a new political crisis was not the result of failure to manage the pandemic, but the specifics lie in the relationship between the coalition partners and ongoing issues related to Serbia and Kosovo's relations with the United States.

More than two months after Kosovar society experienced two crises at the same time, the beginning of June found the country with a new government and an easing of restrictions. But the easing of measures led to increased numbers of infections, and on June 16 a record high was recorded for the largest number of people affected by COVID-19; 141 positive cases out of 397 people tested. This suggests continuity was an issue and partisan politics dominated decision-making.

High standards of journalism

During the pandemic period, the media in Kosovo, especially traditional media, mostly maintained high standards of reporting. They began to pay more attention to COVID-19, especially at the time when the first cases were registered in Albania, a neighbouring country frequented by Kosovars. Television and most online media treated the cases of people affected by the COVID-19 with professionalism, respecting their privacy, and preserved their identity. They also tried to keep society up to date with verified information based on official sources, which was very important at the time as all kinds of information were circulating from a range of dubious sources. Media reported on the number of confirmed cases of Covid-19, the measures imposed by the government, the situation of the Clinic of Infectious Diseases at the University Clinical Centre of Kosovo, the challenges faced by the medical staff or the situation in the municipalities where the cases of those affected with COVID-19 appeared. During this period, the situation in other countries was often reported, sometimes making comparisons between Kosovo and those countries. The media also maintained balance. Even when politicians, in general, shared a consensus on government measures, the media covered the story from several different angles.

Social media usage and disinformation

Political parties in Kosovo have been using Facebook since 2009, and Kurti's LVV was the first party to adopt social media as part of its public communication strategy (Gërguri, 2019). Kurti was noted for his continued use of Facebook during the crisis. Kurti very often addressed the citizens from his Facebook page, and in some cases, even published video messages. Meanwhile, other actors were active on social media, the National Institute of Public Health of Kosovo published daily announcements on those affected by the virus. Hence, Facebook became one of the main platforms for information, but this paved the way for a lot of disinformation to easily reach citizens.

During the pandemic, various verified, unverified, true and false information was disseminated on social media, and their consumption multiplied, due to the public need for information. At first, there was disinformation about the origin of COVID-19, then about vaccines and alternative preventions and cures. Some false notions even became part of the public debate after being distributed by unwary Kosovars. During this period, there was a lack of commitment from institutions and mainstream media to directly combat disinformation, and there were cases when institutions, out of intent to disseminate information more quickly, provided the public with inaccurate information, such as the case of the death of a woman in Istog, who was initially said to have died of COVID-19, but was later found not to have been infected with the virus. Hence keeping the public informed, not misinformed, proved challenging.

Conclusion

Political communication in Kosovo during the pandemic period was more intense due to important political developments which occurred simultaneously to the spread of COVID-19. The overthrow of the government, the formation of a new government, as well as the questioning of Kosovo's good relations with the United States were the main topics of the period when the citizens were also facing the virus and its spread. The political crisis meant that space for COVID-19 in the mainstream media was limited, as mainstream television news focused on political topics. The same happened with the mainstream online media, and there were many cases when the main news on the front page was only for politics.

The overthrow of the government, installation of a caretaker government and formation of a new governing coalition complicated Kosovo's initial response to the crisis. Despite this, the government introduced measures early and would impose containment and quarantine to limit the spread. The declining number of COVID-19 cases precipitated the reopening of the economy. But, as elsewhere, after restrictions were suspended, the number of new cases increased but despite this, and perhaps due to their vocal opposition of Kurti, the new government did not impose new restrictions.

Conflicting political stances and disinformation both prove challenging, and the lack of a coherent position from political leaders and a response from institutions to rebut false notions led to widespread confusion. The media maintained its standards but due to focusing on political machinations did not have the capacity to analyse the disinformation that was disseminated in society. This left a space for disinformation to gain traction. In times of crisis, it is important that citizens receive accurate information, and they act based on that information. Disinformation and partisan disagreements caused many people to expose themselves to risks. Hence the COVID-19 crisis highlights the need during crises for a united political leadership and for professional journalism, both ensuring society is well and accurately informed.

References

Boin, A., Hart, P., Stern, E., & Sundelius, B. (2005). *The Politics of Crisis Management: Public Leadership Under Pressure.* Cambridge University Press.

Brataas, K. (2018). *Crisis Communication. Case Studies and Lessons Learned from International Disasters.* Routledge.

Constitutional Court of the Republic of Kosovo. (2020). Decisions from the review sessions were held on 30 and 31 of March 2020. https://gjk-ks.org/en/decisions-from -the-review-sessions-held-on-30-and-31-of-march-2020/

Eurostat. (2019). Key figures on enlargement countries. https://ec.europa.eu/eurostat/ documents/3217494/9799207/KS-GO-19-001-EN-N.pdf/e8fbd16c-c342-41f7-aae d-6ca38e6f709e

Gërguri, D. (2019). Campaigning on facebook: posts and online social networking as campaign tools in the 2017 general elections in the Republic of Kosovo. *Central European Journal of Communication*, 12(22), 92–109.

Gërguri, D., Qerimi, G., & Blakaj, B. (2020). Coronavirus crisis disinformation on digital platforms: the case of Kosovo. https://medium.com/@DigiComNet/coro navirus-crisis-disinformation-on-digital-platforms-the-case-of-kosovo-c643076af9 11

Halper, Th. (1971). *Foreign Policy Crises: Appearance and Reality in Decision Making.* CE Merrill.

Lilleker, D. (2014). *Political Communication and Cognition.* Palgrave Macmillan.

Ruhrmann, G. (2015). Risk communication. In W. Donsbach (Ed.), *The Concise Encyclopedia of Communication.* John Wiley & Sons.

Shehu, B. (2020). *Kosovë: Dramë politike në kohën e rritjes së pandemisë.* Deutsche Welle (DW). www.dw.com/sq/kosov%C3%AB-dram%C3%AB-politike-n%C3%AB-k oh%C3%ABn-e-rritjes-s%C3%AB-pandemis%C3%AB/a-52895425

Udris, L. (2019). Political communication in and about crises. Potentials of a fragmented field. *Studies in Communication Sciences*, 19(1), 131–152.

29

TURKEY

Declaring war on an epidemic

Elif Kahraman

Political context

The Ak Party has been the ruling party in Turkey since 2002. As an ideological stance, the Ak Party is conservative and right-wing although it describes itself as 'conservative democratic.'[1] Recep Tayyip Erdogan, who is one of the founders of the Ak Party, came to power alone and was initially in power as Prime Minister, and as the President since 2018. In 2018, the parliamentary governance system in Turkey changed into a presidential system. The presidential system gives full executive authority to the President.

> Turkey maintains…a 'strong leader tradition,' which encompasses the 'presidentialisation' of the executive and 'presidential' administration, referring to the greater use of the president's unilateral power over the government, judiciary and bureaucracy in setting respective agendas and steering their implementation through the institutions and actors of the presidential system of government.
>
> *(Bakir, 2020: 5)*

This strong leader tradition impacts policy making and government actions in times of crisis. Considering the COVID-19 crisis in Turkey, the President's executive authority has both positive and negative effects. Positive effects have been seen in the ability to take and implement decisions rapidly. On the other hand, negative effects have occurred as a consequence of the President taking decisions without regard to advice or alternative views. Hence, the approach has been reactive rather than proactive. However, Metropoll Strategical and Social Research Centre's monthly research bulletin *Turkey's Pulse*, in which many areas like economy, agenda and politicians are evaluated, the March

DOI: 10.4324/9781003120254-31

report shows support for Erdogan increased[2] during the struggle with the epidemic.

Chronology

The chronology of COVID-19 for Turkey is divided into three phases: The emergence of COVID-19 when precautions were implemented, the phase after the first case in Turkey was diagnosed and the process of normalisation.

Emergence and the implementation of precautions

While the first cases of coronavirus were diagnosed in China on December 31, 2019, in Turkey, official statements show the first case was diagnosed on March 11, 2020. In pre-COVID-19 Turkey, it was seen that the Ministry of Health and the media started to prepare and forewarn the public. One of the very first actions of the ministry was to establish the Coronavirus Scientific Advisory Board (SAB) on January 10, 2020. 'The SAB is the only procedurally oriented implementation tool composed of medical scientists' (Bakir, 2020: 10). The Board started with 26 members and then in April it increased to 38 members. Regarding the fact that there were no COVID-19 cases in Turkey in January and it was not announced as an epidemic by the World Health Organisation (WHO), this move by the ministry was extremely proactive. In January, the Minister of Health, Dr Fahrettin Koca, discussed suspicious cases whether they were related to COVID-19 or not. The other proactive move was that the Ministry of Health prepared an air ambulance fleet to bring 25 Turkish citizens from Wuhan to Turkey. In addition, Turkish Airlines implemented precautions for cabin crew to wear gloves and masks on flights to and from China, Hong Kong and Taiwan. On January 22, flights to Wuhan were suspended because the virus had spread to countries like the United Kingdom. In addition, 2019-nCov guide was published.

The first television programme appearance of Koca was on January 22 and he informed the people that all necessary precautions were in place at airports including thermal cameras even though WHO had not recommended their use. On January 24, Koca made a press statement stating that medical staff were in place at both ports and airports at all times. Infectious disease control protections were activated for Chinese flights and thermal camera scanning of arriving passengers began. On March 11, the first case was confirmed in Turkey. Measures taken are listed in Table 29.1.

The Process of normalisation

The process of normalisation started gradually at the beginning of May and officially started in June. The important part of the normalisation process was that there have been contradictory views about whether it was too early to normalise.

TABLE 29.1 Turkey chronology

Date		Diffusion of COVID-19	Key official actions	Key communication events
March	11	1 Infection.		The first patient infected with COVID-19 is announced.
	12	2 Infections.	Coronavirus Summit between President and the Ministry of Health.	14 rules against coronavirus are announced.
	13	5 Infections.	Flight restrictions to 11 countries are announced.	
	14	6 Infections.	Ministry of Foreign Affairs established Crisis Management Counter.	
	15	18 Infections.	Citizens coming from abroad, especially Umrah, are taken into quarantine in dormitories.	
	16	47 Infections.	Ministry of Internal Affairs announced Coronavirus circular to governorships.	
	17	Infected: 98. Death toll: 1.		The first death of a patient infected with COVID-19 is announced.
	18	Infected: 191. Deaths: 2.		The President announces economic precautions.
	20	Infected: 670. Death toll: 9.	Non-emergency surgeries are postponed. Foundation and private hospitals are announced as epidemic hospitals.	
	21	Infected: 947. Deaths: 21.	Flight restrictions are extended to 46 countries.	
	22	Infected: 1,236. Death toll: 30.	The curfew starts for citizens aged 65+. Working hours limited. Restaurants allowed to serve takeaway only.	
	23	Infected: 1,529. Death toll: 37.	Distance learning started. Production of national ventilators has been planned.	

(Continued)

TABLE 29.1 (Continued)

Date		Diffusion of COVID-19	Key official actions	Key communication events
	24	Infected: 1,872. Deaths: 44.	New precautions taken for public transport and markets.	
	25	Infected: 2,433. Deaths: 59.	Schools to stay closed until April 30.	
	26	Infected: 3,629. Deaths: 75.		Ministry of Health daily information briefings begin.
	27	Infected: 5,698. Death toll: 92.	Coastal visits banned at weekends.	
	28	Infected: 7,402. Death toll: 108.	Ministry of Internal Affairs announce limited service implementation for bus and flight services.	
	30	Infected: 10,827. Death toll: 168.	Ministry of Internal Affairs announce limited service implementation for taxi services in three metropolitans.	
	31	Infected: 13,531. Death toll: 214.	Several factories suspended production.	The President starts 'We are enough for each other' donation campaign. Numbers of cases in cities shared for the first time.
April	1	Infected: 15,679. Death toll: 277.		
	3	Infected: 20,921. Death toll: 425.	Travel bans to 31 cities. Curfew for under 20s. Mandatory usage of masks in public places.	
	4	Infected: 23,934. Death toll: 501.	Ministry of Internal Affairs announced additional travel restrictions.	
	5	Infected: 27,069. Deaths 574.	Free masks to be distributed to citizens between 20 and 65.	
	6	Infected: 30,217. Death toll: 649.	Selling masks is banned. Economical precautions and support announced.	
	7	Infected: 34,109. Death toll: 725.	The Social Sciences Council is established; COVID-19 is isolated. The President distributed masks and colognes for people above 65.	The Minister: 'We are pioneering in stem cells and plasma treatment.'

Day	Statistics	Event	Statement
8	Infected: 38,226. Death toll: 812.	'Epidemic Isolation Follow-up Project' is announced. Dismissal of employees is banned for 3 months.	
9	Infected: 42,282. Deaths 908.	Free mask distribution is given to the pharmacies.	
10	Infected: 47,029. Deaths: 1,006.	Weekend curfew announced just two hours before start.	
11		Number of intubated patients decreases for first time.	
12	Infected: 56,956. Death toll: 1,198.	The Minister of Internal Affairs offers to resign but the President declines.	
13	Infected: 61,049. Death toll: 1,296.		The Health Minister shares #weovercometogether online campaign encouraging people to stay at home, wearing masks and keeping social distance.
14	Infected: 65,111. Death toll: 1,403.		The Minister: 'Turkey has been the first country having decrease in death increase speed.'
18	Infected: 82,329. Death toll: 1,890.	Life fits into the home application is available.	The Minister of Health: 'Intensive care occupancy rate is 60%, service occupancy rate is 50%.''.
20	Infected: 90,980. Death toll: 2,140.	The four days curfew of April 23–26 is announced. First stage of Istanbul Basaksehir City Hospital opened.	
23		Officials mention gradual normalisation process.	
25	Infected: 107,773. Death toll: 2,706.		The Health Minister shares #iamproudofmycountry online campaign encouraging people to stay home.
27	Infected: 112,261. Death toll: 2,900.	Ministry of Internal Affairs announced 402 people out of 855 had been caught for sharing fake and provocative news about COVID-19 on social media.	The president says, 'The epidemic has reached to the peak point.'
28	Infected: 114,653. Death toll: 2,992.	-The three days curfew on May 1–3 is announced. -The first patient with plasma treatment recovered.	
30	Infected 120,204. Deaths 3,174.	The process of normalisation starts gradually.	

There had been discussions about the need for restarting economic activity and ending curfews. On May 2, Minister Koca mentioned, 'we have begun studies on industrial production appropriate with COVID-19 precautions to continue with safety in the process of normalisation.'[3] Industrial activities started before social and cultural activities, indicating economic concerns dominated the decisions on normalisation. Four days later, Koca announced, 'Turkey has completed the first period in the struggle with coronavirus' adding, 'precaution is a must because the threat continues.'[4] Koca called this the 'controlled social life period' which continued weekend curfews and curfews on national holidays (May 16–19). On May 13, it was announced that the number of patients under intensive care was under 1,000 for the first time. Koca announced, 'We are in the second period of our struggle with coronavirus.'[5] Epidemic risk management strategies were implemented for workplaces and test laboratories were opened in industrial zones in order to prevent infection. Indications were positive, and the Ministry of Education announced that primary and secondary schools planned to continue their education in September. On May 29, mosques were opened and on June 1, public places such as restaurants, cafes, sport clubs, beaches, kindergartens, hotels, museums, airlines and the parliament opened, and the travel ban was removed. And, last of all, on June 21st, wearing masks became mandatory in 48 cities. Hence, with the addition of decisions regarding the social life, the normalisation process had almost completed.

Analysis

In this part, Turkey's officials' political rhetoric and main medium usage, Turkey's strengths and contradictions in the process of crisis are discussed.

Political rhetoric

The rhetoric of government officials has been one of the most important things in the COVID-19 crisis. The media used most were press statements and social media. The main actors have been the Ministry of Health, the President, SAB and the media. In addition, opposition party members, civil society initiatives and experts have been given space, especially in oppositional media. Minister Koca and the President have been among the most visible government officials. Koca made press statements every weekday and spoke live on television for approximately 35 minutes per day with a question and answer session. President Erdogan has given statements approximately twice a week. It is important to mention that the Minister of Health was clear in all the messages, threats, precautions and warnings. He always stayed calm, emphasised his medical identity rather than his political one and always adopted positive rhetoric. During this six-month period, Koca has been consistent with his behaviours, messages and style. While President Erdogan took on the position of leader, it is clear that Koca dominated communication. Drawing on his medical credentials, Koca used expert guidance consistently aiming to inform the public accurately.

The measures imposed were clearly justified and in line with a clear objective which is to inform citizens accurately. Koca was informative and media friendly from the very beginning. The themes that Koca used include 'we should trust our country,' 'the success belongs to all of us' and he shared empty street photographs during the curfew mentioning #ülkemlegururduyuyorum (I am proud of my country). He repeatedly said, 'Trust our health army.' The rhetoric is of national war and struggle against the enemy, COVID-19 with Koca as a commander of the army. Trust in the health system and scientists, the factual nature of information, and transparency are also rhetorical devices that have always been used. When the first death case of coronavirus occurred, Koca said, 'I make this sentence both as the Minister of Health and as a doctor: In our struggle with coronavirus, I lost a patient of mine for the first time.'[6] It is seen that Koca has tried to approach both the press and the public more as a doctor rather than as a minister, and he has tried to approach communication with sympathy and transparency.

In terms of the rhetoric, therefore, the nature of the threat has been reported consistently. But the compliance has been less consistent. While the Minister of Health still continued to warn citizens about the threat, life in Turkey has been normalised for the most part. For example, the restrictions on interprovincial travelling, use of shopping malls, restaurants and cafes were removed while Koca highlighted the importance of precautions.

A new social media campaign was started by the Ministry of Health as #birlikteyenecegiz (we beat it together); accompanying messages included the importance of staying home, wearing masks and keeping social distance. Erdogan has also made several statements and described the new normal as 'mask, distance and hygiene.' When it was announced that the number of patients under intensive care were under 1,000 for the first time, Koca mentioned, 'This success belongs to the 83 million who have fulfilled their responsibilities.'[7]

Strengths

In coping with the crisis, Turkey has shown strengths in some areas. One of the areas is filiation, which is defined as one of the important elements for detecting infected people and their previous contacts.

> The core idea behind filiation as a measure of precaution against the ongoing COVID-19 outbreak was to prevent the disease by interrupting the chain of transmission with a systematical tracing and isolation of susceptible individuals having contact with any confirmed COVID-19 cases.
>
> *(Demirtas & Tekiner, 2020: 354)*

In addition to the filiation, being effective in the treatment of patients, isolation of those infected and ensuring everyone maintains social distance in their daily lives were other areas of strength. On April 14, the fourth week of the epidemic in Turkey, Koca announced that the speed at which the disease was spreading had been taken under control and on the fifth week the numbers dying of COVID-19 had started to slow down. He reemphasised filiation and its importance. He added that Turkey had been the first country to see a decreasing trend in the number of deaths. Koca stated, 'We have two powers: Precaution and treatment. Let's use our powers.' In addition, he claimed Turkey had been successful in-patient treatment and intensive care. On April 18, the Hayat Eve Sigar (Life fits into home) mobile application was introduced by the Ministry of Health. It was designed to provide citizens with a density and risk map that helps them to be careful when out as well as providing information about the current situation overall. On April 20, the first stage of Basaksehir City Hospital was opened, and 100 units of national ventilators were delivered to the hospital.

Turkish citizens arriving both from Europe and Umrah (Islamic pilgrimage) underwent medical examination. Turkish Airlines organised 34 flights and 3,614 Turkish citizens were brought from Europe and placed in quarantine for 14 days in student dormitories run by the state. They were taken from the airport with special buses and transferred to dormitories.

Turkey was thus successful in rescuing its citizens from all over the world. On April 26, a Turkish family living in Sweden asked for help via Twitter and were brought to Turkey by air ambulance fleet. In addition, 32 Turkish citizens in India were brought home in April.

Contradictions

There have, however, been contradictions between official sources during the epidemic. The first issue was the government being late implementing lockdown and some precautions like shutting down mosques and Friday prayers. 'The COVID-19 outbreak is a reminder of the social and cultural impact of medical emergencies' (Alyanak, 2020: 2). The social and cultural life in Turkey changed, but for believers it remained highly important to attend Friday prayers. Hence, the pandemic has affected practising of one of the most important religious duties.

Another issue was with face mask distribution. It is clear that there has been an abundancy of face masks, but sometimes it has been hard to find them due to government actions. Because face mask producers and sellers took advantage of the situation, the government banned the sale of face masks on April 6. The previous day, Erdogan announced that the government would mail five masks every week to citizens between the ages of 20 and 65. This should have been possible for the national postal service (PTT). However, the PTT struggled to meet the need and on April 9, free mask distribution was transferred to pharmacies. That system caused problems and on April 28, it was decided employees would get free masks via their employers. These problems came to an end with the unbanning of selling masks on May 4. The process led to tensions between government, pharmacies and citizens due to the unavailability of masks when needed.

The third issue was the first curfew, which was announced for the weekend in 31 cities on April 10 approximately at 9:45 pm which led to some controversies due to the events afterwards. The problem was that it had been announced two hours before the curfew without previous warning and caused panic. Many citizens rushed out to grocery stores without social distancing and proper usage of masks. In addition, it was claimed that the SAB did not know about the curfew because of the fact that the Minister of Health did not inform them prior to the announcement. In addition, municipalities governed by opposition parties claimed they had also not been informed previously. After those incidents, the Minister of Internal Affairs Suleyman Soylu took full responsibility, admitting he had not foreseen the problems, and consequently resigned, but his resignation was declined by the President.

The fourth contradiction was between the SAB and Turkish Football Federation (TFF) on restarting the football season. TFF decided to restart the football season on May 6. Koca mentioned that TFF had been irresponsible with their decisions because of the fact that SAB had not approved it.

A further contradiction on June 5 led citizens to wonder whether there would be a curfew again at the weekend. First, it was mentioned that there would be no curfew, then Minister Soylu said there would be a curfew and afterwards the President announced that there would be no curfew, due to the fact that Erdogan found it inappropriate for social and economical reasons. Hence, it is clear that there has not always been consensus between the SAB, the ministries and the President.

The last serious contradiction was on May 14 when there was a public difference of opinion between the Ministry of Health and other experts. Minister Koca stated that the infection coefficient ($r0$) was 1.56 whereas other experts claimed that there cannot be a normalisation process without the infection coefficient being under 1. All these served to undermine the credibility of the decision-makers and their decisions.

Conclusion

Turkey pursued proactive and reactive strategies regarding problem solving during the COVID-19 epidemic. Turkey experienced some crises due to the contradictions between officials, distribution of masks and late curfew implementations. On the contrary, polls show that the popularity of President Erdogan has increased. The 'War on epidemic' and related rhetoric dominated the discourse. As a result, it has become obvious that in times of crisis people tend to follow their leaders, as an old saying suggests, 'Do not change horses in midstream.'

Notes

1 See *4. Olağan Büyük Kongre 2023 Siyasi Vizyonu*. www.akparti.org.tr/media/272148 /2023-vizyonu.pdf.
2 See *Türkiye'nin Nabzı – Mart 2020*. http://www.metropoll.com.tr/arastirmalar/turk iyenin-nabzi-17/1846.
3 See *Son Dakika Haberler*. www.hurriyet.com.tr/gundem/son-dakika-haberler-bakan -koca-twitterdan-duyurdu-sanayi-uretimi-icin-normallesme-calismalarini-baslatt ik-41508538.
4 See *Son Dakika*. www.sozcu.com.tr/2020/gundem/son-dakika-bilim-kurulu-to plantisi-sona-erdi-bakan-koca-canli-yayinda-5797772/.
5 See *Gundem*. www.trthaber.com/haber/gundem/bakan-koca-acikladi-kontrollu- sosyal-hayat-donemi-basliyor-482213.html.
6 See *Koronavirüs*. www.aa.com.tr/tr/koronavirus/saglik-bakani-koca-koronavirusle -mucadelemizde-ilk-kez-bir-hastami-kaybettim/1769769.
7 See *Gundem*. www.sadecehaber.com/gundem/bakan-koca-guzel-haberi-verdi-ilk -kez-1000-altina-dustu.html.

References

Alyanak, O. (2020). Faith, politics and the COVID-19 pandemic: The Turkish response. *Medical Anthropology*, 39(5), pp. 374–375, doi:10.1080/01459740.2020.1745482.

Bakir, C. (2020). The Turkish State's responses to existential COVID-19 crisis. *Policy and Society*, 39(3), pp. 424–441, doi:10.1080/14494035.2020.1783786.

Demirtas, T., & Tekiner, H. (2020). Filiation: A historical term the COVID-19 outbreak recalled in Turkey. *Erciyes Medical Journal*, 42(3), 354–358.

30

POLITICAL COMMUNICATION AND COVID-19

Governance and rhetoric in global comparative perspective

Darren Lilleker, Ioana Coman, Miloš Gregor and Edoardo Novelli

The problem we have in mid–September 2020 is that no-one knows what the end game is with COVID-19. What is the magic formula that will allow a return the 'old normal,' one without social distancing, sanitising and wearing face masks? Is it zero cases, or is that a misnomer resulting from ending testing and reporting? Is it a vaccine? It took 25 years for a chicken pox vaccine to be developed. The smallpox vaccine was developed in 1796 but the last known case was in 1977. Flu vaccines are only 40–60% effective and it has never been rolled out universally and does not prevent 99,000–200,000 deaths each year (Paget et al., 2019). Vaccines can be mandated but a significant number of anti-vaxxers refuse proven, tested, well-known vaccines administered for decades with minimal side effects. It seems unlikely people will flock to get a fast tracked, quickly tested vaccine, whose long-term side effects and overall efficacy are at best uncertain. We thus face myriad questions. What if autumn sees more outbreaks as it seems is likely? What if March 2021 is worse than 2020? What if people start to see the risks of 'the new normal' outweighing the risks COVID-19 poses? People manage risk on a daily basis. Driving a car, smoking, drinking and eating unhealthily all pose dangers. In some countries leaving home can be dangerous, particularly for poorer and marginalised communities.

The COVID-19 pandemic remains a crisis of global proportions, impacting every nation however powerful, small or remote. The number of cases by the end of September 2020 was over 30 million and over 1 million lives have been lost. As most economies reopened, people worked and socialised together again; even with social distancing in place this led to a further steady increase of daily cases of 200,000. The current worst hit nations are in the African, and North and South American continents but there are indications of a widespread second wave of infections. Whether the total numbers are an underestimate, due to

DOI: 10.4324/9781003120254-32

many having the virus but being asymptomatic, or due to insufficient access to testing, may never be fully known.

The first wave of COVID-19 was a global test of political leadership and a time when it was crucial for clear, consistent and empathetic political communication. The case studies in this volume test the extent to which this crucial factor was present across a range of diverse regimes and to what extent we can identify notable correlations between the responses of national governments, the nature of the communication environment and the impact of COVID-19 within these countries.

Comparing World Health Organisation (WHO) data across nations for cases and deaths per million of the population, three cases stand out, the United States, India and Brazil. Trump, and Bolsanaro, leaders of two of these nations, denied there was a threat to public health, often contradicted or refuted the arguments of their health officials and gave succour to those who opposed restrictions on movement and refused to wear face masks on civil liberty grounds. India, meanwhile, is shown to have had a chaotic response with sectarian divides hampering a unified national response. Sweden, which never instituted a lockdown, and South Africa, where the social and economic conditions inhibit strict controls being instituted, also stand out.

Global data

Table 30.1 shows, in terms of deaths per million, the UK leads a group of nations which were the first, after China and neighbouring countries, to be hit by the virus. With Spain, Italy and France, the UK demonstrates the fact that many developed countries were ill prepared for the virus and perhaps complacent about its effects. Partially, this may have been the result of the WHO initially likening this to SARS or MERS which had minimal impact beyond a few Middle-Eastern and South-East Asian countries. Universally, we found that even advanced health care systems can be quickly overwhelmed. Vacillation over the point when lockdown was required, if at all in the case of Sweden which also witnessed significant numbers of deaths, based on concerns regarding the impact on the economy, is also a contributory factor. The ability to lockdown efficiently, and/or put in place an effective and widely used system for tracking those with symptoms and tracing their movements, as seen in Germany and South Korea, clearly helped to save lives also. But these broad points do not tell the full story. Drawing on the analytical framework at the start of the volume we explore the similarities and differences across the countries.

Firstly, however, the data shows no clear patterns across all nations, although for some of the countries it would appear decisions over lockdown were crucial. The country with the highest deaths per million is the UK, this was also a country that took one of the longest periods between the first case being reported and implementing lockdown (52 days). The United States remains the worst hit globally, there was no nationwide lockdown, but a series of

TABLE 30.1 Comparative data on cases and lockdowns across our sample nations

Country	First case announced	Number of cases (per mill)	Number of deaths (per mill)	Period between first case and lockdown (days)	Period of lockdown (days)
China	31/12/2019	60	3	24	75
Japan	16/01/2020	214	8	46	74
South Korea	20/01/2020	272	6	No lockdown	n/a
United States	20/01/2020	11,687	427	51 (NY State)	92
France	24/01/2020	2,545	461	48	61
Australia	25/01/2020	506	5	52	15
Germany	27/01/2020	2,427	109	45	29
India	30/01/2020	898	22	54	22
Italy	31/01/2020	4,053	580	42	82
Spain	31/01/2020	5,722	608	42	95
Sweden	31/01/2020	7,773	561	No lockdown	n/a
UK	31/01/2020	4,355	669	52	70
Egypt	14/02/2020	877	44	39	91
Iran	19/02/2020	3,350	177	33	19
Russia	21/02/2020	5,448	88	39	42
Austria	25/02/2020	2,225	79	17	75
Brazil	25/02/2020	10,160	383	15	31
Norway	26/02/2020	1,670	47	15	39
Iceland	28/02/2020	5,396	29	15 (some restrictions)	Ongoing
Eire	29/02/2020	5,229	355	12	67
Czechia	01/03/2020	1,361	34	13	58
Hungary	04/03/2020	453	62	12	44
Poland	04/03/2020	1,088	43	17	26
Ghana	12/03/2020	955	5	18	15
South Africa	12/03/2020	6,659	100	7	43
Kosovo	13/03/2020	0.6	0.1	33	15
Turkey	17/03/2020	2,637	66	4	33

restrictions taken at the state level. New York was slow to lockdown and had the longest period of complete economic shutdown but the situation in many states remains parlous and shutdowns were implemented differentially. Also, one needs to consider that some nations are global travel hubs. London, New York and Paris were badly hit in the early stages of the pandemic, as were hubs for winter tourism like the Italian and Austrian alps. Nations which enjoy less travel were later to witness cases. Patterns of travel as a factor are emphasised by the spread from the ski resorts in Northern Italy and Austria as well as early cases detected within Scandinavian countries. Migration also played a role as seasonal workers returned home from Alpine ski resorts to many Eastern European countries which initially lacked protocols for dealing with the hundreds reaching their borders. Australia, due to it being a destination for Chinese tourists and students, but lacking status as a global travel hub, was able to shut down later and have lower numbers of cases, at least during the first wave. Therefore, when the next pandemic hits, national leaders need to not only look at current infection rates but also consider the likelihood of transmission into a country and rate of spread when considering implementing mitigation measures.

The numbers, however, may not be fully reliable for all nations. Varying levels of effective testing programmes means many cases go undetected. There is also a question regarding the correct registration of deaths in many nations. Estimates for nations where large sections of the population live in poverty, with no proper records, may be unaware of the extent of the spread or impact of the virus within disadvantaged communities. Alternatively, the UK system of recording every death by an individual who has tested positive for COVID-19 within 28 days of their death as being of COVID-19 could inflate figures, although testing is not universal within the nation. Thus, in terms of reliability of figures there are significant questions and it is likely that only South Korea, where an early testing and track and trace system was in place, has a reasonably accurate figure of infections. Therefore, conclusions can only be tentative, particularly as many nations are now experiencing further waves of infections. Therefore, beyond the raw data on figures and strategy, what can the COVID-19 pandemic teach us about managing crises?

Management of the crisis

There is no clear evidence of correspondence between the different political approaches and the policies adopted in order to limit the effects of the pandemic. On a general level, however, we do find that some authoritarian and conservative administrations demonstrated a greater tendency to underestimate the pandemic and to deny the danger represented by COVID-19. This is the case of Trump and Bosonaro, but also of the UK's Boris Johnson. But the authoritarian styles of Orban and Erdogan in Hungary and Turkey seemed to fare much better, suggesting there is not a simple correlation between the style and ideology of a government and the impact experienced during the COVID-19 pandemic. However, analysing the developments across phases of the crisis offer some insights.

Pre-crisis phase

News of a novel coronavirus being detected in Wuhan, China largely came from media, some reporting it as a rumour. For many, the perception was that this was an event of little significance in a distant land despite it being 12–15 hours away by direct flight. Japanese prime minister Shinto Abe closely followed by Korean prime minister Moon, having experienced epidemics previously, were the only leaders to communicate the potential threat that the virus to be designated COVID-19 might pose.

Trump's response, that this posed a minimal threat to his nation, was largely representative of the response of many national leaders. Our studies show that the leaders of France, Italy, Spain, the UK, Egypt, Iran, Russia, Brazil, Hungary and Poland also made early statements that downplayed the threat. However, underestimates can be excused as the first statement from the WHO was to liken the virus to SARS and MERS which had a minimal global impact. This meant that preparations may well have been hindered even in nations with highly developed health systems and effective systems of governance. Reassuring populations further, many of these nations' leaders also declared readiness to deal with an outbreak, and even nations which hinted at the potential calamity an outbreak could bring, as Indian prime minister Modi declared, still claimed they were prepared. It seems that within the pre-crisis phase only Japan, South Korea, Sweden and to some extent Turkey made clear plans to prevent the spread of the virus. Given that China quickly became open about the severity of symptoms and scale of transmission, it is unsurprising their nearest neighbours quickly responded. Furthermore, many of these countries had experienced previous epidemics over recent decades; therefore their quick response could benefit from their experiences. But given the speed of transmission to North America, Europe and Australasia during February, it is surprising that more work was not done in the pre-crisis phase in countries that would have recognised that cases were likely and imminent. Lessons were not learned from the case of Italy, the first European nation to be seriously affected by the virus. In particular, the UK sent no observers and seemed to follow an attitude of exceptionalism,[1] despite cases being detected just a few weeks later. When the situation in Italy became critical and lockdown began, several countries where data showed they were following the Italian trajectory took no measures for some weeks; this indicates clearly the lack of collaboration and coordination at the European level.

Preparation phase

The Politician Prominence Model best explains the norm for the majority of countries. Political leaders took advice from their experts, but personalised command over decision-making and public communication. All nations except Germany, the UK, Sweden, Iran, Iceland, Czechia, Kosovo and Turkey had a highly personalised approach to communication centring credibility on a single actor; for 14 of these cases it was the leader of the nation. Press briefings did involve national leaders, ministers and experts sharing a platform, but largely a single politician took centre stage. Germany, Sweden, Iran, Iceland, Kosovo and Turkey followed the Expert Appointee Prominence Model. Personalisation can ensure clarity of message, which in turn allows for clear framing of the nature of the threat and how citizens should respond. This was not the case in Czechia or the UK where different individuals were dominant at different phases of the pandemic, or where different ministers took turns to deliver daily briefings. While this does not suggest a lack of clarity of message, it does present a fragmented sense of leadership within polities that are normally highly centralised and personalised. Only China demonstrated minimal personalisation.

However, credibility during a pandemic requires health experts be given prominence. Fourteen countries (South Korea, Australia, Germany, India, Italy, Spain, Sweden, the UK, Russia, Norway, Iceland, South Africa, Kosovo and Turkey) gave experts high prominence; a further seven had them appearing at key times or being reference points (Egypt, Iran, Austria, Ireland, Czechia, Poland and Ghana). While there were tensions between experts and government in Japan, these were resolved; however, the experience in the United States, France, Brazil and Hungary saw public and partisan differences of opinion which continued throughout the phases of the crisis. While this may be a contributory factor to the numbers of cases and deaths in the United States and Brazil, the latter being a nation where actual numbers are inaccurate and under-reported, France and Hungary fared well in comparison to similar neighbours despite this. It is worth highlighting that even among experts and scientists there have been differences of opinion, sometimes even radical ones; proof that even science's response to the pandemic has not been prompt and unanimous. In almost all countries, experts became key players in the public debate: protagonists of press conferences, interviewed daily in newspapers and regular guests of talk shows and television programmes. However, they were the bearers of a narrative which in terms of timing, logic and purpose could be very different from those of political institutions. A difference that, especially but not only in the cases of the United States and Brazil, has led to public conflicts between political figures, experts and scientists.

Lockdown plans and the changes required to public behaviour to contain contagion, the widely used strategy of flattening the curve, demonstrated that within many countries there was no clear plan. Our case studies show in France, Australia, India, Italy, the UK, Egypt, Iran, Czechia and Kosovo the statements caused confusion. Whether the national response was unified or federalised partially contributed. Where governments made announcements requesting state or regional governors to act, and they challenged the national line, citizens were left to decide whom to trust. Other national leaders, such as the UK prime minister Johnson, suggested what citizens should do but this was not enforced until instituting a full lockdown. Hence while UK citizens were recommended to avoid large gatherings, sporting events went ahead, pubs and restaurants remained opened and many took the opportunity to party prior to lockdown. The situation was similar in France, where elections were held the day before the lockdown declaration, placing many citizens at risk of infection despite the obvious quick spread of the virus.

The media also played a key role within the phase. In many countries the media stance remained divided between government supporting and oppositional media outlets. Hence overall while some media amplified government messages, other outlets challenged the government narrative. Only the media of South Korea, Germany, Czechia, India, Sweden, Austria, Norway, Iceland, Poland, Ghana and South Africa took a uniformly supportive stance during the pre-lockdown phase, only criticising where governments vacillated or where measures were not implemented appropriately.

The role played by social media was also crucial across many nations. COVID-19 is the first pandemic in an era of global communication where, with few exceptions, the whole planet was connected in real time. Social networks were an exceptional resource utilised for risk communication by most national leaders, as well as a way for citizens to stay connected despite lockdown. However, social media also allowed the spread of an enormous amount of communication only minimally managed by institutional actors and mainstream media, with consequences with regards to the spread of mis/disinformation about the global situation and threats posed within individual nations.

Throughout this phase there was a lack of global cooperation and coordination. While the EU communicated the risk effectively, there was minimal support given to member states forcing each to take a unique approach. This does not mean cooperation was completely lacking, Italy at least during the initial emergency phase received supplies and medical personnel from China, Russia and Albania. But this was ad hoc and due to individual initiatives. The WHO devoted its energies towards the poorest countries, which is understandable, but there is minimal evidence even that WHO guidance was used as a universal rule book. Hence it would appear that national approaches dominated with some lesson learning only and few attempts to institute a global response to the pandemic.

Crisis phase

Most nations instituted a lockdown, the exceptions being South Korea, Sweden and Iceland. In some nations, these started as localised but progressed to being nationwide; even those nations eschewing full lockdown placed restrictions on public gatherings. Five countries saw these measures challenged on constitutional grounds, the United States, France, Spain, Brazil and Kosovo. Within each it was asked whether national governments had the authority to restrict public liberties and impose lockdowns on federal regions. Open disagreements gave greater credence to misinformation circulating across mainstream and social media platforms which questioned the severity of COVID-19 and gave space for conspiracy theories to flourish regarding the true motives of governments for restricting movement. The United States, France, Brazil and Kosovo, along with Japan, Australia, Italy, Egypt, Russia, Czechia, Hungary and South Africa saw conflict between institutions. In the United States and Brazil, the most serious were public contradictions of the advice of health experts by the president. Elsewhere, conflicts were between president and parliament or between ruling and opposition parties. Public disagreements over the necessity or timing of lockdown led to some public non-compliance, a contributory factor noted for the number of cases and deaths in the United States and Brazil. Such conflicts questioned whether governments were right at crucial points when implementing strategies to contain COVID-19.

During lockdown it is argued to be crucial to maintain a dialogue with the people, reminding them of the need to obey the new rules and guidelines, facilitating compliance through support packages as well as imbuing we-ness and self-efficacy to control the spread, as well as providing clear figures to emphasise the threat as well as the success from the strategy taken. Many countries instituted regular press conferences, ten countries making these daily at set times (Germany, Italy, Spain, the UK, Iran, Austria, Iceland, Republic of Ireland, Czechia and Poland), a further seven (Japan, South Korea, Sweden, Ghana, South Africa, Kosovo and Turkey) having them at frequent intervals. The remaining ten countries had a more sporadic approach where a spokesperson would appear on news bulletins or deliver special addresses on key occasions but with no set times or frequency.

Experts played a key communicational role. They stood alongside the political leader and were given full prominence in 12 countries (South Korea, Australia, Germany, Italy, Spain, Sweden, the UK, Egypt, Austria, Iceland, Republic of Ireland and Turkey); only in Hungary, Czechia and Poland did politicians represent science and government. But in most cases science was foregrounded, the exceptions being the United States and Brazil, although where politicians took the lead references to following science had a more rhetoric-laden character. The differential strategies saw high levels of personalisation emphasising the need to identify a universally trusted individual. Under lockdown conditions, most countries managed to develop a unified position among key stakeholders, although where there were conflicts between government and federal systemic levels, politicians and health experts or the government and opposition, these remained a feature of political communication. Hence the difference strategies impacted on public perceptions that the information was credible and the strategy correct.

Despite the highlighted differences between political systems and standing of governments, in general, the COVID-19 crisis increased support for leaders and ruling parties. Attempts by oppositional forces to discredit government actions had little success, outside of systems with severe polarisation such as the United States or Kosovo. Largely, opposition parties had to align themselves with the national interest. The so-called 'rally around the flag' phenomenon imbued we-ness and citizens' trust in their leadership increased. A few leaders took self-contradictory positions towards the pandemic, for example, UK prime minister Johnson within a matter of days of claiming he was unafraid and was shaking hands with COVID-19 patients announced a lockdown. But the trend detected by surveys in almost all countries was the pandemic was of particular advantage to weak governments and leaders.

The most crucial factor was building unity, managing the meaning of compliance and framing the pandemic and role of the public as a national struggle. This was eschewed by some leaders, in the cases of the United States and Brazil adopting an exceptionalist line claiming the virus would not seriously affect the nation or its people. However, other countries quite explicitly defined the meaning of the crisis and placed the public response into that framing. China, where the first cases were discovered, adopted the frame of victimage. An unnatural enemy preyed on the nation and so all citizens must fight it. This was a variant on the framing adopted by France, Italy, Spain, Iran, Russia, Czechia, Hungary, Poland and Turkey. These nations, and to a lesser extent the UK, Austria and Ireland, called citizens to rally around the flag and act in unity against a common enemy. Citizens were thus ascribed the role of combatants or in the case of Iran 'health ambassadors' working together for their nation and one another. Even the softer tone of India's 'don't panic, work together' offered that sense of a nation working as one. In other nations this was a more implicit call, perhaps a recognition that an explicit call for unity was unnecessary.

The framing of COVID-19 as an external threat was important in creating the sense of we-ness that psychologists argue acts as a glue which holds a society together and maintains compliance. Given the origins of the virus, it is perhaps unsurprising that the authoritarian regime in China, with its ability to control the flow of information, raised questions regarding the origins of the new coronavirus. Elsewhere, the threat was external and in many cases leaders put their nations on a war footing: from a holy war or jihad in Iran, joint struggle in Ghana to more mutedly invoking the spirit of Churchill by Johnson in the UK. In particular, the metaphor of war was the main rhetorical tool used by Macron, who punctuated his March 16 televised speech to the nation with the phrase 'nous somme en guerre' (we are at war).[2] Nations where 'we' became exclusive, as opposed to inclusive, witnessed greater problems. The United States, Brazil and Kosovo were sites of political polarisation, aiding the spread and believability of disinformation and fuelling acts of non-compliance. In India where Modi's Hindu nationalism has seen extensive sectarian violence, particularly targeting the large Muslim population, these divisions extended to the pandemic. Therefore, while on the whole nations became united in collective solidarity to combat COVID-19, and their governments gained popular support for their leadership, leaders who stand on platforms which pit sides against one another failed to unite their nations in the face of a health crisis, this perhaps is one factor which leads three large and economically powerful nations (the United States, Brazil and India) to also have the highest death rates per capita.

Such calls for unity and a spirit of inclusive we-ness are particularly required where evidence suggests unpreparedness. Many nations experienced shortages in the provision of personal protective equipment (PPE), hospital beds, having ineffective testing or track and trace systems and failing to implement preventative measures to safeguard the vulnerable in retirement homes. All these factors, which were features of official and media reports within the United States, India, Italy, Spain, the UK, Egypt, Iran, Russia, Brazil, Czechia, Hungary, Ghana, South Africa and Kosovo undermined both the message and the framing. The challenges were particularly problematic within countries that had claimed preparedness during the pre-crises phase: India, Italy, the UK, Egypt, Russia, Brazil, Czechia and Hungary. The power of the unity narrative thus had to overcome evidence that the government was, rhetorically at least, leading the nation into a war with lower chances of victory than were claimed when the war was rhetorically declared. In particular, deficiencies undermined perceptions of governments 'doing it for us.'

Unity narratives were also challenged by misinformation. A range of posts from unknown sources circulated on social media platforms that ranged from offering unproven preventions or cures, claiming the virus had been manufactured deliberately or was linked to 5G technology, or suggesting restrictions were part of a conspiracy which involved national governments or secretive societies such as the masons (in Kosovo), Bill Gates or even the Bilderberg group.[3] The governments of some countries, in particular Germany and Ireland, took measures to combat false claims, as did the UK's state broadcaster the BBC. In most cases, the more spurious claims had minimal impact on the overall national mood. The most serious cases were found where misinformation was actually provided by the national government to rebut challenges to their narrative. In China the government initially quashed health reports and accused a doctor of undermining the state and party. Trump meanwhile contradicted the advice of his United States Chief Medical Officer declaring he was protecting himself from COVID-19 by taking the unproven drug hydroxychloroquine while also questioning face mask wearing. Similar discourse was promoted by Brazil's President Jair Bolsonaro. Elsewhere, Australia's prime minister was found to misinform citizens, as were the leaders of Czechia and South Africa although these cases were more signs of incompetence than strategic. The regime in Egypt endorsed a number of conspiracy theories invoking a long-standing trope about forces of evil undermining national unity, a similar approach was adopted by Iranian president Rouhani. Hungary's Orban firstly claimed migrants were the cause of the virus spreading, later also pointing the finger at transnational actors. In open media environments, such wild and spurious claims undermine the credibility of a unified message and are problems for a range of areas of political communication. Where governments deliberately misinform, trust in institutions is undermined. This situation can lead to increased non-compliance with containment measures and for compliance to be determined by partisanship as has been the case in the United States and Brazil. The slow or lack of a response from the WHO to quell false information did not help the situation either.

A further way in which government credibility was undermined was the need to perform policy U-turns. China firstly had to reverse their policy of suppression of information, to national and international opprobrium. US president Trump had to declare a state of emergency after downplaying the threats, agree to state-wide lockdowns and support the wearing of face masks after decrying their value. The governments of Iran and Brazil also had to publicly reverse their position on the threat posed as the virus took hold. Kosovo faced severe challenges that led to the fall of the government and a whole new approach being adopted. Elsewhere, when policies had to be adapted, it depended on clear communication of both the policy and the case for the measures. Shifting curfew times in Egypt and South Africa led to confusion but largely these issues were more related to the changes to lockdown or the easing of measures.

Despite or because of government failings, civil society initiatives acted as buffers against the worst effects of lockdown. Brazilian activists engaged in extensive work providing food and medical advice within the favelas. Even in highly developed nations like the United States and the UK, food banks have increased activities to support those vulnerable during the closure of the economy. These are the most dramatic examples of a range of activities that involved volunteers helping to shield vulnerable family members or neighbours. On a more basic level, there were also a range of activities where communities kept in touch with one another through acts of solidarity. Chinese residents in Wuhan under lockdown were shown waving across the streets and displaying signs in their windows. Italians showed their musical skills, performing arias from their balconies. Many countries also engaged in doorstep clapping for those working on the frontline in hospitals, showing them playing their part supporting the 'war' effort. Social media was used to orchestrate these and other supportive civil society initiatives, such as using hashtags to organise information or showing support to others. The #wearetogether hashtag was used in a variety of national contexts. In many nations, people also helped with production and distribution of homemade face masks for more vulnerable members of society.

Normalisation phase

As Table 30.1 shows, lockdown periods varied in length and the extent to which countries' citizens returned to some forms of normality differed according to the severity of impact experienced. With citizens yearning for normality while also being scared for their own and the health of more vulnerable loved ones, there was never a point when being right, credible and empathetic was more necessary. Support for normalisation measures became very polarised in the United States and France; within the former it remains a highly partisan issue relating to the positions Trump adopted in opposition to medical advice. Elsewhere, there were a range of mixed responses with the challenge of saving lives being balanced against potentially catastrophic economic effects from remaining under lockdown. It would appear from our case studies that Australia, Germany, Italy, Spain, Austria, Czechia, Poland and Turkey witnessed a smooth transition. These nations saw general agreement regarding the implementation and timing of easing restrictions and alternative views were marginal only. Other nations witnessed greater consternation with some seeing easing as being introduced too early while others called for a quicker normalisation process.

Credibility during the normalisation phase appears heavily reliant on the prominence given to science and to health experts. The marginalised position of science in Japan, India, the UK, Iran and Russia led some to suspect that the economy was prioritised over public health. More seriously conflicting and partisan use of science in the United States, Ireland, Hungary, South Africa and Kosovo led to further challenges in maintaining some containment measures. One of the most controversial issues that caused confusion was when and where to use face masks. While this became a partisan issue in the United States, the UK saw civil liberty protests against face mask wearing and confusion reigning in Norway. Frequent changes to WHO recommendations provided succour to critical voices. The confusion was fuelled by conflicting information on the capacity of face masks to protect the wearers, the sorts of face coverings that were most appropriate and the inconsistencies in policy on where they should be worn. Credibility became a serious issue around this issue with a serious impact on compliance.

Strategies to frame normalisation were also far less widespread. While China hailed victory, other countries offered less compelling narratives. The Iranian government called on citizens to keep fighting. The UK meanwhile used 'Stay Alert'; Ireland 'Safety First.' However, an empathetic tone was taken in attempts to balance the concerns of citizens who needed to return to work as well as those concerned for their health. Failures to frame normalisation, develop an empathetic tone and to demonstrate competence are evidenced in those nations where normalisation became chaotic and poorly managed. Evidence of this is found in the United States as states veer between full and partial lockdown while others have emerged from at least the first wave of infections. Major reversals of strategy also had to be enacted in India, Spain, the UK, Brazil, Czechia, South Africa and Kosovo. Hence while many countries had to adjust strategy, as was the case during the crisis phase, how change was communicated was of crucial importance to avoid descent into chaos. It appears of little surprise that the countries evidencing incoherent strategies are also those that have an increasing number of cases, Kosovo being the outlier due to it not having large numbers of international traffic or centres of high habitation.

Misinformation and disinformation also played a crucial role during normalisation, perhaps more so than during the crisis phase. The United States, India, UK, Egypt, Brazil, Czechia, Hungary, South Africa and Kosovo all suffered from competing narratives becoming widespread. Aside from confusing or contradictory statements from national institutions which dogged progress in some countries, notably the United States and Brazil, the competing perspectives on face coverings, fears over vaccines containing microchips, conspiracy theories relating to track and trace systems and stories that people are getting infected by COVID-19 testing pervaded to undermine national government initiatives. While many governments did offer an appropriate response, where institutions were contributing to the misinformation environment conspiracy theories were able to gain credence and have the same credibility as the advice given by the health experts.

Unfortunately, normalisation cannot be globally uniform, due to the differing situations each nation finds themselves in. One of the major challenges with this pandemic from a crisis standpoint is that normally a crisis ends after the normalisation phase and you enter a phase in which you can evaluate the response, learn lessons and start preparing better in case a similar crisis hits in the future.

However, with COVID-19 we are repeating the cycle (at different speeds) with a second wave currently emerging across many European countries. This gives little time for the political or economic systems to recover, the time for reflection, and so insufficient time for a second preparation phase.

Political communication during a pandemic

The crisis is ongoing, but we can reflect on its management, the political communication strategies and what the situation indicates for our discipline. Firstly, political communication during the pandemic adopted a highly personalised approach. In most cases, the prime minister or president became chief communicator and figurehead for the nation and its response. In some nations, key ministers or medical experts gained prominence. But in all nations COVID-19 confirmed the trend towards personalisation and the importance, in particular during an emergency of this scale, to have a central figure who has at least majoritarian support across political factions and from key media outlets, able to deliver a unifying message and being seen to lead the response. But personalisation within this context does not have to simply be a factor of political leadership, ministers or experts who were thrust into the spotlight due to their role or expertise were able to win public trust. The flipside of this phenomenon is that where there were prominent figures who disagreed and conflicted on the framing of the crisis and the appropriate response that should be taken, this is reflected in the outcomes in terms of public unity as well as the scale of the impact of COVID-19.

Secondly, we confirm the importance of mediatisation in explaining the effectiveness of political communication strategies. Mediatisation is exacerbated as a consequence of the new media system and is one of the causes of the personalisation of political communication (Altheide, 2020). The COVID-19 pandemic hence further stresses the importance of media in the management of a crisis. In particular, where a national government enjoyed the support of main media outlets, and there was minimal open oppositional rhetoric, the public largely got behind governments and adhered to the measures implemented. The pandemic also saw media which normally criticise government become more supportive, at least during the first weeks of the crisis phase when strict measures were instituted. This could be the result of two factors: an awareness of the need for national unity and the fact that changes and new measures were announced so quickly that media were less able to analyse the measures, offer a plurality of views, and so became information conduits. However, this does not suggest that governments and media became entirely united in a national effort even when leaders called for unity and put the nation on a war footing. In several nations, we detect differences between the communication strategies and agendas of political and state institutions on one side, and media and information systems on the other. Also, across the phases of the crisis the different perspectives offered by political institutions and media became accentuated, resulting in conflict between media and political institution over the public agenda. Hence although many societies are mediated societies, meaning media are the most important source of information and political institutions must adhere to media logic in order to gain positive coverage (Stromback, 2008), there remain battles at points when political logic is expected to be reasserted. During crises one might expect political logic to dominate, and through the use of scheduled press conferences and control over information this was indeed the case; politicians could determine what information was released when and in what form. However, where media has maintained independence from the state, it was able to follow its own logic and normal working practices forcing political actors to adhere to the requirements of the media. This adds to our understanding of the complex relationship which exists between politics and media, showing that complexity extends even to times of national crisis.

However, the role of mainstream media is challenged. Our study confirms the systemic change in political communication and the roles of traditional media as a range of social media actors played an important role in the diffusion of information. Chadwick (2017) shows how media have become interdependent, information flows down from state actors and up from society via social media to create greater celerity of information and hybridity over control of the message. Therefore, control over the narrative and agenda is no longer possible, rather there is a collective effort in shaping interpretations of official statements and a range of alternative voices increasing the plurality of opinion. This is especially visible where there are clear systemic divisions characterised by political polarisation and oppositionalism where a range of competing and conflicting voices contribute to the information flow.

Despite this we cannot confirm that across all nations the pandemic was experienced concurrently with high instability and change in the public and political consensus. While this trend has been observed as being exacerbated with the advent of the hybrid media system, despite heavy usage of social media in most cases, we did not find a highly changing public opinion and a fluctuating consensus. Rather we found the so-called 'rally around the flag' phenomenon a dominant theme across most nations, with increased support given to the leader. Only where there were weak or unpopular leaders and systemic democratic problems (Kosovo, France, the United States, Brazil) did we find attempts at building unity work only among certain factions. In fact, to an extent COVID-19 saw partisanship be replaced by a sense of collective unity. The situation was unable to heal serious rifts, but where democratic processes were taking a natural course, such as in the Republic of Ireland, even a leader who had lost an election and was in their twilight moments as national leader was able to command the support of their nation. But there are some caveats to add here. Firstly, support was contingent on the way the country was perceived to have handled the first wave, through the preparation, crisis and normalisation phases. Secondly, support was contingent on trust in the leader prior to the pandemic. Long-standing support for German Chancellor Angela Merkel ensured her strong position despite recent political challenges. However, where there is high political polarisation, for example in the Czech Republic, political preferences in polls hardly changed despite the fact the first wave of COVID-19 was handled well. So, some leaders remained polarising despite having provided good leadership during the pandemic.

Finally, we turn to the role of social media within societies. Political communication literature initially highlighted the benefits for connectedness and greater plurality offered by social media (Keen, 2007). However, more recent research has focused on the more negative impacts of digital technologies, as a flow of misinformation has affected communication environments (Morozov, 2011). The COVID-19 pandemic was accompanied by information overload, mainly widespread through social networks, which offered an opportunity for the spread of misinformation, and so the characterisation of there being an infodemic accompanying the pandemic is true. However, it is not possible to confirm that misinformation and disinformation have been seriously problematic or the main outcome of the greater use of social media. Most people across all countries had the potential to be exposed to misinformation, but where this gained purchase within public debates there were also public divisions between political factions, low trust in the government, polarised politics and media and the open challenging of experts and the science. So, misinformation went viral in places where we detect the presence of the broader factors that exacerbate lower trust in political institutions and make for a post truth environment (Lilleker, 2018). Hence, despite the worries regarding misinformation, the evidence suggests it featured within discourse online but impacted nations with different levels of intensity and consequences dependant on the political context and whether disinformation was a recognised issue in the country before the pandemic, for example, many Central European countries have faced problems of disinformation for years.

We argue digital technology played a very positive role during the pandemic. Firstly, it enabled a lot of economic and social activity to continue. The pandemic ushered in an increased virtualisation of life which is now routinised and may be irreversible. Digital technology modified the ways most people work, study, pray, socialise, communicate etc. Secondly, linked to the more social routines which started to take place online, social media was used to connect local communities, for the purposes of mutual support and aid for the vulnerable, friends and families. Within these spaces, initiatives such as the 'clapping for carers' or 'sanitary claps' as well as the performances from balconies began. Due to trends witnessed during recent elections, we may be forgiven for expecting social media to play a negative role by providing the conditions for the spread of a climate of mistrust, criticism of institutions and a degraded political debate. But, in actual fact, social media's most important functions were positive, promoting solidarity and linked to we-ness initiatives. Therefore, we suggest that social media platforms should be viewed as apolitical and amoral; they are able to have positive and negative impacts on society depending on systemic stability and social unity. However, within the context of crises and lockdowns more people engaged in 'sanitary clapping' than the sharing of misinformation in the majority of nations.

The lessons of COVID-19

We found largely that political communication within the context of a crisis such as the COVID-19 pandemic, a more personalised politics is appropriate, alongside a coherent message and a unifying frame. Political leaders must promote and embody 'we-ness' abandoning partisan positions and oppositionalism. This is because the nation must come together and act as one, for one another. The media's function as informer is crucial, but this does not mean abandoning its function of holding government to account. We see the traditional battle for the agenda continue, however governments which command widespread support and provide clear and transparent messages avoid intensely critical coverage. These factors, along with successes in mitigating the worst effects of a pandemic, ensure governments increase their support. Social media can be problematic if politics is polarised, where politics and science conflict or where there are long-standing issues with misinformation. But largely, digital technology played a key role in ensuring economic and social life continues in some form and proved crucial for maintaining social cohesion.

The major failure the crisis exposes is the absence of global or even regional leadership. The WHO failed to recognise the threat and promote early measures to reduce the spread of the virus. The EU failed to bring member states together and develop a co-ordinated approach. Hence national leaders, some beset by internal instability, were left to manage the crisis as best they could. In a globalised world, where each country's approach is visible, this can undermine the measures taken by any actor who does not follow that of their neighbour. Our analysis shows the world was ill prepared for this crisis, some leaders handled it well, some were lucky, others allowed politics to dominate. Cumulatively, this analysis offers lessons for political communication as a discipline and a practice.

Concluding thoughts

Social media offers interesting insights into community initiatives, the sharing and caring cultures that grew during the crisis, as well as the anxieties that many feel during the weft and wane of the spread of COVID-19 across their nation and the world. One meme[4] circulating as the second wave began in Europe captured many questions ordinary people were asking; these were highlighted at the start of this chapter. The meme ends with a statement that many will perhaps feel intuitively:

> I understand that there is a minuscule possibility I could die...I understand I could possibly pass it to someone else...but I can pass any virus onto

someone else. I'm struggling to see where or how this ends. We either get busy living or we get busy dying.

The anxieties captured in this meme reflect a hidden impact of COVID-19, the impact on the mental health and well-being of populations. The questions raised are ones no national leader, medical officer or the WHO have answers to. That is the serious problem. Will it disappear like so-called Spanish flu, will we become naturally immune, how many will die before either happen, how many deaths globally are of COVID-19 or just attributed to it for administrative purposes. The myriad unknowns lead ordinary people to assess what they should think and do. The uncertainty and anxiety fuels searches for alternative perspectives and provides succour for conspiracy theories. People are searching for something to believe in, to get answers to questions that are genuinely unanswerable.

There are also bigger questions which require political answers. What about the inequalities COVID-19 has exposed? Many in developed nations cannot afford to self-isolate as their economic conditions prevent it. Many lack the luxury of access to open spaces, family, friends. Many are in danger of becoming homeless, due to a fall in their income, making them further isolated and vulnerable. These disparities will continue and increase the chances of mental and physical illness. The disparities are even higher in nations where many already experience fragile existences, from the favelas of Brazil to the shanty towns of South Africa or the refugee camps on the Syrian borders. We-ness requires there to be one community that face the challenges of COVID-19 on an equal footing. While the richest and poorest are equally susceptible to the virus, the poor have less opportunities to protect themselves. Vulnerability is not just a factor of age or health; it is felt deeply across societies by those less economically secure. Feeling vulnerability means feeling less equal, discriminated against, it increases fear, it increases the likelihood of seeking alternative explanations, preventative solutions, the potential for failing to comply with restrictions or even rebelling. The future is thus uncertain. Given the polarisation that has swept many nations, during the age of anxiety, a term used to characterise the decade leading up to 2020 (Öniş, 2017), which is exacerbated by many political projects, we need political communication to unify, to build a more global we as there are many future disasters we must face as a single community.

Notes

1 www.bbc.co.uk/news/extra/dj3jonuhi1/coronavirus-year-of-the-mask
2 www.lemonde.fr/politique/article/2020/03/17/nous-sommes-en-guerre-face-au-c oronavirus-emmanuel-macron-sonne-la-mobilisation-generale_6033338_823448 .html
3 www.bbc.com/news/53191523
4 www.worldofwellness.co.uk/uploads/1/1/1/8/11187633/mulligan.pdf

References

Altheide, D. L. (2020). Media Logic and Media Psychology. In J. van den Bulck (Ed.), *The International Encyclopedia of Media Psychology*, Wiley, 1–15.

Chadwick, A. (2017). *The Hybrid Media System: Politics and Power*. Oxford University Press.

Keen, A. (2007). *The Cult of the Amateur*. New York.

Lilleker, D. (2018). Politics in a Post-Truth Era. *International Journal of Media & Cultural Politics*, 14(3), 277–282.

Morozov, E. (2011). *The Net Delusion: How Not to Liberate the World*. Penguin UK.

Öniş, Z. (2017). The Age of Anxiety: The Crisis of Liberal Democracy in a Post-Hegemonic Global Order. *The International Spectator*, 52(3), 18–35.

Paget, J., Spreeuwenberg, P., Charu, V., Taylor, R. J., Iuliano, A. D., Bresee, J., ... Viboud, C. (2019). Global Mortality Associated with Seasonal Influenza Epidemics: New Burden Estimates and Predictors from the GLaMOR Project. *Journal of Global Health*, 9(2). www.ncbi.nlm.nih.gov/pmc/articles/PMC6815659/

Strömbäck, J. (2008). Four Phases of Mediatization: An Analysis of the Mediatization of Politics. *International Journal of Press – Politics*, 13(3), 228–246.